Science and Practice of Pressure Ulcer Management

Editor Marco Romanelli

Coeditors Michael Clark, George Cherry,
Denis Colin, and Tom Defloor

Science and Practice of Pressure Ulcer Management

With 52 Illustrations
including 34 Color Plates

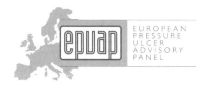

EUROPEAN
PRESSURE
ULCER
ADVISORY
PANEL

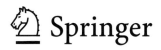 Springer

Marco Romanelli, MD, PhD
Department of Dermatology
University of Pisa
Pisa
Italy

Michael Clark, PhD
Wound Healing Research Unit
University of Wales College of
   Medicine
Cardiff, UK

George Cherry, D.Phil (Oxon)
Clinical Faculty
Oxford Medical School
University of Oxford
Oxford, UK

Denis Colin, MD, PhD
Centre de l'Arche
Le Mans
France

Tom Defloor, RN, PhD
Nursing Science
Ghent University
Ghent
Belgium

British Library Cataloguing in Publication data
A catalogue record for this title is available from the British Library.

Library of Congress Control Number: 2005923439

ISBN 10: 1-85233-839-3   Printed on acid-free paper
ISBN 13: 978-1-85233-839-8

Printed in the United States of America   (BS/MVY)

9 8 7 6 5 4 3 2 1

Springer Science+Business Media
springeronline.com

Foreword I

I consider it a great privilege to have been asked to write the foreword for this book. The European Pressure Ulcer Advisory Panel (EPUAP) is less than 10 years old having been founded in 1997. I had the honour of being the first president of this group and have been amazed and delighted at the progress and achievements the panel have made since that time. The progress is remarkable, not only because it is a truly European group consisting of a wide range of clinical and academic interests but also because it has retained its focus on the prevention and treatment of pressure ulcers.

The officers and board should be congratulated in developing a range of educational and research opportunities in this important but often neglected aspect of clinical practice. Not only have they organised a series of successful annual conferences that have been held in a number of a European countries but they have developed a number of other exciting initiatives. These have included setting up working groups, developing guidelines, undertaking prevalence studies and research projects. The latest addition to these activities is the publication of this book which I am confident will rapidly become the standard textbook for all interested in this subject—not only in Europe but on a global scale.

The editors of this book—who are all internationally known for their work in this area—are all key individuals in the success of the EPUAP. They have pulled together a comprehensive review of this subject written by a range of experts from different professional backgrounds representing many European countries. This is no mean feat and they should be congratulated on their vision and determination.

The 22 chapters address key issues in this condition and range from updates in research through to epidemiological aspects on to assessment of patients and equipment. The book also debates local wound care either by conservative or surgical methods, complications such as infection onto issues around developing and implementing guidelines and the increasingly important subject of litigation in this area. Many special interest groups claim to be working in a 'Cinderella' area but few conditions other than pressure ulceration can really justify that description. In an increasingly diverse world the challenges of providing pressure ulcer care in developing countries are different but no less challenging than those of providing care in so called developed or advanced healthcare systems. It is perhaps surprising that in such advanced healthcare systems some cancer can be cured, heart disease can be prevented and organs can be transplanted but many patients in such systems can not guarantee that they will receive prompt and appropriate interventions to prevent or treat pressure ulceration. The challenge to all caring for such patients is considerable but this book provides a reference source for anyone who needs to understand the basis of many aspects of patient care in this area. In addition, the colour section provides excellent clinical illustrations that demonstrate a number of key points in pressure ulceration.

This subject is receiving increasing attention from a number of professional, governmental and legal directions. The importance, cost and ability to use aspects of this clinical problem as an indicator of the quality of health care delivery is to be encouraged but how robust is the research base, the development of standards of clinical care and consistency of healthcare practices in pressure ulceration on a local national and international basis?

This book will not replace all of the work needed to address these problems but it will provide a strong foundation from which we can build our understanding of this condition for improved standards of care to patients in what has been a long standing but neglected clinical challenge.

I congratulate the editors, authors and publishers for remaining focused on their task—to provide the best and most comprehensive and up to date review of this subject. I commend this book to you as an essential companion to help you improve standards of care for your patients.

Keith Harding, MD

Foreword II

One of the outcomes of advancing medical technology is that people are living longer. As life is extended, the complex issue of managing persons with chronic diseases becomes increasingly important. The increased number of persons with chronic wounds such as pressure ulcers is already being realized. The health-care burden of managing these chronic wounds can only be lessened if effective prevention programs are aggressively implemented and evidence-based management protocols are developed and followed.

The information contained in this book provides the critical elements for developing effective, evidence-based protocols for the prevention and management of pressure ulcers. What this book cannot provide is the commitment required to create an environment where the development of a pressure ulcer on a person is unacceptable. Protocol development is only one component of a comprehensive program for prevention and management of pressure ulcers. Everyone involved in patient care from administration to bedside provider has to make the commitment that pressure ulcers will not occur in their facility.

This book is a tremendous resource, but it needs to be used effectively. In the United States, the government sponsored the development of evidence-based guidelines on prevention and management of pressure ulcers. These guidelines became available in the early nineties. Since their publication, the prevalence of pressure ulcers in the United States has not changed at the national level. However, in those facilities that chose to use the guidelines to develop and implement new protocols for prevention and management of pressure ulcers, the incidence of pressure ulcers was reduced to zero or to a very low level.

The information in this book can be used to prevent new pressure ulcers from developing, and rapidly healing those that have unfortunately already developed. The only thing missing is the commitment to make change. I hope that everyone who reads this book makes the personal commitment to prevent pressure ulcers from occurring and to optimize the management of those that occurred at a different facility.

George T. Rodeheaver, PhD
Founding Member and Past President
National Pressure Ulcer Advisory Panel

Acknowledgments

The European Pressure Ulcer Advisory Panel is grateful to the following corporate sponsors which have helped make the publication of this book possible:

Frontier Therapeutics Ltd
Gaymar Industries
KCI Europe B.V.
Nutricia Healthcare
Smith & Nephew

Contents

Contributors   xiii

1 **Pressure Ulcer, the Scale of the Problem**
   Theo Dassen, Antje Tannen, and Nils Lahmann   1

2 **Pressure Ulcer Patients' Quality of Life from a
   Nurse's Perspective**
   Helvi Hietanen   7

3 **Recent Advances in Pressure Ulcer Research**
   Dan Bader and Cees Oomens   11

4 **Etiology and Risk Factors**
   Mark Collier and Zena Moore   27

5 **Pressure Ulcer Classification**
   Carol Dealey and Christina Lindholm   37

6 **Risk Assessment Scales for Predicting the Risk of
   Developing Pressure Ulcers**
   *Joan-Enric Torra i Bou, Francisco Pedro García-Fernández,
   Pedro L. Pancorbo-Hidalgo, and Katia Furtado*   43

7 **Equipment Selection**
   Jacqueline Fletcher   59

8 **Pressure Ulcer Prevention and Repositioning**
   *Tom Defloor, Katrien Vanderwee, Doris Wilborn, and
   Theo Dassen*   67

9 **Skin Care**
   Sue Bale, Janice Cameron, and Sylvie Meaume   75

10 Pressure Ulcers and Nutrition: A New
    European Guideline
    Joseph Schols, Michael Clark, Giuseppe Benati,
    Pam Jackson, Meike Engfer, Gero Langer, Bernadette Kerry,
    and Denis Colin   85

11 Clinical and Instrumental Assessment of Pressure Ulcers
    Diego Mastronicola and Marco Romanelli   91

12 Pressure Ulcers and Wound Bed Preparation
    Vincent Falanga   99

13 Conservative Management of Pressure Ulcers
    Elia Ricci, Andrea Cavicchioli, and Marco Romanelli   111

14 Surgical Management of Pressure Ulcers
    Jens Lykke Sørensen, M.J. Lubbers, and Finn Gottrup   119

15 Debridement of Pressure Ulcers
    Andrea Bellingeri and Deborah Hofman   129

16 The Role of Bacteria in Pressure Ulcers
    R. Gary Sibbald, Paul Chapman, and
    Jose Contreras-Ruiz   139

17 Litigation
    Courtney H. Lyder   163

18 The Development, Dissemination, and Use of Pressure
    Ulcer Guidelines
    R.T. van Zelm, Michael Clark, and Jeen R.E. Haalboom . . .   169

19 Developing a Research Agenda
    Denis Colin   177

20 The European Pressure Ulcer Advisory Panel: A Means of
    Identifying and Dealing with a Major Health Problem
    with a European Initiative
    George W. Cherry   183

21 Pressure Ulcer Prevention and Management in the
    Developing World: The Developed World Must
    Provide Leadership
    Terence J. Ryan   189

22 Innovation in Pressure Ulcer Prevention
    and Management
    Keith G. Harding and Michael Clark   197

Index   205

Contributors

Dan Bader, BSc MSc PhD, MIPEM, DSc
Professor of Medical Engineering
Department of Engineering
Queen Mary University of London
London, UK

and

Professor of Soft Tissue Remodelling
Biomedical Engineering Department
Eindhoven University of Technology
Eindhoven, The Netherlands

Sue Bale, PhD, BA, RGN, NDN, RHV, PG Dip, Dip Nursing
Professor
Associate Director of Nursing
Grange House
Llanfrechfa Grange Hospital
Cwmbran, UK

Andrea Bellingeri, RN
Secretary of Italian Nurse Association for the Study of Wound
Italian Nurse Society on Wound study (AISLeC)
Pavia, Italy

Giuseppe Benati, MD
Unita Operativa di Medicina Geriatrica
Ospedale Morgagni Pierantoni
Forli, Italy

Cinzia Brilli, RN
Tissue Viability Nurse
Azienda Ospedaliera Universitaria Pisana
Pisa, Italy

Janice Cameron, MPhil, RGN, ONC
Clinical Nurse Specialist in Wound Management
Department of Dermatology
Oxford Radcliffe Hospitals NHS Trust
Churchill Hospital
Headington, Oxford, UK

Andrea Cavicchioli, RN
Tissue Viability Nurse
Azienda Unità
Sanitaria Locale di Modena-Osp. Estense
Modena, Italy

Paul Chapman, BScPT
Medical Student
University of Manitoba
Winnipeg, Manitoba, Canada

George W. Cherry, DPhil (Oxon)
Secretary Treasurer EPUAP
Clinical Faculty
Oxford Medical School
University of Oxford
Oxford, UK

Michael Clark, PhD
Senior Research Fellow
Wound Healing Research Unit
University of Wales College of Medicine
Cardiff, UK

Denis Colin, MD, PhD
Centre de l'Arche
Le Mans, France

Mark Collier, BA, RNT, RCNT, ONC, RN
Lead Nurse/Consultant-Tissue
  Viability
United Lincolnshire Hospitals
Pilgrim Hospital
Boston, Lincolnshire, UK

Jose Contreras-Ruiz, MD
Wound Care Fellow
Dermatology Daycare/Wound Healing
  Centre
Sunnybrook and Women's College
  Health Sciences Centre
Toronto, Ontario, Canada

and

Dermatologist Hospital General "Dr
  Manuel Gea Gonzalez"
Toriello Guerra, Mexico

Theo Dassen, RN, PhD
Professor Dr
Institut für Medizin-/Pflegepädagogik
  und Pflegewissenschaft
Universitätsklinikum Charité
Berlin, Germany

Carol Dealey, PhD, MA, BSc (Hons),
  RGN, RCNT
Research Fellow
School of Health Sciences
University of Birmingham
Edgbaston, Birmingham, UK

Tom Defloor, RN, PhD
Nursing Science
Ghent University
Ghent, Belgium

Meike Engfer, PhD
Clinical Nutrition Adviser
Numico Clinical Nutrition
Schiphol, The Netherlands

Vincent Falanga, MD, FACP
Professor of Dermatology and
  Biochemistry
Boston University School of Medicine
Chairman, Department of
  Dermatology
Roger Williams Medical Center
Providence, Rhode Island, USA

Jacqueline Fletcher, BSc, RGN, PgCert,
  ILTM
Principal Lecturer
School of Nursing and Midwifery
University of Hertfordshire
Hatfield, Hertfordshire, UK

Katia Furtado, RN
Centro de saúde da Penha de França
Lisbon, Portugal

Francisco Pedro García-Fernández, RN
Quality, Research and Formation
  Manager
Complejo Hospitalario de Jaén
Jaén, Spain

Finn Gottrup, MD, DMSci
Professor
Department of Plastic Surgery
Odense University Hospital
Odense C, Denmark

Jeen R. E. Haalboom, MD, PhD, EPUAP
Professor of Internal Medicine
University Medical Centre
Utrecht, The Netherlands

Keith G. Harding, MB ChB, MRCGP,
  FRCS
Professor
Department of Surgery
Wales College of Medicine
Cardiff University
Cardiff, Wales, UK

Helvi Hietanen, RN
Head Nurse
Department of Plastic Surgery
Tōōlō Hospital
HUCH Helsinki University Central
  Hospital
Finland

Deborah Hofman, BA Hons, RGN, Dip
  Nurse
Clinical Nurse Specialist
Department of Dermatology
Churchill Hospital
Headington, Oxford, UK

Pam Jackson, MPhil, BSc, RGN, RHV, RNT, RCNT, ILT
Senior Lecturer
University of Southampton
Southampton, UK

Bernadette Kerry, RGN, RPN, PGD, Dip
Tissue Repair and Wound Management
Midland Health Board
Tullamore, Co. Offaly, Ireland

Nils Lahmann, RN, BA
Institut für Medizin-/Pflegepädagogik und Pflegewissenschaft
Universitätsklinikum Charité
Berlin, Germany

Gero Langer, MScN (EU), RN
Coordinator of the German Centre for Evidence-based Nursing "sapere aude"
Martin Luther University
Halle-Wittenberg, Germany

Christina Lindholm, RN, PhD
Professor
Department of Health Sciences
Kristianstad University
Sweden

M.J. Lubbers
Department of Surgery
AMC University Hospital
Amsterdam, The Netherlands

Courtney H. Lyder, ND
Professor
University of Virginia
McLeod Hall
Charlottesville, Virginia, USA

Diego Mastronicola, MD
Consultant Dermatologist
Department of Dermatology
University of Pisa
Pisa, Italy

Sylvie Meaume
Hôpital Charles Foix
Ivry sur Seine
France

Zena Moore, RGN, MSc, FFNMRCSI
Lecturer
Faculty of Nursing and Midwifery
Royal College of Surgeons in Ireland
Dublin 2, Ireland

Cees Oomens, PhD
Associate Professor
Biological Engineering Department
Eindhoven University of Technology
Eindhoven, The Netherlands

Pedro L. Pancorbo-Hidalgo, PhD, RN
Professor of Medical-Surgical Nursing
School of Health Sciences
University of Jaén
Las Lagunillas S/N, Jaén, Spain

Elia Ricci
Consultant Surgeon
Wound Healing Unit
Casa di Cura San Luca
Torino, Italy

Marco Romanelli, MD, PhD
Department of Dermatology
University of Pisa
Pisa, Italy

Terence J. Ryan, BM BCh, DM, MA, FRCP
Emeritus Professor of Dermatology
Oxford University
Department of Dermatology
Churchill Hospital
Headington, Oxford, UK

Joseph Schols, MD, PhD
Department Tranzo
Tilburg University
The Netherlands

R. Gary Sibbald, MD, FRCRC, MEd
Department of Medicine
University of Toronto
Toronto, Ontario, Canada

Jens Lykke Sørensen, PhD
Clinical Director
Department of Plastic Surgery
Odense University Hospital
Odense C, Denmark

Antje Tannen, RN, MA
Institut für Medizin-/Pflegepädagogik
   und Pflegewissenschaft
Universitätsklinikum Charité
Berlin, Germany

Joan-Enric Torra i Bou, RN
Clinical Manager
Advanced Wound Care Division
Smith and Nephew Spain
Sant Joan Despi, Barcelona, Spain

Katrien Vanderwee, RN, MA
PhD Student
Nursing Science
Ghent University
Ghent, Belgium

R.T. van Zelm
Advisor
Dutch Institute for Health Care
   Improvement
Utrecht, The Netherlands

Doris Wilborn, RN, MA
Nursing Science
Humboldt-University
Berlin, Germany

1 Pressure Ulcer, the Scale of the Problem

Theo Dassen, Antje Tannen, and Nils Lahmann

Introduction

The main goal of this chapter is to provide information about the frequency of pressure ulcers. However, in doing this it becomes evident that the chapter title—the scale of the problem—sh 'd really be amended to the problem of the scale. Due to the different rates (prevalence, incidence), different grades/stages of pressure ulcers (1, 2, 3, 4) body sites, different settings (hospital, nursing home, at home) and differ wa of data collection it is almost impossible to find comparable data about the scale of this phenomenon in human beings. Therefore, this chapter should be regarded more as a guide on how to deal with data on pressure ulcers obtained from the literature. First, information is provided about the use of rates and their application to pressure ulcers. Then some suggestions are given about how to interpret the figures from the literature.

Rates

Measures of frequencies in a disease are usually expressed as rates.[1] Those rates are fractions or proportions that consist of three elements: a numerator, a denominator, and a time period. In this case the numerator is the number of people suffering from pressure ulcers. The denominator is the population that was selected as the number of possible occurrences (e.g. all patients in a hospital). The time period can be one moment in time or another well-defined period (for instance a year). In pressure ulcer research it is common practice to express the rate as a percentage, which means per hundred cases. The numerator is divided by the denominator and then multiplied by 100. For example, ten persons out of a thousand suffer from a pressure ulcer; this is: $10/1000 \times 100 = 1\%$.

The difference between prevalence rates and incidence rates is important. Pressure ulcer prevalence refers to the number of people with pressure ulcer as a proportion of the total population under investigation. Prevalence rates include all old and all new cases. If only the new cases are counted this is called the incidence.

So far, it does not appear complicated to provide comparable data about pressure ulcer, but the problem is that an exact definition is necessary for both parts, numerator and denominator, to make the calculated rates coherent.[2] Every author uses a definition for both, but there is standardization. This leads to publications with rates ranging from 5% to 50% or sometimes even less or more. It is not clear whether there are indeed different rates or if these are the result of differences in the way the numerator and/or denominator have been defined.

Another aspect is the time period. If a prevalence rate is measured at one moment in a given period of time it is called a point prevalence. A period prevalence refers to the condition over a specified period of time. It is obvious that incidence rates are always calculated for a period. It is important in both cases that the chosen period of time is the same when comparing rates from different publications.

Numerator Confusion

When looking at a definition of pressure ulcer it becomes obvious that the numerator can vary depending on the project. In other chapters of this book this is discussed in more depth. According to the definition of the European Pressure Ulcer Advisory Panel (EPUAP)[3] a pressure ulcer can be located anywhere on the skin of the body and is a discoloration of the skin (with nonblanchable erythema), but it can also be an extensive destruction with tissue necrosis, damage to the muscle, bone or supporting structures with or without full-thickness skin loss. This means the numerator can include a red, damaged area of skin at the elbow and also a deep hole in the skin of the sacrum. Is it sensible to combine all these in a single classification? Yes and no! If we know that 10% of all patients in a hospital have a pressure ulcer we obtain information about this phenomenon. However, without a classification of the pressure ulcer according to grades and body sites this information cannot be used for any kind of policy. For this reason researchers divide the numerator into grades (or stages) and body sites. Table 1.1 shows an example of a division according to body sites, which is derived from a study conducted by EPUAP.[4]

This table shows that more than 25% of all pressure ulcers are located on the sacrum. This is supported by several other studies.[5,6] However, the sites of pressure ulcers in children are different. The occipital region of the scalp in infants and toddlers and the sacrum in children are prevalent sites of pressure ulcer formation.[7]

Approximately one third of the pressure ulcers are located on the heel, which is also supported by the literature.[8,9] So far it could be concluded that about half of the pressure ulcers are located on either the sacrum or the heel. What about the rest? Table 1.1 shows that the division of pressure ulcers at other body sites varies

Table 1.1. Pressure ulcer prevalence rates at different body sites (% of total prevalence)

Location	Belgium	Italy	Portugal	Sweden	UK	Total
Sacrum	25.6	40.9	26.9	25.3	37.5	532
Heel	34.9	31.9	33.9	30.0	26.2	484
Ischium	12.2	7.6	2.7	11.6	13.7	186
Ankle	3.6	9.1	10.2	24.5	6.4	149
Elbow	14.3	0.0	6.9	3.0	10.3	143
Hip	9.3	10.6	19.3	5.6	5.8	136
Total	301	132	186	233	778	1630

Source: Based on Clark et al.[4]

depending on the country. For instance, the pressure ulcer rate on the hip was about 5% in the UK and about 20% in Portugal. In the Swedish sample nearly 25% of pressure ulcers were located on the ankle compared to less than 5% in Belgium. These variations in pressure ulcer rates at particular body sites are found also in the literature.[10]

As well as different body sites the numerator can also include different grades or stages. Grade 1 (nonblanchable erythema) accounts for almost half of all pressure ulcers, as several studies show.[11] The measurement of grade 1 in people with dark skin is a special problem. The most severe form of pressure ulcer is grade 4 in the EPUAP classification. It was 2.5% in the study from which Table 1.1 was derived. In other studies it is reported at rates from 3% to 10%.[12]

As mentioned above, four grades and at least seven body sites result in more than 28 combinations that can be part of the numerator. Unfortunately, this is not the only problem regarding the numerator. The fact that some people have more than one pressure ulcer is another complication. In a prevalence study conducted in the Netherlands, 13.2% of the patients had one ulcer, 4.7% had two ulcers, and 3.5% had three or more.[13] This means that a person sustaining a new pressure ulcer, which is to be counted in an incidence study, could have already had one. A grade 1 pressure ulcer could also develop into a grade 2 ulcer, which is of course still regarded as a pressure ulcer, but should it be recorded as a new or as an old one? In other words: the difference between prevalence and incidence in pressure ulcers is increasingly complicated. Suggestions on how to deal with this problem are given by EPUAP[14] but not every researcher necessarily agrees with the solutions given.

This part of the chapter has shown that dealing with pressure ulcers is similar to dealing with fruit: there are various sorts with different characteristics, sometimes appearing individually and sometimes in a group of several. This has to be taken into account when calculating or comparing prevalence or incidence rates.

Denominator Complications

In order to calculate the prevalence or incidence rate of pressure ulcers the nominator must be divided by the denominator. In the case of prostate hypertrophy people with this condition form the numerator and all males in the sample are the denominator. Why are women not included in the denominator as well? Naturally, because they cannot have this disease and the denominator should consist only of persons "at risk." This confronts us with a serious problem when calculating prevalence rates of pressure ulcers. If, for example, we have all patients in a hospital as the denominator, this would mean we are dealing with a denominator that also includes people "not at risk." It is quite simple to find crude prevalence rates in the literature for entire institutions such as hospitals.[15,16] Even if they were all grade 4 pressure ulcers on the heel, the question with which denominator the calculation was made would still arise. Only those figures are comparable that use the same definition of the population "at risk." But how can it be defined? In some studies, e.g. the above-mentioned EPUAP survey, the Braden score (see Chapter 6) was used to divide the sample into "at-risk" and "not-at-risk" groups. In the literature there are several examples of investigations using this solution. There is only one problem, namely the cutoff point. For instance, in a comparison of pressure ulcers in the Netherlands and Germany the authors used a Braden score of 20 as the cutoff.[17] In clinical practice a cutoff point of 16 or 18 is more common. Naturally, the differences in choosing a cutoff point are permitted but they complicate the comparison of results from the literature with clinical practice.

Due to the different cutoff points the number of at-risk individuals varies considerably. The rate increases if the denominator is smaller. This means that a high prevalence rate could be the result of a well-defined risk group. Or, conversely, a low prevalence rate could be the result of a widely defined risk group (e.g. all patients of the hospital). It should be remembered that the prevalence of prostate hypertrophy would be only half the size if all women were included in the denominator as well.

About one third of the hospital population and two thirds of the nursing home population were at risk when using a Braden score of 20 as the cutoff point. In a nationwide study in Germany[18] this proportion remained stable over some years. The above-mentioned comparison between Germany and the Netherlands revealed a different number of "at-risk" patients, with more than 50% in the Dutch hospitals. The EPUAP survey also showed (cutoff = 16) different proportions "at risk," from about 34% in Belgium to 23% in Italy. It is not the intention of this chapter to discuss the risk assessment but to show that calculating prevalence rates by using total populations of institutions will inevitably lead to figures that are not comparable. A highly sophisticated solution, called the case mix method, involves correction for all kinds of factors that can influence the occurrence of a pressure ulcer.[19] It is only practicable if all the information is available, which is, however, not always the case.

Apart from the difficulty of defining the risk group the denominator give rise to another serious problem—the influence of the nonresponse. Researchers have to respect ethical rules when using people's data for a scientific purpose. This means that permission has to be obtained from each patient in the hospital as a basic condition for using their data for the calculation of a prevalence or incidence rate. One of the side effects is that not every patient agrees to participate in the study.

Prevalence research can be classified as descriptive research. This is research that aims to generalize the results for a whole target group. In this case the target group could comprise all at-risk patients in a hospital or all at-risk residents in a nursing home. A high external validity is necessary for this kind of research.[20] It means that the sample under investigation should reflect the target group. This will not be the case in practice. Nonresponse rates can influence the prevalence significantly, as Table 1.2 illustrates. A measured prevalence of 19.7% could in fact be lower (15.2%) or higher (38.1%) depending on the nonresponse rate.[21] In this example the lowest rates were calculated on the assumption that all the at-risk people in the nonresponse portion *did not have* a pressure ulcer. The highest rates were calculated on the assumption that all the at-risk people in the nonresponse portion *had at least one* pressure ulcer.

Table 1.2. Example of measured and calculated (lowest and highest) pressure ulcer prevalence rates

Institution	Response %	Measured %	Lowest %	Highest %
Nursing home	79.6	12.5	10.0	30.3
Hospital	75.6	24.2	18.3	42.7
Total	76.6	19.7	15.2	38.1

Source: Based on Dassen et al.[18]

Solution of the Problem

It was established that the calculated rates can differ considerably depending on different definitions of the numerator and/or the denominator. This is a well-known problem that often occurs when using statistics. Tukey expressed it as follows: "Far better an approximate answer to the right question, which is often vague, than an exact answer to the wrong question, which can always be made precise."[22] This statement shows us that a question like "what is the pressure ulcer prevalence in this hospital" is wrong. A correct question would be "How many patients on intensive care wards have a pressure ulcer grade 2, 3, 4 on the sacrum?" An example of the answer then is "58% of all people who had a pressure ulcer."[23] This answer is not precise but it tells us that a pressure ulcer on this part of the body is not an exception. It can become more informative if the prevalence and the definition of the risk group are known. In this case, the answer was 21% of people who scored 20 or lower on the Braden scale. This means that about 12% of the people "at risk" had a pressure ulcer grade 2, 3, or 4 on the sacrum.

Another example is the number of pressure ulcers in dead bodies that were inspected prior to cremation. A difference in grade 4 was found in a comparison between Berlin (2.3%) and Hamburg (0.9%).[24] Here the population was defined as "all dead bodies that were brought to the crematorium." Again a specific group was selected and a clear distinction between grades and body sites was used to present the data.

Finally

The problem of prevalence and incidence of pressure ulcers was discussed without obtaining a precise answer to the question of the scale of the problem as mentioned in the title of this chapter. Naturally, it is not intended to evade this question. The reason quite obviously is that there are almost no comparable data. A prevalence rate of 10% in one publication can be quite different from 10% in another publication. Depending on the definition of the numerator and the denominator a prevalence or incidence rate can include different information. A clear distinction between prevalence and incidence is nearly impossible owing to factors such as multiple pressure sores in the same patient and progression to higher grades in an existing pressure ulcer.

Therefore, information regarding findings from different publications is more interesting and safer. Most studies revealed more grade 1 than grade 4 pressure ulcers. Several studies mention the sacrum and the heels as those body sites with the most frequently occurring pressure ulcers. In children other parts of the body (occipital region of the scalp) are more predominant.

Special groups such as intensive care patients or patients on geriatric wards are affected by pressure ulcers to a larger extent than are hospital patients on other wards.

Finally, it can be stated that pressure ulcers are found more often in geriatric patients than in younger patients, more often in intensive care wards than in lower care wards, and more often on the heel or the sacrum than on other body sites. Furthermore, it is known that a grade 1 pressure ulcer occurs in about 50% of patients with pressure ulcers and the higher the grade the lower the proportion of all pressure ulcers. Comparable figures concerning the prevalence or incidence of pressure ulcers in human beings are not known.

References

1. Mulhall A. Epidemiology nursing and healthcare. A new perspective. Basingstoke: Macmillan; 1996.
2. Fletcher R, Fletcher S. Clinical epidemiology. The essentials, 4th edn. Baltimore: Williams & Wilkins; 2005.
3. EPUAP. Pressure ulcer treatment guidelines. http://www.epuap.org.
4. Clark M, Bours G, Defloor T. Summary report on the prevalence of pressure ulcers. EPUAP Review 2002; 4:49–56.
5. Ash D. An exploration of the occurrence of pressure ulcers in a British spinal injuries unit. J Clin Nurs 2002; 11:470–478.
6. Eriksson E, Hietanen H, Asko-Seljavaara S. Prevalence and characteristics of pressure ulcers. A one-day patient population in a Finnish city. Clin Nurse Spec 2000; 14:119–125.
7. Curley M, Razmus I, Roberts K, Wypij D. Predicting pressure ulcer risk in pediatric patients: the Braden Q Scale. Nurs Res 2003; 52:22–33.
8. Schue R, Langemo D. Prevalence, incidence, and prediction of pressure ulcers on a rehabilitation unit. J Wound Ostomy Continence Nurs 1999; 26:121–129.
9. Levett D, Smith S. Survey of pressure ulcer prevalence in nursing homes. Elder Care 2000; 12:12–16.
10. Williams D, Stotts N, Nelson K. Patients with existing pressure ulcers admitted to acute care. J Wound Ostomy Continence Nurs 2000; 27:216–226.
11. Halfens R, Bours G, Ast W van. Relevance of the diagnosis "Stage 1 pressure ulcer": an empirical study of the clinical course of stage 1 ulcers in acute care and long-term hospital populations. J Clin Nurs 2001; 10:748–757.
12. O'Brien S, Wind S, Rijswijk L van, Kerstein M. Sequential biannual prevalence studies of pressure ulcers at Allegheny-Hahnemann University Hospital. Ostomy Wound Manage 1998; 44:78–89.
13. Bours G, Halfens R, Wansink S. Landelijk prevalentie onderzoek Decubitus, Resultaten zesde jaarlijkse meting 2003. Universiteit Maastricht, 2003.
14. Defloor T, Bours G, Schoonhoven L, Clark M. Draft EPUAP statement on prevalence and incidence monitoring. EPUAP Review 2002; 4:13–15.
15. Thoroddsen A. Pressure sore prevalence: a national survey. J Clin Nurs 1999; 8:170–179.
16. Pearson A, Francis K, Hodgkinson B, Curry G. Prevalence and treatment of pressure ulcers in northern New South Wales. Aust J Rural Health 2000; 8:103–110.
17. Tannen A, Dassen T, Bours G, Halfens R. A comparison of pressure ulcer prevalence: concerted data collection in The Netherlands and Germany. Int J Nurs Stud 2004; 41(6):607–612.
18. Dassen T, et al. Pflegeabhängigkeit, Sturzereignisse, Inkontinenz, Dekubitus, Erhebung 2003. Humboldt-Universität zu Berlin, 2003.
19. Bours G, Halfens J, Berger P. Development of a model for case-mix adjustment of pressure ulcer prevalence rates. Med Care 2003; 41:45–55.
20. Polit D, Beck Ch. Nursing research, principles and methods. Philadelphia: Lippincott; 2004.
21. Lahmann N, Halfens R, Dassen T. Prevalence of ulcers in Germany, submitted for publication.
22. Tukey J. Cited in: Silverman W, Where's the evidence, Debates in modern medicine. (Chapter 2: Does a difference make a difference.) Oxford: Oxford Medical Publications, 1998.
23. Heinrichs P, Dassen T. Zahlen zur Prävalenz des Dekubitusgeschwürs in der Intensivpflege. Crit Care 2004; 115–119.
24. Troike W, Schneider V. Zur Prävalenz von Decubitalulcera, Ergebnisse einer Stichprobe bei der zweiten Leichenschau in drei Berliner Krematorien. Berl Ärzte 2000; 12:28–30.

2 Pressure Ulcer Patients' Quality of Life from a Nurse's Perspective

Helvi Hietanen

Part of a nurse's work is to assist patients with their physical, spiritual, and social needs if patients are unable to satisfy these needs on their own. Hygiene and skin condition, including nutritional balance, are significant factors in preventing pressure ulcers. The occurrence of pressure ulcers has an important influence on the patient's quality of life in many ways. According to the literature,[1-5] factors influencing the pressure ulcer patient's quality of life, and which can be influenced by nursing, include skin condition, cost-effective wound care, comfortableness of the mattress, quality of sleep, high-quality auxiliary devices, and treatment of pain including appropriate care practices.[6,7] In addition, the nursing staff's motivation, competence, and skills in effective methods[8-10] influence the success of preventive measures.

The patient's wellbeing, feeling of comfort in bed, and quality of sleep can be promoted by selecting an appropriate mattress for the patient, taking the known risk factors of ulceration into account. Experience has shown that even though the patient is informed about the beneficial effects of an alternating pressure mattress, the patient may not be willing to test such a mattress. Reasons for this decision may be the patient's previous negative experiences or beliefs. For some patients, even the most silent machinery is experienced as annoying and affecting the quality of sleep. On the other hand, the spasticity of a patient with a spinal cord injury may be activated, a very skinny and small patient may feel as though they are "drowning" in the mattress, and an extremely obese or tall and large patient might experience the dimensions of the mattress as uncomfortable. Consequently, the patient's own wishes and experiences of special mattresses must always be taken into account. Sometimes, the best solution is to allow patients to bring their own special mattress for the hospital stay.

In some cases, the patient's quality of life and motivation improve if the patient becomes aware of the costs arising from pressure ulcers and the effects of these ulcers.[11-13] Regrettably, young patients especially often only understand the actual risk of having a pressure ulcer when the first ulcer occurs. In the research data of the Helsinki University Hospital[14] over half of the patients with pressure ulcers were patients with spinal cord injury. Thus, in particular young patients with a spinal cord injury should have peer support and practical examples in their own language. The care staff should create ways, together with the patients, by which the best possible preventive methods for pressure ulcers can be offered.[15,16] This requires personnel who have appropriate education, competence, and motivation for high-quality nursing.[17] In her doctoral dissertation "Pressure Ulcer Risk Assessment in Long-term Care. Developing an Instrument," Lepistö[18] concludes that staff are aware of the need to prevent pressure ulcers in high-risk patients, for example bedridden patients, but that prevention of other patients' pressure ulcers is more difficult.

However, not all pressure ulcers can be prevented. Treatment of pressure ulcers, preventing infections, and preventing an infection from spreading are a very important part of nursing. Pressure ulcers are usually located in difficult places, which is unpleasant for the patients, and it is impossible for them to treat these ulcers themselves. The patients might easily feel like "prisoners" of the ulcers and isolate themselves, being anxious about the bandages becoming soaking wet or odors coming through.[9] Nurses are required to have expertise in selecting the most economical bandages that will also have a positive effect on patients' quality of life, allowing patients to lead as normal a life as possible. In western countries, there are hundreds of products from which to choose. However, the problem is that the products are usually very expensive and knowledge of their effects is based mainly on recommendations generated through experience and information given by the manufacturers. Whenever possible, the most economical treatment should be selected if its effect is as good as the more expensive alternative. In treatment of chronic wounds, no differences have been observed in healing of the wounds when the use of sterile and factory clean techniques, including sterile wound cleaning, and the use of drinking water have been compared.[19] However, using drinking water is significantly cheaper. A pressure ulcer in itself causes significant additional costs for the patient in addition to human suffering.

A Practical Example of the Methods Used for Prevention of a Plastic Surgery Patient's Pressure Ulcers

The patient's risk of having a pressure ulcer is individually evaluated. There is no risk evaluation indicator in regular use but the risk evaluation is based on experience, research, and the most recent available knowledge including following up of the incidence of pressure ulcers and common agreements. For example, the European Pressure Ulcer Advisory Panel (EPUAP) prevention and treatment guidelines have been utilized in teaching.

All patients coming for corrective surgery of pressure ulcers or patients who already have a pressure ulcer when they are hospitalized, including all immobile patients, will have an alternating pressure mattress preoperatively at the hospital. If the number of mattresses is not sufficient on the ward, it is possible to rent them and they are available within a few hours. The patient's nutritional imbalance is primarily treated with dietary supplements. Those patients who are not allowed to change their position freely in bed postoperatively will have a mattress of this kind at latest in the recovery room. The nurse receiving the patient evaluates his or her need of special mattresses and other auxiliary devices when the patient enters the hospital. In addition to written instructions, regular training is organized in prevention of pressure ulcers, for example use of auxiliary devices and correct lifting techniques. It has also been commonly agreed that a physiotherapist and several nurses participate for the first few times in moving those patients who need a lot of help. The physiotherapist guides the patient but also shows the nursing staff how to use the best methods. Following up the incidence of pressure ulcers is an issue of utmost importance. If a pressure ulcer occurs during the patient's stay on the ward, the reasons why it may have occurred are examined together with the patient at the earliest possible opportunity. An open discussion on the ward which includes the nursing staff, the physicians, and the surgery personnel has decreased the incidence of pressure ulcers. On the other hand, when the issue has become public so to say, it seems to have improved the nursing personnel's motivation to implement high-quality nursing.

References

1. Grindley A, Acres J. Alternating pressure mattresses: comfort and quality of sleep. Br J Nurs 1996; 5(21):1303–1310.
2. Ballard K. Pressure-relief mattresses and patient comfort. Prof Nurse 1997; 13(1):27–32.
3. Buckle P, Fernandes A. Mattress evaluation—assessment of contact pressure, comfort and discomfort. Appl Ergon 1998; 29(1):35–39.
4. Bader GG, Engdal S. The influence of bed firmness on sleep quality. Appl Ergon 2000; 31(5):487–497.
5. Kaufman MW. The WOC nurse: economic, quality of life, and legal benefits. Dermatol Nurs 2001; 13(3):215–219, 222.
6. Eriksson E, Hietanen H, Asko-Seljavaara S. Prevalence and characteristics of pressure ulcers. A one-day patient population in a Finnish city. Clin Nurse Spec 2000; 143(3):119–125.
7. Meaume S, Gemmen E. Cost-effectiveness of wound management in France: pressure ulcers and venous leg ulcers. J Wound Care 2002; 11(6):219–224.
8. Yang KP. Relationships between nurse staffing and patient outcomes. J Nurs Res 2003; 11(3):149–158.
9. Gunningberg L, Lindholm C, Carlsson M, Sjoden PO. Reduced incidence of pressure ulcers in patients with hip fractures: a 2-year follow-up of quality indicators. Int J Qual Health Care 2001; 13(5):399–407.
10. Lepistö M, Erksson E, Hietanen H, Asko-Seljavaara S. Patients with pressure ulcers in Finnish hospitals. Int J Nurs Pract 2001; 7(4):280–287.
11. Harding K, Cutting K, Price P. The cost-effectiveness of wound management protocols of care. Br J Nurs 2000; 9(19 Suppl):S6, S8, S10 passim.
12. Hirshberg J, Rees RS, Marchant B, Dean S. Osteomyelitis related to pressure ulcers: the cost of neglect. Adv Skin Wound Care 2000; 13(1):25–29.
13. Kaufman MW. The WOC nurse: economic, quality of life, and legal benefits. Dermatol Nurs 2001; 13(3):215–219, 222.
14. Juutilainen V, et al. 2004. In: Haava, WSDY. Helsinki. Article Painchaava, p. 186–187.
15. Baier RR, Gifford DR, Lyder CH, et al. Quality improvement for pressure ulcer care in the nursing home setting: the Northeast Pressure Ulcer Project. J Am Med Dir Assoc 2003; 4(6):291–301.
16. Dukich J, O'Connor D. Impact of practice guidelines on support surface selection, incidence of pressure ulcers, and fiscal dollars. Ostomy Wound Manage 2001; 47(3):44–53.
17. Langemo DK, Melland H, Hanson D, et al. The lived experience of having a pressure ulcer: a qualitative analysis. Adv Skin Wound Care 2000; 13(5):225–235.
18. Lepistö M. Pressure Ulcer Risk Assessment in Long-term Care. Developing an Instrument. Turun yliopisto. Hoitotieteen laitos; 2004.
19. Stotts NA, Barbour S, Griggs K, et al. Sterile versus clean technique in postoperative wound care of patients with open surgical wounds: a pilot study. J Wound Ostomy Continence Nurs 1997; 24(1):10–18.

3 Recent Advances in Pressure Ulcer Research

Dan Bader and Cees Oomens

Introduction

The concept of scientific research aimed at both the prevention and treatment of pressure ulcers has been evident in the literature for at least four decades. Indeed in 1975 a seminal conference entitled Bed Sore Biomechanics was organized at Strathclyde University, the proceedings of which were published in a book, *Bed Sore Biomechanics*,[1] which included an impressive list of contributions from a variety of scientific and medical disciplines. The book contained a number of critical messages concerning the factors associated with the absolute levels of prolonged pressure at the patient–support interface that can cause tissue breakdown. In particular, the time of prolonged pressure[2] and the presence of shear forces[3,4] were both clearly established as important factors. In addition, the effects of a number of external mechanical stimuli on tissue using animal models were described, the damage being assessed using histological methods.

Given this knowledge base it may be worth asking what has been achieved in the last 25 years as prevalence rates have remained unacceptably high as described in other chapters. This is, at least, partly due to the limited fundamental knowledge related to the etiology of the clinical condition. Thus, the design and application of preventive aids and risk assessment techniques are still dominated by subjective measures or, at best, based on a relatively small amount of data focusing on skin, which are largely outdated or misinterpreted.

A striking example is the traditionally quoted value for capillary closure pressure of 32 mmHg (4.3 kPa) that is still frequently used as a threshold for tissue damage. This value was based on the measured pressure in the skin capillaries within the nail folds[5] and thus represents a measure of localized interstitial pressure not relevant to areas at risk of pressure-induced damage. Its use is totally inappropriate as a threshold value for interface pressures at load-bearing sites. Interface pressures at the contact area between skin and supporting surfaces in excess of this value are assumed to produce a degree of ischemia that, if applied for a sufficient period of time, may lead to tissue breakdown.[6,7] Ignoring factors other than pressure-induced ischemia for tissue breakdown in pressure ulcers, capillary closure depends on local pressure gradients across the vessel wall and not just on interface pressures at skin level. Hence interface pressures well above capillary pressures can be supported by the soft tissues before blood flow is seriously impaired.[8] An interesting observation reported by Husain[9] was that localized interface pressures obliterated more vessels in the skin and subcutaneous tissue than in the muscle, while the latter was severely damaged and the skin and subcutis were not. Later studies also demonstrated that muscle tissue is more susceptible to mechanical loading than skin.[6,10]

In order to be able to reduce the prevalence of pressure ulcers it is essential to improve and expand understanding of the etiology in terms of both basic science and clinical experience. A more rigorous analysis of existing data is postulated followed by a hierarchical research approach in which the effects of mechanical loading on the different functional units of soft tissue are studied. This chapter evaluates the current research achievements and proposes new avenues which can provide the necessary scientific evidence to enable the development of successful prevention strategies.

Interface Pressure Measurements

It has long been recognized that the field of bioengineering can play a major role in the research activity. Perhaps its most established activity in pressure sore research has involved the development of a range of pressure monitoring systems, to supersede the previous gold standard, the Talley-Schimedics single cell system (described by Reswick and Rogers[2]). One such advance was the Oxford Mk I/II, later the Talley Pressure Monitoring system, employing an array of 96 sensors.[11] This system has been replaced by other more numerous sensor arrays with associated elegant software to display pressure profiles, produced by companies such as Tekscan, FSA, and Novel. Such monitoring systems are clearly valuable in both research and clinical settings, either in assessing the performance of one product (often new) against its competitors or in the comparison of a range of support products with an individual patient. However, it is well recognized that pressure measurements alone are not able to either alert the clinician to areas of tissue that are particularly vulnerable to the initiation of ulcers or provide insight into many fundamental aspects of the clinical problem, such as etiology or identification of susceptible subjects.

Such a conclusion could be supported by examining the pressure profile of a patient with motor neuron disease who reported to a seating clinic with persistent tissue breakdown in an area marginally distal to the left ischial tuberosity.[12] Close examination revealed some asymmetry in the pressure distribution (Figure 3.1), but no obvious high peak pressures or high pressure gradients under the left ischium compared to the right. However, the measurement of local transcutaneous gas tensions was significantly different on the two sides (Figure 3.1). Thus it appeared that the measured interface pressures of up to 73 mmHg (9.7 kPa) were sufficient to reduce the tissue oxygen from an inherently compromised level under the left ischium, but were not able to produce the same effect on the tissue under the right ischium, which had higher unloaded oxygen levels. This led to a series of studies which evaluated the effects of pressure and time on skin tissue viability.

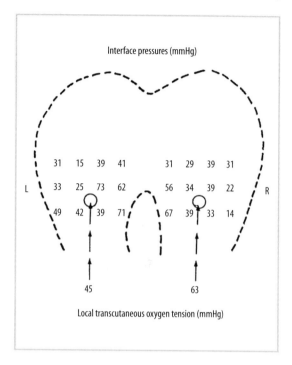

Figure 3.1 Interface pressure profile under the ischia of a patient with recurrent tissue breakdown under the left ischium. (Based on Bader and Chase.[12])

Evaluation of Tissue Status under External Loading

Over the last two decades, a number of techniques have been proposed to indicate the viability, or status, of soft tissues subjected to periods of loading. These techniques have been, to date, largely restricted to examining the response of skin layers to mechanical loading, and include measurements of blood flow in the skin using laser Doppler fluxmetry[13] and reflective spectrophotometry.[14,15] Advances in the latter technique have enabled distinct absorption spectra to be identified for oxygenated and deoxygenated blood in skin. The authors claimed that a number of other skin biomolecules, such as melanin and collagen, can also be distinguished.[15] However, the most common technique employed to measure skin viability involves transcutaneous gas tensions ($TcPO_2$ and $TcPCO_2$), which to ensure maximum vasodilation have to be measured at elevated skin temperatures.[8,16–19]

One such study examined the effects of cyclic loading on the tissue viability of healthy and debilitated subjects.[8] Two distinct responses were observed as shown in Figure 3.2. The normal response yielded a rapid and complete tissue recovery to unloaded $TcPO_2$ levels and the apparent effect of the applied load diminished with successive cycles. By contrast, in some cases recovery was not fully achieved within a prescribed period and subsequent loading had a cumulative effect on the diminution of $TcPO_2$ levels. It is this latter group who must be considered to be at particular risk of developing pressure ulcers.

The technique has also been employed specifically to investigate patients both in the acute phase[20] and in the subacute phase of spinal cord injury.[21] The latter study employed an assessment criterion for tissue viability based on the

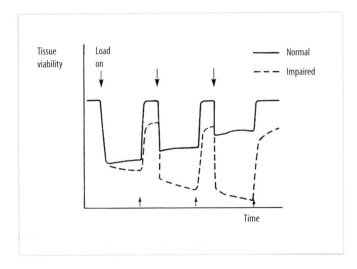

Figure 3.2 A schematic representation of two distinct responses with respect to the viability of soft tissues subjected to repeated loading. Arrows up (down) represent start of applied loading (recovery) period. (Based on Bader and Chase.[12])

percentage time at which the TcPO$_2$ and TcPCO$_2$ values were within acceptable levels when subjects were seated on prescribed support cushions. Clear relationships were indicated between depressed levels of TcPO$_2$ and elevated levels of TcPCO$_2$, at associated high values of interface pressure.[21] In addition, it was reported that changes in tissue viability do occur during a 12-month period, although a subpopulation, involving paraplegic subjects with flaccid paralysis, remain highly susceptible to the development of pressure ulcers.

This research activity spawned the routine use of these objectives measures to assess all patients with spinal cord injury at a specialized seating clinic.[18] This recent paper questioned the efficiency of short-term pressure lifts in restoring the tissue oxygen levels following prolonged seated periods. Indeed the authors recommend the use of alternative pressure relief strategies tailored to individual patients. Although yielding solid practical education for both patients and carers, these and related studies have still yielded no clear guidelines as to the precise relationship between compromised tissue gas levels for a set time period and the onset of progressive tissue breakdown that will ultimately result in a pressure ulcer.

Tissue Biochemistry

An alternative biochemical approach to assessing tissue status is to examine the metabolite levels in localized soft tissue areas subjected to pressure ischemia and subsequent reperfusion. These metabolites can be transferred via the sweat glands, which are simple tubular glands, and can be collected at the skin surface. Sweat is a hypotonic solution of sodium and chloride ions in water, together with other constituents including lactate, urea, and potassium, these metabolites accounting for about 95% of the osmotically active substances in sweat.[23]

In one of the few relevant studies, Hagisawa and colleagues[24] used a bulky system to chemically induce sweat production. By contrast, a series of studies by the author and colleagues[25–28] collected thermally induced sweat by absorption on thin pads, made from filter paper, attached to the skin surface. This collection system provided minimal distortion and proved ideal for use at a loaded tissue support interface. One such study compared sweat collected during periods of loading at the ischium and sacrum with sweat collected during unloaded periods at adjacent tissue sites.[25] The study revealed that tissues subjected to partial ischemia, specifically produced by a uniaxial indenter system, yielded a general increase in concentrations of sweat lactate, chloride, urea, and urate associated with a decreased sweat rate. Following the removal of loading, the levels of both sweat metabolites tended to be restored to basal levels.

In a separate study,[29] sweat was collected at two adjacent sites, one loaded and one unloaded, at the sacrum of a number of able-bodied subjects. Three distinct pressures were applied. Estimations were made of both the absolute values of sweat metabolite concentrations and the ratios of the concentration at both loaded and unloaded tissue sites, thus eliminating the wide variation between subjects. As an example, the ratio for lactate is presented as a function of the three applied pressures in Figure 3.3. It is evident that there is a significant increase in sweat lactate ratios at applied pressures of 40 mmHg (5.3 kPa) and above. Indeed a linear regression model applied to the lactate data, using the Spearman correlation coefficient, revealed statistical significance at the 5% level. Similar trends were also apparent with sweat urea, urate, and chloride.[28] In addition, the absolute lactate concentrations for the three pressures were pooled as loaded data in conjunction with unloaded data to yield two separate relationships with the inverse of sweat rate. The data sets yielded significant linear trends, although both slopes and intercepts of the models associated with the loaded data were higher than those for the unloaded controls.[30]

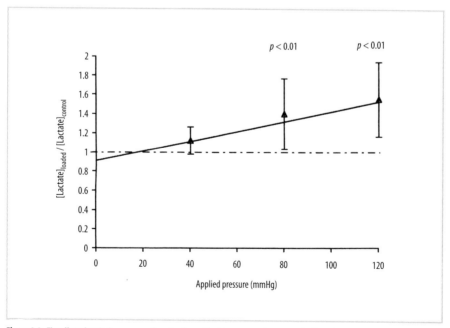

Figure 3.3 The effect of applied pressure on the ratio of sweat lactate concentration as a result of sacral loading in a group of able-bodied subjects. Linear model $y = 0.0046x + 0.975; r = 0.48, p < 0.01$.

The study was extended by employing two independent techniques in combination to assess the soft tissue response to applied pressure in a group of able-bodied subjects, to establish baseline data.[29] The methods involved the simultaneous measurement of the local tensions of oxygen and carbon dioxide ($TcPO_2$ and $TcPCO_2$) and the collection and subsequent analysis of metabolite concentrations of sweat samples. Adjacent loaded and unloaded sites on the sacrum were tested to allow for between-subject variation. Several parameters were selected from each of the techniques and their interrelationships were examined. Results indicated that oxygen levels ($TcPO_2$) were lowered in soft tissues subjected to applied pressures of between 40 mmHg (5.3 kPa) and 120 mmHg (16.0 kPa).[29] At the higher pressure levels, this decrease was generally associated with an increase in carbon dioxide levels well above the normal basal levels of 45 mmHg (6 kPa). By comparing selected parameters, a threshold value for loaded $TcPO_2$ could be identified, representing a reduction of approximately 60% from unloaded values, as indicated in Figure 3.4a. Above this threshold level there was a significant relationship between this parameter and the loaded/unloaded concentration ratios for both sweat lactate and urea.[29] Given that tissue oxygen and sweat lactate reflect different aspects of tissue ischemia, this degree of reduction (60% in median oxygen tension) may represent a critical level for the development of tissue damage. The study also related the lactate ratio to the percentage time at which $TcPCO_2$ exceeded 50%. Figure 3.4b indicates the presence of two distinct clusters of data. For example, when the carbon dioxide parameter exceeded 37%, the lactate ratios were well in excess of unity. Differences could be attributed to the degree of pressure-induced tissue ischemia. Thus under conditions of mild ischemia elevated levels of tissue carbon dioxide may be released from loaded areas in a normal manner, resulting in $TcPCO_2$ values below 50 mmHg, whereas in severe conditions, both sweat lactate and $TcPCO_2$ will be elevated (Figure 3.4b).

Sweat lactate is generally thought to be derived from the sweat gland itself.[23,31] During normal metabolism, oxidative phosphorylation is believed to be the main metabolic pathway of the eccrine sweat gland.[32] However, under conditions of ischemia and/or in anaerobic conditions, glycolysis becomes the main metabolic pathway resulting in the formation of lactate. This explains the elevated lactate concentrations observed in the sweat collected from the loaded experimental site and suggests that a sufficient degree of ischemia was induced in the sacral tissue during the two loading periods.

Sweat urea is believed to be derived mainly from serum urea by the passive diffusion across the glandular wall and cell membrane, although it is still unknown whether it is also produced by the sweat gland.[32] Urea is the main product of protein metabolism and can thus be an indicator of tissue damage if elevated levels are found in bodily fluids, such as urine or blood. Prolonged periods of ischemia can lead to muscle damage, resulting in an increased serum urea level which, in turn, can result in enhanced concentrations of sweat urea.[32] These findings as evidenced in the published study[29] suggest that the tissue was compromised during the loading period. It was strongly proposed by the authors that such an approach, using a series of parameters, might prove useful in identifying those subjects whose soft tissue may be compromised during periods of pressure ischemia.

Current work by the authors suggests that monitoring sweat lactate and urea alone is not sufficient to give a full indication of the tissue status, particularly during reperfusion.[30] Sweat purines, specifically uric acid, xanthine, and hypoxanthine, are undoubtedly useful markers or "finger prints," as they provide an

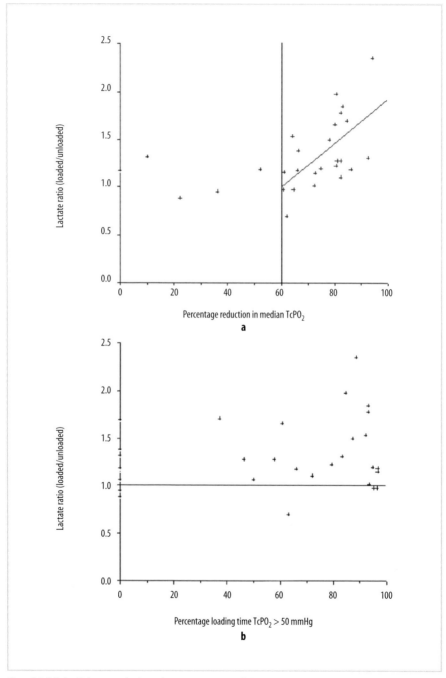

Figure 3.4 Relationship between ratio of sweat lactate concentration and (**a**) percentage reduction in transcutaneous gas tension (TcPO$_2$) and (**b**) percentage of time for which transcutaneous carbon dioxide tension (TcPCO$_2$) exceeded 50 mmHg, as a result of sacral loading on individual subjects. (Based on Knight et al.[29])

indication of the metabolic status of the tissue during both ischemia, when there is energy depletion, and reperfusion and, as such, may be of significant potential use to identify patients at risk of developing pressure ulcers. It is clear that the use of a combination of biochemical markers is required to monitor the status of soft tissues.

Internal Mechanical Environment

Although it is well acknowledged that pressure sores are primarily caused by sustained mechanical loading of the soft tissues of the body, prevention of the sores by reducing the degree of loading alone remains difficult. This is mainly due to the fact that the underlying pathways whereby mechanical loading leads to tissue breakdown are poorly understood. It is not clear how global, external loading conditions are transferred to local stresses and strains inside the tissues and how these internal conditions may ultimately lead to tissue breakdown.

As mentioned in the introduction, surface or interface pressures are not representative of the internal mechanical conditions inside the tissue, which are most relevant for tissue breakdown. This is especially the case when tissue geometry and composition are complex and surface pressures result in highly inhomogeneous internal mechanical conditions, as is the case adjacent to bony prominences. Nonetheless, in order to study the response of various tissue layers to mechanical loading the local mechanical environment within these layers needs to be known. There are options available to measure the internal mechanical state, although they inevitably involve invasive techniques such as a wick catheter.[33,34] Sangeorzan et al.[34] reported that the values for interface and intersitial pressures were not equivalent and were highly dependent on the nature of the intervening soft tissues. Thus the thickness, tone, and mechanical integrity of subcutaneous tissues, and the proximity of bony prominences will influence this relationship. A more recent investigation of elderly subjects during a single surgical procedure, namely the fixation of a fractured neck of femur, examined the response of tissues adjacent to the lateral aspect of the proximal thigh. Results indicated that skin interface pressures were dissipated within the depth of the tissues resulting in reduced internal stresses.[35] Indeed linear models of the data suggested interstitial stresses ranging between 29% and 40% of the applied interface pressures, as illustrated in Figure 3.5. This highlights the protective nature of tissues to attenuate the effects of sustained pressure.

An alternative approach to investigate the transition from global external loads to local internal stresses and strains involves the use of computer models, in particular using finite element analysis (FEA).[36–39] This approach, which models the complex geometries and material behavior of the human buttocks, is often unfamiliar to experimentalists and clinical and nursing staff. In the study by Todd and Tacker,[37] the seated positions were simulated, thereby manipulating boundary conditions of the model. These authors concluded that there was no clear correlation between interface pressures and the local mechanical conditions. Oomens and co-workers[40] created a finite element model of a human subject sitting on a cushion, which incorporated three different tissues, overlaying the human ischial tuberosities, simulated by an undeformable bony indenter. The soft tissues, namely the muscle, fat, and skin, were modeled as nonlinear viscoelastic materials. Figure 3.6 clearly shows the inhomogeneous mechanical condition of the various tissue layers and areas of high internal stresses in the deeper fat and muscle layers.

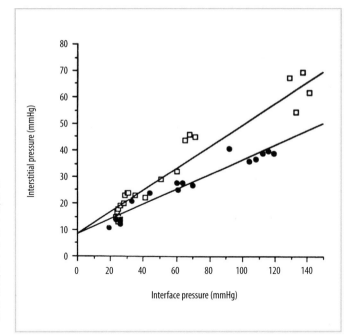

Figure 3.5 The relationship between interface pressures and interstitial pressures within the soft tissues adjacent to the greater trochanter of two surgical patients undergoing hip screw fixation of an intertrochanteric femoral fracture. Slopes of two linear models are 0.28 and 0.41, $r > 0.96$ in both cases. (Based on Bader and White.[35])

However, any extrapolation of results from these computer analyses to the clinical setting must be undertaken with extreme caution. Specifically these models are dependent on the lack of reliable material properties for soft tissues, which can be influenced by many systemic and local factors, such as temperature and nutritional status. Thus, although several studies have examined uniaxial and biaxial properties of skin parallel to its surface, there are few reported studies examining the compressive properties of the soft tissue composite. Such studies have been

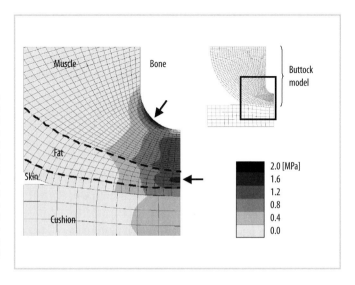

Figure 3.6 Simplified computer model of axisymmetric deformed buttock (*top right*) demonstrating the differential response of the separate soft tissue layers (*left*) during sitting of an 80 kg male subject on a foam cushion. Values indicate Von Mises stresses, representing distortional energy. Note the areas of high stress in the subcutaneous fat and muscle layers (*arrows*). (Based on Oomens et al.[40])

hampered by the lack of appropriate non-invasive techniques that can characterize material properties of tissue under load. For example, ultrasound has offered
much potential for many years but has, as yet, not proved reliable, although more
sophisticated systems involving elastography in association with ultrasound
imaging might prove successful in the future. Other imaging technologies
involving infrared spectroscopy and magnetic resonance imaging/spectroscopy
(MRI/MRS) may also provide valuable data under loading conditions for both
healthy tissues and where tissue status is compromised. Indeed in recent studies
Gefen and colleagues[41,42] have determined mechanical stiffness of soft tissues
under load, using routine MRI scans. An increased mechanical stiffness was also
reported corresponding to mixed tissue specimens around human ulcers compared to control values.[43]

Mechanisms of Pressure Ulcer Development

Conventional wisdom on the pathogenesis of pressure ulcers has focused on the
effects of pressure-induced ischemia on skin tissues. Although important there are
other major considerations, as outlined in a recent viewpoint article,[44] involving
the lymphatic system, interstitial transport, underlying tissues particularly the
muscle, ischemia–reperfusion injury, and sustained deformation of cells. Several
seminal papers associated with each of these mechanisms have been highlighted
in Table 3.1. Although known for several decades, these mechanisms have not been
fully explored often due to technical reasons. As an example, the obliteration of
lymphatic flow due to external pressure was measured in an animal limb, using a
radioactive tracer.[48] Clearly, this experimental approach could not be adopted in a
human model. In a similar manner, ischemic and reperfusion damage is traditionally evaluated using histological techniques, which are both time-consuming
and do not permit real-time assessment of damage.

Overall the theories focus on different functional units of soft tissue, involving
cells, the interstitial space with extracellular matrix, and blood and lymph vessels.
These units are affected by mechanical loading to varying degrees and hence have
different relevance for tissue breakdown. Most probably each of them contributes
to the causation of pressure ulcers, although their individual and combined role in

Table 3.1. The pathophysiology of pressure ulcers: soft tissue response to mechanical loading

Mechanism	Consequences	Key papers
1. Localized ischemia	Capillary perfusion decreases with mechanical loading Lack of local vital nutrients	Daniel et al.[6]—animal model Kosiak[7]—animal model Dinsdale[4]—animal model Herrman et al.[45]—animal model
2. Impaired interstitial fluid flow and lymphatic drainage	Accumulation of metabolic waste products	Krouskop et al.[46]—hypothesis Reddy et al.[47]—theoretical model Miller and Seale[48]—animal model
3. Reperfusion injury	Restoration of blood flow may lead to toxic levels of oxygen free radicals	McCord[49]—hypothesis Peirce et al.[50]—animal model Unal et al.[51]—animal model
4. Sustained deformation of cells	Local cell damage and death	Ryan[52]—theoretical model Landsman et al.[53]—cell model Bouten et al.[54]—cell model

tissue breakdown will undoubtedly vary depending on the nature of the mechanical insult and patient characteristics such as illness or age,[55] which affect soft tissue properties and hence the liability to tissue breakdown.

Hierarchical Approach

A hierarchical approach has recently proposed[44] in which the effects of loading are studied using different, yet complementary, model systems with increasing complexity and length scale and incorporating one or more functional tissue units. Thus, in vitro models, ranging from the single cell (µm scale) to cell-matrix constructs (mm scale) and individual tissue layers (mm–cm scale), might be used to study the relationship between cell deformation and cell damage as well as the influence of the surrounding extracellular matrix and three-dimensional tissue architecture on this relationship. The role of tissue (re)perfusion and lymph flow as well as the interaction between tissue layers in bulk tissue might further be assessed using in vivo studies with animal models or human subjects.

The different length scales of these models can be coupled to multiscale computer calculations that enable the prediction of the internal microscopic mechanical environment within a given model from global, macroscopic loading conditions, such as interface pressures (and vice versa). In this way relationships between, for instance, cell deformation and cell damage[54] can be extrapolated to the level of bulk tissue to give clinically relevant predictions on tissue breakdown.

Recent Focus on Pressure-Induced Muscle Damage

Muscle tissue is particularly susceptible to sustained compression. Compression-induced muscle breakdown predominantly occurs in muscle layers associated with bony prominences, eventually leading to gross tissue degeneration in the form of deep pressure ulcers.[8,21,57–59] This breakdown starts at the cellular level with nuclear pyknosis and disintegration of the contractile proteins and the cell membrane, followed by inflammatory reactions.[6,7,10,60,61] Although it is clear that both the magnitude and the duration of compression affect the cellular breakdown, the underlying pathways whereby tissue compression leads to injury of the cell remain poorly understood. Moreover, most of the mechanisms detailed in Table 3.1 ignore the direct effects of cellular deformation due to prolonged tissue compression, which have recently been suggested as an important trigger for pressure ulcer development.[52–54]

The earlier study[52] was extended to study cellular breakdown in response to sustained cell deformation, independently of other factors, such as blood perfusion. It utilized a three-dimensional in vitro system, incorporating cultured muscle cells seeded in an agarose gel construct. The feasibility of this system to induce prolonged cell deformation during gross construct compression was recently demonstrated by the authors.[54] Strain applied to the translucent agarose gel results in deformation of the muscle cells to an elliptical form, which can be quantified using confocal laser scanning microscopy. Identical cylindrical cores cut from the agarose/cell suspension were subjected to two separate compressive strains, 10% and 20%. The strain was applied for time periods ranging from 0.5 to 12 hours, using a specially designed loading apparatus.[62] After each compression period, sections taken from the central horizontal plane of the individual constructs were stained using both histological and fluorescent probes, to assess the proportion of damage. It was found that constructs subjected to the higher strain values demonstrated significantly higher values of nonviable cells for equivalent time points compared to the unstrained constructs, as illustrated in Figure 3.7. These findings imply a relationship between the duration of applied compression and damage to muscle cells seeded in the gel. Such an approach might be useful in establishing damage threshold levels at a cellular level. The model was extended further by developing a more physiological tissue equivalent muscle,[63] by suspending premature muscle cells in a collagen scaffold. The muscle cells fused into a branched network of multinucleated, contractile myofibers by the application of appropriate biochemical and mechanical cues. Results indicated that cell death was evident within 1–2 hours at clinically relevant straining percentages.

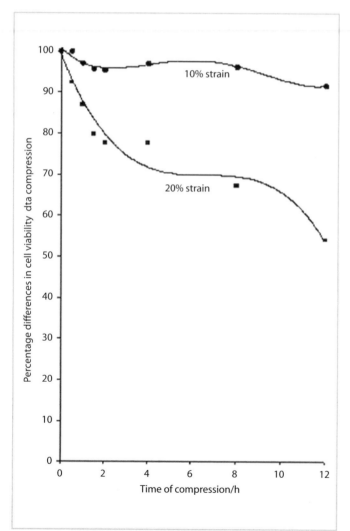

Figure 3.7 THE effects of prolonged static compression at two applied strains on the viability of muscle cells seeded in agarose constructs, as indicated by histological assessment.

In addition, the uniform distribution of dead cells throughout the muscle constructs suggested that sustained deformation was the principal cause of cell death. A hybrid approach was then adopted by the authors in which these experimental data were used in the derivation of a damage law.[64] In particular, the evolution of damage was predicted in a single microstructural unit, which could be extrapolated to the macroscopic scale. A damage evolution parameter, D, was defined, which accumulates with time when the dimensionless strain energy density parameter, U, in a cell is higher than a cell tolerance parameter, α. The authors proposed a damage evolution equation:

$$D = \int_0^t \beta(U - \alpha)dt,$$

where both α and β are material parameters that can be determined from the in vitro experiment. Although limited at the present time to qualitative insight into tissue damage, this multilevel finite element approach has future potential as a quantitative predictor of damage in patient-related simulations.

The advent of new technologies that are sensitive to changes throughout the soft tissue composite provide new opportunities for the examination of animal models,[50,51,60] despite their limitations associated with intrinsic biological variation, ethical issues, and inadequate experimental controls. As an example, Bosboom et al.[60] examined the ability of MRI to assess local muscle damage after prolonged transverse loading. The tibialis anterior muscle (TA) and overlying skin of a rat were compressed between an indenter and tibia. A very large pressure, equivalent to 1875 mmHg (250 kPa), was applied for 2 hours. Histological examination, using a semi-automated image-processing program, and in vivo T2-weighted MRI were performed 24 hours after the completion of the loading session. Figure 3.8 (see color section) illustrates the damage in transverse histological slices (below) and the associated MR images for three sets of experiments. In each case, the location of damage coincided well in the two assessment techniques. However, the inter-animal variability in damage is evident. Current work has involved a modified MR-compatible loading apparatus to produce more reproducible tissue damage and learn more about the influence of deformation of the tissue and the influence of reperfusion.[65]

A large variety of imaging techniques have been developed that can be applied to assess structure, function, and metabolism of skeletal muscle. These include tagging MRI and perfusion MRI, which can be used to measure local tissue deformation and tissue perfusion, respectively. In addition, MR spectroscopy could be applied to examine the biochemical status of the tissue.

Final Comments

After a stagnant period of research on pressure ulcers and their etiology, there is now real hope of a resurgence of progress, largely associated with the applicability of new technology allied to the well-established financial implications of the costs of the clinical problem to the health of individual nations. This can only be achieved by research teams, medical doctors, carers, and organizations such as the European Pressure Ulcer Advisory Panel (EPUAP) lobbying the appropriate agencies to release valuable research funds.[66]

Acknowledgments

The author (DLB) is grateful to a large number of clinical colleagues and students, who have worked with him in Oxford and London. In addition, since 2000, he has had the wonderful opportunity to collaborate with his joint author at the Technical University of Eindhoven, with valuable contributions and support from Carlijn Bouten and Frank Baaijens, and the team of enthusiastic research students.

References

1. Kenedi RM, Cowden JM, Scales JT. Bed sore biomechanics. Basingstoke: Macmillan; 1976: 1–357.
2. Reswick JB, Rogers JE. Experiences at Rancho Los Amigos Hospital with devices and techniques to prevent pressure sores. In: Kenedi RM, Cowden JM, Scales JT (eds) Bed sore biomechanics. Basingstoke: Macmillan; 1976: 301–310.
3. Reichel S. Shearing force as a factor in decubitus ulcers in paraplegics. JAMA 1958; 116:762.
4. Dinsdale SM. Decubitus ulcers: role of pressure and friction in causation. Arch Phys Med Rehabil 1974; 55:147–152.
5. Landis EM. Micro-injection studies of capillary blood pressure in human skin. Heart 1930; 15:209–228.
6. Daniel RK, Priest DL, Wheatley DC. Etiologic factors in pressure sores: an experimental model. Arch Phys Med Rehabil 1982; 62:492–498.
7. Kosiak M. The etiology of pressure sores. Arch Phys Med Rehabil 1961; 42:19–29.
8. Bader DL. The recovery characteristics of soft tissue following repeated loading. J Rehabil Res Dev 1990; 27:141–150.
9. Husain T. An experimental study of some pressure effects on tissues, with reference to the bed sore problem. J Pathol Bacteriol 1953; 66:347–358.
10. Nola GT, Vistnes LM. Differential response of skin and muscle in the experimental production of pressure sores. Plast Reconstr Surg 1980; 66:728–733.
11. Bader DL, Hawken MB. Pressure distribution under the ischium of normal subjects. J Biomed Eng 1986; 8(4):353–357.
12. Bader DL, Chase AP. The patient-orthosis interface. In: Bowker P, Bader DL, Pratt D, et al. (eds) Biomechanical basis of orthotic management. Oxford: Butterworth-Heinemann; 1993: 58–69.
13. Schubert V, Fagrell B. Post-occlusive reactive hyperaemia and thermal response in the skin microcirculation of subjects with spinal cord injury. Scand J Rehabil Med 1991; 23:33–45.
14. Hagisawa S, Ferguson-Pell M, Cardi M, Miller SD. Assessment of skin blood content and oxygenation in spinal injured subjects during reactive hyperaemia. J Rehabil Res Dev 1994; 31:1–14.
15. Ferguson-Pell M, Hagisawa S. An empirical technique to compensate for melanin when monitoring skin microcirculation using reflectance spectrophotometry. Med Eng Phys 1995; 7:104–110.
16. Newson TP, Rolfe P. Skin surface PO_2 and blood flow measurements over the ischial tuberosities. Arch Phys Med Rehabil 1982; 63:553–556.
17. Bader DL. Effects of compressive load regimens on tissue viability. In: Bader DL (ed) Pressure sores—clinical practice and scientific approach. Basingstoke: Macmillan Press; 1990: 191–201.
18. Colin D, Saumet JL. Influence of external pressure on transcutaneous oxygen tension and laser Doppler flowmetry on sacral skin. Clin Physiol 1996; 16:61–72.
19. Colin D, Loyant R, Abraham P, Saumet JL. Changes in sacral transcutaneous oxygen tension in the evaluation of different mattresses in the prevention of pressure ulcers. Adv Wound Care 1996; 9:25–28.
20. Bogie KM, Nuseibeh I, Bader DL. Transcutaneous gas tensions in the sacrum during the acute phase of spinal cord injury. Eng Med 1992; 206:1–6.
21. Bogie KM, Nuseibeh I, Bader DL. Early progressive changes in tissue viability in the seated spinal cord injured subject. Paraplegia 1995; 33:1441–1447.
22. Coggrave MJ, Rose LS. A specialist seating assessment clinic: changing pressure relief practice. Spinal Cord 2003; 41:692–695.
23. Van Heyningen R, Weiner JS. The effect of arterial occlusion on sweat composition. Physiology 1952; 116:404–413.

24. Hagisawa S, Ferguson-Pell M, Cardi M, Miller SD. Biochemical changes in sweat following pressure ischaemia. J Rehabil Res Dev 1988; 25:57–62.
25. Polliack AA, Taylor RP, Bader DL. The analysis of sweat during soft tissue breakdown following pressure ischaemia. J Rehabil Res Dev 1993; 30(2):250–259.
26. Polliack AA, Taylor RP, Bader DL. Sweat analysis following pressure ischaemia in a group of debilitated subjects. J Rehabil Res Dev 1997; 34(3):303–308.
27. Taylor RP, Polliack AA, Bader DL. The analysis of metabolites in human sweat: analytical methods and potential application to investigation of pressure ischaemia of soft tissues. Ann Clin Biochem 1994; 31:18–24.
28. Knight SL. Non-invasive techniques for predicting soft tissue status during pressure induced ischaemia. PhD thesis, Queen Mary, University of London; 1997.
29. Knight SL, Taylor RP, Polliack AA, Bader DL. Establishing predictive indicators for the status of soft tissues. J Appl Physiol 2001; 90:2231–2237.
30. Bader DL, Wang Y-N, Knight SL, et al. Biochemical status of soft tissues subjected to sustained pressure. In: Bader DL, Bouten CVC, Colin D, CWJ Oomens (eds) Pressure ulcer research: Current and future perspectives. Springer-Verlag; 2005 (in press).
31. Sato K. The physiology, pharmacology and biochemistry of the eccrine sweat gland. Rev Physiol Biochem Pharmacol 1977; 79:51–131.
32. Sato K, Dobson RL. Glucose metabolism of the isolated eccrine sweat gland. J Clin Invest 1973; 5:2166–2174.
33. Dodd KT, Gross DR. Three-dimensional tissue deformation in subcutaneous tissues overlying bony prominences may help to explain external load transfer to the interstitium. J Biomech 1991; 24:11–19.
34. Sangeorzan BJ, Harrington RM, Wyss CR, et al. Circulation and mechanical response of skin to loading. J Orthopaed Res 1989; 7:425–431.
35. Bader DL, White SH. The viability of soft tissues in elderly subjects undergoing hip surgery. Age Ageing 1998; 27:217–221.
36. Chow CC, Odell EI. Deformation and stresses in soft body tissues of a sitting person. J Biomech Eng 1978; 100:79–86.
37. Todd BA, Tacker JG. Three dimensional computer model of the human buttocks in vivo. J Rehabil Res Dev 1994; 31(2):111–119.
38. Oomens CWJ, Van Campen DH, Grootenboer HJ. A mixture approach to the mechanics of skin. J Biomech 1987; 9:877–885.
39. Zhang JD, Mak AFT, Huang LD. A large deformation biomechanical model for pressure ulcers. J Biomech Eng 1997; 119:406–408.
40. Oomens CWJ, Bressers OFJT, Bosboom EMH, et al. Can loaded interface characteristics influence strain distributions in muscle adjacent to bony prominences? Comput Methods Biomech Biomed Eng 2003; 6:171–180.
41. Gefen A, Megido-Ravid M, Azariah M, et al. Integration of plantar foot stiffness measurements in routine MRI of the diabetic foot. Clin Biomech 2001; 16:921–925.
42. Linder-Ganz E, Gefen A. Stiffening of muscle tissue under bony compression is a key factor in the formation of pressure sores. In: 25th International Conference of the IEEE Engineering in Medicine and Biology Society, Cancun, Mexico; 2003.
43. Edsberg LE, Cutway R, Anain S, Natiella JR. Microstructural and mechanical characterisation of human tissue at and adjacent to pressure ulcers. J Rehabil Res Dev 2000; 37: 463–471.
44. Bouten CVC, Oomens CWJ, Baaijens FPT, Bader DL. The aetiology of pressure sores: Skin deep or muscle bound? Arch Phys Med Rehabil 2003; 84:616–619.
45. Herrman EC, Knapp CF, Donofrio JC, Salcido R. Skin perfusion responses to surface pressure induced ischemia: Implication for the developing pressure ulcer. J Rehabil Res Dev 1999; 36:109–120.
46. Krouskop TA. A synthesis of the factors that contribute to pressure sore formation. Med Hypotheses 1983; 11:255–267.
47. Reddy NP, Patel H, Krouskop TA. Interstitial fluid flow as a factor in decubitus ulcer formation. J Biomech 1981; 14:879–881.
48. Miller GE, Seale J. Lymphatic clearance during compressive loading. Lymphology 1981; 14:161–166.
49. McCord JM. Oxygen-derived free radicals in postischaemic tissue injury. N Engl J Med 1985; 312:159–163.
50. Peirce SM, Skalak TC, Rodeheaver GT. Ischemia-reperfusion injury in chronic pressure ulcer formation: a skin model in the rat. Wound Repair Regen 2000; 8:68–76.

51. Unal S, Ozmen S, Demir Y, et al. The effect of gradually increased blood flow on ischaemia-reperfusion injury. Ann Plast Surg 2001; 47(4):412–416.
52. Ryan TJ. Cellular responses to tissue distortion. In: Bader DL (ed) Pressure sores: Clinical practice and scientific approach. Basingstoke: Macmillan Press; 1990: 141–152.
53. Landsman AS, Meaney DF, Cargill RS 2nd, et al. High strain rate tissue deformation. A theory on the mechanical aetiology of diabetic foot ulcerations. J Am Podiatr Med Assoc 1995; 85:519–527.
54. Bouten CVC, Lee DA, Knight MM, Bader DL. Compressive deformation and damage of muscle cell sub-populations in a model system. J Biomech Eng 2001; 29:153–163.
55. Bliss MR. Aetiology of pressure sores. Rev Clin Gerontol 1993; 3:379–397.
56. Crenshaw RP, Vistnes LM. Decade of pressure sore research: 1977–1987. J Rehabil Res Dev 1989; 262:63–74.
57. Harman JW. The significance of local vascular phenomena in the production of ischaemic necrosis in skeletal muscle. Am J Pathol 1948; 24:625–641.
58. Bouten CVC, Stijnen JM, Oomens CWJ, et al. Interstitial fluid pressure measurement during compressive loading of the rat tibialis anterior muscle. ASME Bioengineering Conference, BED-35; 1997: 491–492.
59. Makelbust J. Pressure ulcers: Etiology and prevention. Nurs Clin North Am 1987; 22:359–375.
60. Bosboom EMH, Bouten CVC, Oomens CWJ, et al. Quantification and localisation of damage in rat muscles after controlled loading; a new approach to the aetiology of pressure sores. Med Eng Phys 2001; 23:195–200.
61. Caplan A, Carlson B, Faulkner J, et al. Skeletal muscle. In: Woo SL-Y, Buckwalter JA (eds) Injury and repair of the musculoskeletal soft tissues. Park Ridge, IL: American Academy of Orthopedic Surgeons; 1988: 213–291.
62. Lee DA, Bader DL. Compressive strain at physiological frequencies influence the metabolism of chondrocytes seeded in agarose. J Orthop Res 1997; 15:181–188.
63. Breuls RGM, Bouten CVC, Oomens, et al. Compression induced cell damage in engineered muscle tissue: An in vitro model to study pressure ulcer aetiology. Ann Biomed Eng 2003; 31:1357–1364.
64. Breuls RGM, Bouten CVC, Oomens CWJ, et al. A theoretical analysis of damage evolution in skeletal muscle tissue with reference to pressure ulcer development. J Biomech Eng 2003; 125:902–909.
65. Stekelenburg A, Oomens CWJ, Bader DL. Compression induced tissue damage; animal models. In: Bader DL, Bouten CVC, Colin D, Oomens J (eds) Pressure ulcer research: Current and future perspectives. Springer-Verlag; 2005 (in press).
66. Bouten CVC, Bosboom EMH, Oomens CWJ. The aetiology of pressure sores: A tissue and cell mechanics approach. In: Van der Woude LHV, Hopman MTE, Van Kemenade CH (eds) Biomedical aspects of manual wheelchair propulsion. Amsterdam: IOS Press; 1999: 52–62.

4 Etiology and Risk Factors

Mark Collier and Zena Moore

Introduction

Despite an increased number of publications being dedicated to issues relevant to the etiology, prevention, and development of pressure ulceration—especially during the past decade—recent prevalence studies undertaken throughout Europe[1] indicate that there is still much work to be undertaken and that pressure ulceration is a real problem both for patients and for the healthcare systems in which those patients are being cared for.

This chapter seeks to explore the etiology of pressure ulceration, relating the same to known pathophysiological effects likely to be experienced by the patient, and also highlights some of the known risk factors that may predispose an individual to pressure ulcer development—as supported by available current literature.

While it is acknowledged that there is still much to discover about the etiology of pressure ulceration, most of the evidence to date focuses on the relationship between external pressures applied to a patient's skin and tissues not adapted to these pressures, as well as the effects of the same on the local microcirculation.[2,3]

Pressure Defined

Bennett and Lee defined pressure as a perpendicular load or force exerted on a unit of area such as the sacrum.[4] This gravitational force is also often referred to as compression. The average pressure exerted on the skin can be calculated using the following formula:

$$\text{Pressure} = \text{Body weight/Skin contact area}$$

or by the use of pressure-sensitive equipment.[5]

In addition to the overall concept of pressure, other differing forms of pressure have also been highlighted—those of shear and friction.

Shear (a Stretching Force)

Shear is a mechanical stress that is parallel to a plane of interest.[4] When a high level of shear is present, then the amount of external pressure necessary to produce vascular occlusion is only about half the amount when shear is not present.[6] When trying to describe various clinical examples of shear, many authors have noted that when the head of the bed is elevated there is automatically a greater compressive force placed on the sacral tissues than when the bed is in the flat position.[7-9] It is thought that the shear ulcer may typically develop as a result of the patient's sacral skin adhering to the bed linen (in the sitting position); the deep fascia moves in a downward direction with the skeletal structure as a result of gravitational forces, while at the same time the sacral fascia remains attached to the sacral dermis. This effect can be minimized if the patient support surface is covered with a vapor-permeable two-way stretch cover that helps to reduce moisture build-up at the interface.[10] However, if the effects of shear are prolonged or exacerbated by the presence of moisture, regional stretching of the microcirculation of the skin may occur. If this is left unchecked it can lead to the avulsion of local capillaries and arterioles, increasing the possibility of the development of some localized tissue necrosis.

Although shear can be differentiated from pressure (compression), it has been previously highlighted that it is difficult to create pressure without shear and shear without pressure.[11]

Friction

Friction occurs when two surfaces move across one another,[12] for example when a patient undertakes a sliding transfer from a bed to a wheelchair. Friction itself is not thought to be a primary factor in the development of pressure ulcers. However, it can exacerbate the stripping of broken epidermis or be the cause of an initial break in the skin, which may then be compounded by the effects of pressure and shear forces. If the surface on which the patient is being supported is moist, it has been shown that the friction coefficient will rise and if great enough will actually lead to adherence of the patient's skin to the damp surface,[13] thereby resulting in an increase in any associated shearing effects.

In summary, then, the physical parameters that must be considered when thinking of the etiology of pressure ulcers are:

- pressure/compression,
- shear,
- friction,
- humidity of the patient's skin (may increase risk of adherence as previously described).

Transmission of Pressure

Any external pressure measured at an interface will be transmitted from the body surface (the skin) to the underlying skeletal anatomy (the bone), compressing all of the intermediate tissues. The resultant pressure gradient has been described as the McClemont "cone of pressure,"[14] in which external pressures can increase by three to five times at the point of greatest pressure experienced, such as at a bony surface. For example, an external interface pressure of 50 mmHg could rise to as much as 200 mmHg at a bony prominence such as an ischial tuberosity.

With pressure being distributed in this way it should become apparent that any external skin blemishes, however minor, identified as a result of the use of a pressure ulcer/wound classification tool such as those of Torrance[15] and Collier[16] amongst others,[17] may be indicating that necrosis of the underlying tissue is already becoming established. It is therefore important that all practitioners are able to distinguish between a normal and abnormal physiological response and if the latter is suspected that they initiate the further assessment of the same with available technology such.[18,19]

The Normal Physiological Response to Pressure

The previous information should be considered in the light of research[20] that has shown that the pressure in the capillary bed in healthy medical student volunteers ranges between 12 and 32 mmHg (Figure 4.1—see color section). Landis in 1930 suggested that a value of 32 mmHg was the mean capillary pressure at its arterial inflow—using a micro-injection technique—and other studies suggested that if this pressure is exceeded then capillary occlusion occurs—predisposing to tissue damage.[21,22] However, in 1941 Landis revised his work—using an amended technique—identifying that a more realistic figure to be considered as the capillary closing pressure should be between 45 and 50 mmHg, over which threshold damage was likely to ensue. It should be remembered, though, that any pressures measured may have different effects on different parts of the body depending on the local bone, muscle, and skin structure.

This information becomes clinically relevant when interface pressures between the skin and the standard National Health Service contract mattress have been reported as between 70 and 100 mmHg over the main bony prominences and the interface pressure between the skin and a commercially available pressure-reducing replacement mattress[5] has been shown to be between 30 and 40 mmHg when measured on an "average" individual lying in the supine position.[23]

The capillary loops in the skin run vertically to the surface and are coiled at their bases, thereby limiting the risk of occlusion as a result of direct pressure. However, in the subcutaneous tissue, the blood vessels lie mainly in the parallel planes of the deep fascia and follow the paths of ligaments and nerves. This renders them very vulnerable to distortion and occlusion as a result of pressure from both external sources and the underlying bony structures.[24] Prolonged pressure may cause ischemic changes at and around the point of occlusion. If this occlusion is prolonged, the result is both anoxia and a build-up of circulating metabolites. A release of pressure, however, produces a large and sudden increase in blood flow, as the anoxia and metabolites act on structures within the circulatory system, such as precapillary sphincters. This increase in blood flow may be as much as 30 times the resting value and the bright red flush, which is often noted, is referred to as reactive or blanching hyperemia,[25] a normal response! As little as 5 seconds of external pressure can provoke a physiological reaction that may last between one third and three quarters of the period of ischemia.[26] If the lymphatic vessels of the dependent tissue remain intact and excess interstitial fluid is removed, then it is said that permanent tissue changes will not progress.[12] *Blanching hyperemia* has been described as the distinct erythema caused by reactive hyperemia which when light finger pressure is applied will blanch (change color—whiten), indicating that the patient's microcirculation is generally intact. *Nonblanching hyperemia*—an abnormal physiological response—is detected when the color of the erythema remains when light finger pressure is applied, indicating a degree of microcirculatory disruption often associated with other clinical signs such as blistering, induration (alteration in texture of the skin), and edema.[15]

Note: The vessels in the subcutaneous tissues also give rise to the perforators that also supply the skin, and so deep vessel obstruction is likely to result in both cutaneous and subcutaneous ischemia if the period of occlusion is sustained. The results of transcutaneous oxygen assessments have suggested that perfusion of the skin is affected more greatly by subcutaneous pressure than by external interface pressures only.[27]

In order to accurately recognize both blanching and nonblanching hyperemia, it is important for the assessing practitioner not only to fully understand the definition of a pressure ulcer, but also to understand the pathophysiology of reactive hyperemia as has been reported elsewhere.[28]

Although the fragile nature of the microcirculation has been acknowledged, this does not take account of the protective function of collagen. It appears that if tissue collagen levels are not depleted, this helps to prevent disruption to the microcirculation by buffering the interstitial fluid from external pressures, thereby maintaining the optimum hydrostatic pressure.

Risk Factors

In order to identify which individuals are at risk of pressure ulcer development, it is first necessary to understand what is meant by risk. Risk has been defined as the probability of an individual developing a specific problem, such as a pressure ulcer.[29] Interventions employed to combat risk are often expensive and healthcare resources are not infinite; therefore, it is important for all practitioners to accurately identify those patients who need prevention strategies.

Many authors have attempted to identify the factors that influence the development of pressure ulcers and have summarized these factors into risk assessment tools for use in clinical practice.[30-33] This has proved a difficult task, as it is known that there are a vast number of potential risk factors. Indeed this is borne out in a review of 100 pressure ulcer articles by Gosnell,[34] where a possible 126 risk factors were identified.

Despite the apparent lack of clarity regarding what precisely predisposes an individual to risk, what appears to be central is that pressure ulcers will only develop if the individual cannot withstand the adverse effects of pressure, shear, and friction[35] as previously discussed. This ability had been defined by Braden and Bergstrom[33] as the person's "tissue tolerance," which they suggest is affected by both intrinsic and extrinsic factors. Whereas it is acknowledged that there are numerous potential risk factors it has been postulated that some specific factors play a key role in the development of pressure ulcers, namely mobility, age, nutrition, skin condition, and perfusion.[36,37] Mobility, age, and nutrition will form the basis of discussion in the remainder of this chapter.

Mobility

The role of mobility/immobility in pressure ulcer development has been an important area of interest to those involved in pressure ulcer prevention for many years. This is brought to mind when one considers that much of the expense related to this area of patient care revolves around the use of equipment based upon removing or reducing interface pressures caused by prolonged periods of immobility.

Healthy individuals regularly change their position while seated or recumbent. Indeed, Keane[38] suggested that the minimum physiological mobility requirement (MPMR) to maintain healthy tissue, while lying on a soft mattress, is one gross postural change every 11.6 minutes. This MPMR is based on observations of average individuals' repositioning frequencies during sleep. Allman[39] agrees that the association between limited activity and mobility remains an important consideration as highlighted in the seminal work of Exton-Smith and Sherwin.[40] In this study, the authors found that the amount of spontaneous nocturnal movement of elderly individuals was positively related to the development of pressure ulcers. Furthermore, as the number of movements increased the number of pressure ulcers decreased. Patients who made 50 or more movements had no pressure ulcers, whereas 90% of patients who made 20 or fewer movements developed ulcers.[39]

Pressure, from lying or sitting on a particular part of the body, results in oxygen deprivation to the affected area.[38] There is a responding painful stimulus that motivates the individual to move if this feedback mechanism has not been impaired as a result of previous injury for example; failure to reposition will result in ongoing oxygen deprivation and inevitable tissue damage.[35] The amount of damage that ensues is partly influenced by the individual's level of adipose tissue and the type of surface they are lying on.[38] Importantly, the duration of pressure sustained is also affected by a number of factors. The primary concern is the individual's ability to feel pain and the secondary concern is the individual's actual physical ability to move or reposition themselves.[35]

Using regression techniques, Papanikolaou et al.[41] estimated the probability of pressure ulcer occurrence in patients with reduced mobility, compared with those without reduced mobility. The odds ratio (OR) was identified as 5.41 ($p = 0.001$, CI 2.00–14.63). Odds ratio is a way of comparing whether the probability of a certain event is the same for two groups. In this case, because the odds ratio is greater than one, this would suggest that reduced mobility increases the likelihood of pressure ulcer development.[29]

This study is supported by the earlier work of Mino et al.[42] who found a four-fold greater relative risk (RR) for the development of pressure ulcers in patients who are unable to turn over in bed (RR 4.09). Relative risk is calculated by dividing the risk of an event in one group (pressure ulcers, in those incapable of turning in bed) by the risk of the event in the other group (pressure ulcers, in those capable of turning in bed).[29]

The relationship between pressure ulcer development and immobility has also been noted by Berlowitz et al.[43] (OR 1.1) and Lindgren et al.[44] (OR 0.53, $p = 0.011$). Although these studies have been conducted on different groups of patients, in different healthcare settings, they do suggest that prolonged periods of immobility will increase an individual's risk of developing pressure ulcers. Therefore, the levels of activity and mobility appear to be important factors to consider in assessing an individual's risk of pressure ulcer development.

Age

The association between age and pressure ulcer development is of value to explore in today's healthcare climate. Demographic forecasts suggest that in 50 years there will be three times more elderly people living in the world.[45] Indeed, by the year 2050, it is estimated that the elderly will comprise almost 17% of the global population compared to 7% in 2002.[45] The older population appear to be at greater risk of pressure ulcer development due to the likelihood of underlying neurological and cardiovascular problems.[46] Furthermore, as a consequence of aging, the skin undergoes a number of pathological changes.[37] These changes alter the elastin and collagen content of the skin, reducing its elasticity and resilience, which in turn lowers the skin's protective mechanism against the adverse effects of shear and friction.[35]

The precise association between age and pressure ulcer development has been explored by Margolis et al.[47] In this UK study the authors identified an incidence of 0.57–0.60 g/l per 100 person-years, over a 3–9 month period among elderly patients (>65 years) attending general medical practice services.[47] Pressure ulcers of stage 2 or more were included in the data, as defined by Margolis.[48] Increasing age was noted to heighten the likelihood of pressure ulcer development and this was found to be statistically significant ($p < 0.001$).

A relationship between age and pressure ulcer development was also found in an incidence study conducted in 116 acute care facilities in the USA.[49] In this study the incidence of pressure ulcers was noted to be 7%. Grade 1–4 pressure ulcers were included as per the NPUAP grading[50] and most pressure ulcers were observed to be of grade 1 or grade 2 damage (91%). Seventy-three percent of ulcers developed in those over 65 years of age, with the most common anatomical sites affected being the sacrum/coccyx and the heels.

Other authors have noted the association between increasing age and pressure ulcers; for example, Halfens et al.[51] identified an odds ratio of 2.68, and found this to be statistically significant ($p < 0.001$). Furthermore, Casimiro et al.,[52] Young et al.,[53] and Baumgarten et al.[54] found odds ratios of 1.03, 1.3, and 6.0 respectively, linking age with pressure ulcer development. These findings have been confirmed by Bergstrom et al.,[55] who identified an odds ratio of 0.91 using logistic regression, and this again was noted to be statistically significant ($p < 0.001$).

Therefore, it is reasonable to assume that the older the individual the greater the risk of pressure ulcer development. However, this information should not be interpreted blindly as any individual of any age can develop a pressure ulcer if their condition is sufficiently poor.[46] Therefore, although the older population are a high-risk group, one should also be alert for other vulnerable individuals.

Nutrition

The precise role of nutrition in the development of pressure ulcers remains a subject of debate.[56] However, despite this uncertainty, there remains a great interest in this area and thus it is of value to explore the subject further. It appears that, primarily, poor nutrition leads to increased muscle wasting and soft tissue loss, increasing the prominence of bony points.[57] This in turn compounds the adverse effects of prolonged immobility. Furthermore, collagen production is influenced by nutritional status and adequate synthesis and deposition is needed for tissue strength.[37] Adequate tissue strength is required in order to protect the individual from the negative effects of pressure, shear, and friction forces.[35]

Anthony et al.[58] suggest that the serum albumin levels of individual patients have been traditionally the focus of wide research, including its potential role in pressure ulcer development. Working on the basis that serum albumin is the most common method of assessing nutritional status, Anthony et al.[58] set out to explore its relevance as a predictor of pressure ulcer risk. Serum albumin levels were recorded for 773 patients, over the age of 65 years, admitted without a pressure ulcer to an acute hospital setting. The patients were expected to have a hospital stay of greater than 7 days and all had Waterlow pressure ulcer risk scores recorded. A statistically significant difference ($p < 0.001$) was noted regarding the serum albumin levels of those patients who went on to develop a pressure ulcer when compared to those who did not. The authors conducted further statistical analysis, using logistic regression, and serum albumin levels remained a statistically significant consideration ($p = 0.009$). The odds ratio was calculated at 0.9465 (adjusted), suggesting that reducing the serum albumin level by 10 would increase the individual's risk of pressure ulcer development by two thirds.[58] Despite the limitations of the study, such as the restriction of the population to only the elderly and the purposive method of sampling, the authors do demonstrate a link between albumin and pressure ulcer risk. Furthermore this link has also been noted by Mino et al.,[42] who identified that the relative risk for the development of pressure ulcers in patients with hypoalbuminemia was 5.9 and this was found to be statistically significant ($p < 0.001$).

In a study by Margolis et al.[47] that looked at pressure ulcer risk in community patients, 0.4% of the population were noted to be suffering with malnutrition. When pressure ulcer rates for those with malnutrition were compared with rates for those without malnutrition, the authors noted that the relative risk was 3.06. The role of malnutrition in pressure ulcer development has also been explored by Baumgarten et al.[54] In a sample of 9400 elderly patients with hip fractures, 6% were noted to be suffering from cachexia or malnutrition. Of those who were poorly nourished, 19.6% developed a pressure ulcer, compared to 8.1% in the group who were nutritionally stable. The odds ratio for pressure ulcer development in the cachexia or malnourished group was 1.1 (adjusted).

Although there is a body of evidence suggesting that there is an association between pressure ulcer development and nutritional status, what remains unclear is the precise mechanism by which malnutrition affects this development.[35] One needs to bear in mind factors such as general wellness, ability to eat, quality and availability of food, and psychosocial factors, all which influence nutritional intake. As nutrition may impact on the individual's ability to withstand the adverse effects of pressure shear and friction, an emphasis on improving the intake of food and fluids is essential.[56]

Conclusion

Issues relevant to pressure ulcers remain a major challenge in today's healthcare settings. Knowledge of both the etiology and risk factors associated with pressure ulcer development is the key to successful prevention strategies. Although there are a vast number of potential risk factors there are a few (Table 4.1) that have been reinforced in the literature as being of considerable importance. Mobility, age, and nutrition have been discussed in this chapter and have been found to be positively associated with the development of pressure ulcers. It is therefore important that due consideration be given in particular to these risk factors when planning pressure ulcer prevention strategies/interventions.[36] It is also important, however, to

Table 4.1. Summary of 'evidence-based' risk factors

Risk factors	References
Intrinsic factors:	
Acute illness	Torrance,[15] Malone,[59] McSorley and Warren,[60] Barrow and Sikes[61]
Pyrexia	
Medication	
Extremes of age	Bliss,[46] Margolis et al.[47]
Level of consciousness	Summer et al.,[62] Philips[63]
Mobility/immobility	Exton Smith and Sherwin,[40] Allman[39]
Nutrition	Anthony et al.,[58] EPUAP[56]
Sensory impairment	Raney[64]
Extrinsic factors:	
Pressure/shear/friction	Collier,[5] Bennett and Lee,[4,6] Berecek,[7] Bridel,[11] Krouskop,[12] McClemont[14]
Exacerbating factors:	
Skin moisture	Flam,[65] Norton et al.[66]
Sleep	Torrance,[67] Kelly et al.,[68] Grindley and Acres[69]

Source: After Collier.[10]

highlight that there may be other factors impacting on the individual and therefore, each person should be assessed for their potential risk as this forms the basis for individualized care planning.

References

1. Clark M, Bours G, Defloor T. Summary report on the prevalence of pressure ulcers. EPUAP Review 2002; 4(2):49–56.
2. Barbenel J, Jordan MM, Nicol S, Clark M. Incidence of pressure sores in the Greater Glasgow Health Board Area. Lancet 1977; ii:548–550.
3. Bader D, Gant CA. Effects of prolonged loading on tissue oxygen levels. In: Spence V, Sheldon C (eds) Practical aspects of blood flow measurements. London: Biological Engineering Society; 1985: 82–85.
4. Bennett L, Lee B. Shear versus pressure as causative factors in skin blood flow occlusion. Arch Phys Med Rehabil 1986; 60:309–314.
5. Collier M. Pressure reducing mattresses. J Wound Care 1996; 5(5):207–211.
6. Bennett L, Lee B. Pressure versus shear in pressure sore formation. In: Lee B (ed) Chronic ulcers of the skin. New York: McGraw Hill; 1985: 39–55.
7. Berecek K. Etiology of pressure sores. Nurs Clin North Am 1975; 10:157.
8. Brown MM, Boosinger J, Black J, Gaspar T. Nursing innovation for prevention of decubitus ulcers in long-term facilities. Plast Surg Nurse 1985; 5(2):57–64.
9. Reichel S. Shearing forces as a factor in decubitus ulcers in paraplegics. JAMA 1958; 116:762.
10. Collier M. Fundamental concepts. Resource file: Mattresses and beds. London: EMAP; 1999:1–8.
11. Bridel J. The aetiology of pressure sores. J Wound Care 1993; 2(4):230–238.
12. Krouskop T. Mechanisms of decubitus ulcer formation—a hypothesis. Med Hypotheses 1976; 4(1):37–39.
13. Lowthian PT. Underpads in the prevention of decubitus. In: Kenedi R, Cowden JM, Scales JT (eds) Bedsore biomechanics. London: Macmillan; 1976: 141–145.
14. McClemont E. Pressure sores. Nursing 1984; 2(21) Suppl.
15. Torrance C. Pressure sores: aetiology, treatment and prevention. London: Croom Helm; 1983.
16. Collier M. Assessing a wound—RCN Nursing Update Unit 29. Nurs Stand 1994; 8(49) Suppl: 3–8.
17. European Pressure Ulcer Advisory Panel. Guide to pressure ulcer grading. EPUAP Review 2001; 3(3):75.
18. Collier M. Pressure ulcer development and principles for prevention. In: Glover D, Miller M (eds) Wound management: Theory and practice. London: NT Books; 1999.

19. Longport Incorporated. Applications of ultrasound biomicroscopy in wound care; 2003 (www.longportinc.com).
20. Landis E. Microcirculation studies of capillary blood pressure in human skin. Heart 1930; 15: 209–228.
21. Barton A, Barton M. The management and prevention of pressure sores. London: Faber; 1981.
22. Daniel R, Priest D, Wheatley D. Etiologic factors in pressure sores: an experimental model. Arch Phys Med Rehabil 1981; 62:492–498.
23. Scales J, Lowthian P, Poole A, Ludman W. Vaperm patient support system: a new general-purpose hospital mattress. Lancet 1982; ii(8308):1150–1152.
24. Bliss M. Aetiology of pressure sores. Clin Gerontol 1993; 3:379–397.
25. Lamb J, Ingram C, Johnson T, Pitman R. Essentials of physiology. London: Blackwell Scientific; 1980.
26. Lewis T, Grant R. Observations upon reactive hyperaemia in man. Heart 1925; 4(1):37–39.
27. Sangeorzan B, Harrington R, Wyss C, et al. Circulatory response of skin to loading. J Orthop Res 1989; 7:425–431.
28. Collier M. Blanching and non-blanching hyperaemia. J Wound Care 1999; 8(2):63–64.
29. Deeks J, Higgins J, Riis J, Silagy C. Module 11: Summary statistics for dichotomous outcomes data. In: Alderson P, Green S (eds) Cochrane Collaboration open learning material for reviewers. Version 1.1. Chichester: John Wiley; 2002: 87–102.
30. Gosnell DJ. An assessment tool to identify pressure sores. Nurs Res 1973; 22:55–59.
31. Lowthian P. Pressure sore prevalence. Nurs Times 1979; 75:358–360.
32. Waterlow J. A risk assessment card. Nurs Times 1985; 81(48):49–56.
33. Braden B, Bergstrom N. A conceptual schema for the study of the etiology of pressure sores. Rehabil Nurs 1987; 12(1):8–16.
34. Gosnell DJ. Pressure sore risk assessment part 2: analysis of risk factors. Decubitus 1988; 2(3): 40–43.
35. Defloor T. The risk of pressure sore: a conceptual scheme. J Clin Nurs 1999; 8:206–216.
36. National Institute for Clinical Excellence. Pressure ulcer prevention: Clinical Guideline No. 7. London: NICE; 2003.
37. Nixon J. Pressure sores. In: Morison MJ, Ovington LG, Wilkie K (eds) Chronic wound care, a problem-based learning approach. London: Mosby; 2004: 227–245.
38. Keane FX. The minimum physiological mobility requirement for man supported on a soft surface. Paraplegic 1978; 16:383–389.
39. Allman RM. Pressure ulcer prevalence, incidence, risk factors and impact. Clin Geriatr Med 1997; 13(3):421–436.
40. Exton-Smith AN, Sherwin RW. The prevention of pressure sores: significance of spontaneous bodily movements. Lancet 1961; 2(7212):1124–1126.
41. Papanikolaou P, Lyne PA, Lycett EJ. Pressure ulcer risk assessment: application of logistic analysis. J Adv Nurs 2003; 44(2):128–136.
42. Mino Y, Morimoto S, Okaishi K, et al. Risk factors for pressure ulcers in bedridden elderly subjects: Importance of turning over in bed and serum albumin level. Geriatr Gerontol Int 2001; 1:38–44.
43. Berlowitz DR, Brandeis GH, Morris JN, et al. Developing a risk-adjustment model for pressure ulcer development using the minimum data set. J Am Geriatr Soc 2001; 49(7): 866–871.
44. Lindgren M, Unosson M, Fredrikson M, Ek AC. Immobility—a major risk factor for the development of pressure ulcers among hospitalised patients: a prospective study. Scand J Caring Sci 2004; 18:57–64.
45. US Census Bureau. International population reports WP/02, global population profile, 2002. Washington DC: US Government Printing Office; 2004.
46. Bliss M. Geriatric medicine. In: Bader DL (ed) Pressure sores: Clinical practice and scientific approach. London: Macmillan; 1990: 65–80.
47. Margolis DJ, Bilker W, Knauss J, et al. The incidence and prevalence of pressure ulcers among elderly patients in general medical practice. Ann Epidemiol 2002; 12:321–325.
48. Margolis DJ. Definition of a pressure ulcer. Adv Wound Care 1995; 8:8–10.
49. Whittington K, Patrick M, Roberts J. A national study of pressure ulcer prevalence and incidence in acute care hospitals. J Wound Care Nurs 2000; 24(4):209–215.
50. National Pressure Ulcer Advisory Panel. Pressure ulcer prevalence, cost and risk assessment: consensus development conference statement. Decubitus 1989; 2:24–28.
51. Halfens RJ, van Achterberg T, Bal RM. Validity and reliability of the Braden scale and the influence of other risk factors: a multi-centre prospective study. Int J Nurs Stud 2000; 37:313–319.

52. Casimiro C, Garcia-de-Lorenzo A, Usan L. Prevalence of decubitus ulcer and associated risk factors in an institutionalised Spanish elderly population. Nutrition 2002; 18:408–414.
53. Young J, Nikoletti S, McCaul K, et al. Risk factors associated with pressure ulcer development at a major Western Australian teaching hospital from 1998 to 2000; Secondary data analysis. J Wound Care Nurs 2002; 29:234–241.
54. Baumgarten M, Margolis D, Berlin JA, et al. Risk factors for pressure ulcers among elderly hip fracture patients. Wound Repair Regen 2003; 11:96–103.
55. Bergstrom N, Braden B, Kemp M, et al. Multi-site study of incidence of pressure ulcers and the relationship between risk level, demographic characteristics, diagnoses and prescription of preventive interventions. J Am Geriatr Soc 1996; 44(1):22–30.
56. European Pressure Ulcer Advisory Panel. Report from the guideline development group. EPUAP Review 2003; 5(3):80–82.
57. Eachempati S, Hydo LJ, Barie PS. Factors influencing the development of decubitus ulcers in critically ill surgical patients. Crit Care Med 2001; 29(9):1678–1682.
58. Anthony D, Reynolds T, Russell L. An investigation into the use of serum albumin in pressure sore prediction. J Adv Nurs 2000; 32(2):359–365.
59. Malone C. Intensive pressures. Nurs Times 1992; 88(Suppl):3–8.
60. McSorley P, Warren D. The effects of propranolol and metoprolol on the peripheral circulation. BMJ 1978; ii:1598–1600.
61. Barrow T, Sikes C. Decubitus ulcers in rheumatic fever treated with cortisone. JAMA 1951; 147: 41–42.
62. Summer W, Curry P, Haponikm E, et al. Continuous mechanical turning of intensive care unit patients shortens length of stay in some diagnostic related groups. J Crit Care 1989; 4:45–53.
63. Philips P. Obesity and weight reduction programmes. Geriatr Med 1981; 11(6):53–57.
64. Raney J. A comparison of the prevalence of pressure sores in hospitalised ALS and MS patients. Decubitus 1989; 2(2):48–49.
65. Flam E. Skin maintenance in the bedridden patient. Ostomy Wound Manage 1990; May/June: 48–54.
66. Norton D, McLaren R, Exton-Smith A. An investigation of geriatric nursing problems in hospital. Edinburgh: Churchill Livingstone; 1975.
67. Torrance C. Sleep and wound healing. Surg Nurse 1990; 3(3):16–20.
68. Kelly M, Coverdale S, Williams S, et al. Easing the pressure. Nurs Times 1995; 91(22):72–76.
69. Grindley A, Acres J. Alternating pressure mattresses: comfort and quality of sleep. Br J Nurs 1996; 5:1303–1310.

5 Pressure Ulcer Classification

Carol Dealey and Christina Lindholm

Introduction

Pressure ulcer classification is a method of determining the severity of a pressure ulcer. A classification system describes a series of numbered stages or grades each determining a different degree of tissue damage. The deeper the ulcer and the more extensive the tissue damage the higher the grade number, as illustrated in Table 5.1. Pressure ulcer classification is a valuable tool for prevalence and incidence surveys as well as clinical practice and research.

The first author to publish a pressure ulcer classification system was Shea.[1] Since then, numerous systems have been developed with varying numbers for grades ranging from a 0–5 grade classification to a 1–7 grade classification. The most complex system is the Stirling Grading System, which has 0–4 grades with up to four subscales within some of the grades; thus a deep necrotic infected ulcer would be labeled as 4.131.[2] A review by Hitch[3] identified ten different classification systems and a later review by Haalboom et al.[4] found a further four systems. Probably the most widely used classification is that developed by the National Pressure Ulcer Advisory Panel (NPUAP)[5] and later adopted by the European Pressure Ulcer Advisory Panel (EPUAP) with some minor textual changes (e.g. NPUAP refers to stages and EPUAP to grades; see Table 5.1).[6] Figures 5.1–5.4 (see color section) show examples of each of the EPUAP grades with line drawings to show diagrammatically the degree of tissue damage.

The major weakness of all classification systems is the lack of evidence to support their use, the most important factor being inter-rater reliability. Healey[7] studied inter-rater reliability amongst 109 nurses when using three classification systems (Stirling,[2] Torrance,[8] and Surrey[9]) and found that although none of the systems showed a high level of reliability, it was significantly lower in the most complex scoring system (Stirling). Healey also found that there was greater reliability in reporting the grades of severe ulcers compared with the less severe grades. Russell and Reynolds compared the reliability of the Stirling and EPUAP classification systems when used by 200 specialist and nonspecialist nurses and again found that the Stirling classification system was less reliable than the simpler EPUAP system.[10] Russell and Reynolds conclude that classification of pressure ulcers is not easy. Sharp concurs and suggests that such is the complexity of some classification systems that they require a level of expertise beyond the capability of general nurses.[11] Certainly, education is essential to ensure high levels of inter-rater reliability.[10]

Table 5.1. EPUAP pressure ulcer classification system

Grade	Definition
1	Nonblanchable erythema of intact skin. This may be difficult to identify in darkly pigmented skins
2	Partial thickness skin loss involving epidermis and/or dermis: the pressure ulcer is superficial and presents clinically as an abrasion, blister or shallow crater
3	Full-thickness skin loss involving damage or necrosis of subcutaneous tissue that may extend down to, but not through, underlying fascia: the pressure ulcer presents clinically as a deep crater with or without undermining of adjacent tissue
4	Extensive destruction tissue necrosis, or damage to muscle, bone or supporting structures with or without full-thickness skin loss

Defloor and Schoonhoven describe the validation process for an educational tool using the EPUAP classification to grade photographs of pressure ulcers.[12] In the first stage of the process nine specialists were asked to review the clarity of 67 photographs and grade the ulcers. Eleven unclear photographs were eliminated. In the second phase 44 experts were asked to grade the pressure ulcers in the 56 remaining photographs and their findings were compared with the original nine experts. A high level of agreement was found between all the experts. However, the authors consider that it is likely that there would be less agreement amongst those with little experience.

Controversies in Pressure Ulcer Classification

There are a number of controversies relating to pressure ulcer classification that may well be linked to reliability. They are listed below and each will be discussed in turn.

- Grade 1 ulcers
- Assessing dark skin
- Reverse grading
- Identifying incontinence lesions

Grade 1 Ulcers

Russell has stressed the difficulties in defining early skin damage.[13] A reaction to temporary closure of the dermal capillaries is called reactive hyperemia, clinically seen as a bright flush or reddened area that blanches under light pressure. It is thought to last from 30 minutes to 48 hours.[14,15] At this stage, damage to the underlying tissues has not yet occurred.

Shea provided the definition of a grade 1 ulcer as a persistent reddened area that does not blanch.[1] This definition was later supported by Versluysen and Yarkony et al.[14,15] Dinsdale put forward an alternative definition of a grade 1 pressure ulcer as persistent redness for more than a 24-hour period.[16] Lyder states that blanching erythema indicates that tissue damage has not yet occurred.[17] Hence, this must precede pressure ulcer development and thus nonblanching erythema should be taken as a true presentation of a grade 1 ulcer. Lyder also set up criteria for assessing a grade 1 pressure ulcer. Hitch considered that there is consensus on Lyder's criteria for a grade 1 ulcer.[3] Lyder's criteria have subsequently been adapted by Russell[13] and are shown in Table 5.2.

Table 5.2. Criteria for grade 1 pressure ulcers

Skin area that ranges from pale pink to bright red in color
Skin area that is nonblanching (blanchable erythema being a precursor to a grade 1 pressure ulcer)
Skin area that is warmer or cooler to touch
Skin area with erythema that does not resolve within 2 hours
Skin area that possibly has edema or induration that is ill defined when palpated
Skin area with epidermis intact

Source: Russell.[13] Reproduced by kind permission of MA Healthcare Ltd.

Assessing Dark Skin

Darkly pigmented skin creates problems because early skin changes are difficult to see.[13] Meehan demonstrated that patients with dark skin had a larger percentage of high-grade ulcers and the least number of stage 1 ulcers.[18] Since nonblanchable erythema is difficult to detect in the darkly pigmented skin, palpation has been recommended.[19] Observation of localized heat has also been suggested.[13]

The NPUAP convened a task force to review the definition of stage 1 pressure ulcer and determine the adequacy of this definition in assessing individuals with darkly pigmented skin. Following a comprehensive review of the literature and peer review by attendees at the Fifth NPUAP Conference in February 1997, the National Task Force on Darkly Pigmented Skin and Stage 1 Pressure Ulcers drafted the following new definition for stage 1 pressure ulcers, which was approved by the NPUAP Board of Directors in 1998:

A Stage I pressure ulcer is an observable pressure related alteration of intact skin whose indicators as compared to the adjacent or opposite area on the body may include changes in one or more of the following:

skin temperature (warmth or coolness), tissue consistency (firm or boggy feel) and/or sensation (pain, itching).

The ulcer appears as a defined area of persistent redness in lightly pigmented skin, whereas in darker skin tones, the ulcer may appear with persistent red, blue, or purple hues.[20]

Reverse Grading

As the use of pressure ulcer classification systems became established in clinical practice a number of misconceptions also crept in. One was the assumption that pressure ulcers will first present as a grade 1 and then naturally progress through to grade 4 without preventative measures, even though there is no evidence to support this belief. The other was the practice of reverse grading or describing a healing ulcer as progressing from a grade 4 to a grade 3 and so on back to grade 1. There is no logic in this practice as the tissues in a healing wound do not equate to the tissues as they were before pressure damage occurred. Thus a healing grade 4 pressure ulcer, which initially penetrated through to muscle, does not first replace the muscle tissue and then the dermis but gradually fills with granulation tissue. This topic was the subject of considerable debate in the USA[21,22] and led to the NPUAP making a position statement on the subject.[23] Within the position statement the NPUAP state that:

> Pressure ulcer staging is only appropriate for defining the maximum anatomical depth of tissue damage.

We support that viewpoint. If a pressure ulcer presents as a grade 3 it must always be described as such. However, it is also important to monitor healing and describe it clearly. Dealey described different ways in which wound healing could be evaluated.[24]

Incontinence Lesions

Persistent incontinence can cause erythema, maceration, and excoriation of the skin, which can be mistaken for a pressure ulcer, as can be seen in Figure 5.5 (see color section). Until recently there has been little discussion of this problem in the literature.[25] Schnelle et al. monitored the impact of incontinence on the skin and found a high incidence of blanchable erythema, particularly in the perineal region.[26] They consider it to be a marker for increased risk of pressure ulcers and other skin disorder, but it seems reasonable to postulate that an unskilled observer may consider such incontinence lesions to be grade 1 pressure ulcers. Incontinence lesions can be identified in the following ways:

- They are unlikely to occur over bony prominences.
- They may be more purple than red in appearance.
- The skin may be swollen or edematous.
- The skin may also be macerated and/or excoriated.
- The patient is incontinent or suffers from diarrhea.

Education is essential to alert staff to the possibility of incontinence lesions and learn how to differentiate them from superficial pressure ulcers.

Conclusions and Recommendations

Pressure ulcer grading is a useful tool for defining the severity of pressure ulcers. However, it is obvious that education is essential in order to ensure that grades are correctly identified and that incontinence lesions are not mistaken for pressure ulcers. The EPUAP provides access to a very useful educational program via its website (www.epuap.org.uk). The PUCLAS program was developed at the University of Ghent, Belgium. It provides both educational material and a self-assessment quiz. It is currently available in nine languages—English, Dutch, Finnish, French, German, Italian, Portuguese, Spanish, and Swedish—and may be freely used for personal or educational purposes. This is a great opportunity for individuals to improve their own assessment skills. Wide use of such educational tools could substantially improve the accuracy of pressure ulcer grading in the clinical area.

References

1. Shea JD. Pressure sores, classification and management. Clin Orthop 1975; 112:89–100.
2. Reid J, Morison M. Classification of pressure sore severity. Nurs Times 1994; 90(20):46–50.
3. Hitch S. NHS Executive Nursing Directorate—Strategy for major clinical guidelines—prevention and management of pressure sores, a literature review. J Tissue Viability 1995; 5(1):3–24.
4. Haalboom JRE, van Everdingen JJE, Cullum N. Incidence, prevalence and classification. In: Parish LC, Witkowski JA, Crissey JT (eds) The decubitus ulcer in clinical practice. London: Springer; 1997.
5. Agency for Health Care Policy and Research. Pressure ulcers in adults: prediction and prevention. Rockville, MD: AHCPR; 1992.
6. EPUAP. Guidelines on the treatment of pressure ulcers. EPUAP Review 1999; 2:31–33.
7. Healey F. The reliability and utility of pressure sore grading scales. J Tissue Viability 1995; 5(4): 111–114.
8. Torrance C. Pressure sores: aetiology, treatment and prevention. Beckenham: Croom Helm; 1983.
9. David J, Chapman RG, Chapman EJ. An investigation of the current methods used in nursing for the care of patients with established pressure sores. Harrow: Nursing Practice Research Unit; 1983.
10. Russell L, Reynolds T. How accurate are pressure ulcer grades? An image-based survey of nurse performance. J Tissue Viability 2001; 11(2):67–75.
11. Sharp A. Pressure ulcer grading tools: how reliable are they? J Wound Care 2004; 13(2):75–77.
12. Defloor T, Schoonhoven L. Inter-rater reliability of the EPUAP pressure ulcer classification system using photographs. J Clin Nurs 2004; 13(8):952–959.
13. Russell L. Pressure ulcer classification: defining early skin damage. Br J Nurs 2002; (Suppl) 11(16):33–41.
14. Versluysen M. Pressure sores: causes and prevention. Nursing 1986; 5(3):216–218.
15. Yarkony GM, Kirk PM, Carlsson C, et al. Classification of pressure ulcers. Arch Dermatol 1990; 126(9):1218–1219.
16. Dinsdale SM. Decubitus ulcers: Role of pressure and friction in causation. Arch Phys Med Rehabil 1974; 62:492–498.
17. Lyder CH. Conceptualization of the stage 1 pressure ulcer. J ET Nursing 1991; 18(5):162–165.
18. Meehan M. National pressure ulcer prevalence survey. Adv Wound Care 1994; 7(3):27–38.
19. Young T. Classification of pressure sores: 1. Br J Nurs 1996; 5(7):438–446.
20. NPUAP. Stage I assessment in darkly pigmented skin. NPUAP, 1998 (http://www.npuap.ord/positn4.htm).
21. Maklebust J. Policy implications of using reverse staging to monitor pressure ulcer status. Adv Wound Care 1997; 10(5):32–35.
22. Xakellis G, Frantz R. Pressure ulcer healing: what is it? What influences it? How is it measured? Adv Wound Care 1997; 10(5):20–26.
23. National Pressure Ulcer Advisory Panel. The facts about reverse staging in 2000. The NPUAP Position Statement, 2000 (www.npuap.org/positn5.htm).
24. Dealey C. Care of Wounds 3rd ed. Oxford: Blackwell Publishing; 2005.
25. Defloor T. Drukreductie en wisselhouding in de preventie van decubitus. [Pressure reduction and turning in the prevention of pressure ulcers]. PhD thesis, Ghent University, 2000.
26. Schnelle JF, Adamson GM, Cruise PA, et al. Skin disorders and moisture in incontinent nursing home residents: intervention implications. J Am Geriatr Soc 1997; 45(10):1182–1188.

6 Risk Assessment Scales for Predicting the Risk of Developing Pressure Ulcers

Joan-Enric Torra i Bou, Francisco Pedro García-Fernández, Pedro L. Pancorbo-Hidalgo, and Katia Furtado

Introduction

Currently, pressure ulcers are an important health problem, both for people with pressure ulcers and their caregivers and for health institutions and professionals. Therefore it is evident, with the knowledge acquired, that the best strategy to cope with this problem is to prevent it, since the majority of pressure ulcers (up to 95% according to some authors[1]) can be avoided, if the appropriate preventive measures are applied with adequate resources and within the correct context (such as clinical practice guidelines).

Nevertheless, pressure ulcer prevention is not costless, because it implies high expenditure, in equipment and human resources.[2,3] Thus there is a need to find assessment tools that can determine which patients require preventive measures and to what extent, and which patients can be spared these measures. It is feasible for experienced nurses to do the selection and apply preventive measures, according to their own clinical judgment. The issue is whether there are risk assessment tools that could be used (especially by less trained nurses or those who lack experience in managing these patients) that have the same success (or more) in detecting risk as expert clinical judgment. This is the main reason why different risk assessment scales have been proposed as tools to assess patients' risk of developing pressure ulcers.

We could define a pressure ulcer risk assessment scale (PURAS) as a tool that establishes a point scale according to a group of parameters regarded as risk factors for the development of pressure ulcers.

PURAS could be beneficial for patients. For example, Hodge et al.[4] and Bale et al. 1995[5] demonstrated that patients assessed using the Norton scale, received 76% more preventive measures than a control group not systematically assessed, and moreover that the allocation of pressure-relieving surfaces was optimized according to risk factors, thus reducing incidence. However, there is not a general use of assessment scales nationally or internationally. In the first national pressure ulcer prevalence study in Spain,[6] with professionals who answered a questionnaire about epidemiological data and preventive measures, a systematic use of PURAS was found in 72.8% of cases in hospital care, 60.31% in residential settings, and 59.5% in primary healthcare.

It is necessary to be aware of the usefulness of PURAS and what they are being used for. Simply using a PURAS without introducing the appropriate protocol on prevention, which would support the necessary preventive measures according to their risk staging, has no effect on the reduction of pressure ulcer incidence. The use of scales must be followed by other preventive methods which would be much more effective if adequately prescribed according to the patient's risk. Therefore, PURAS must be settled in a protocol context for healthcare, extracted from evidence-supported procedures as developed by clinical practice guidelines, which in turn are a result of the best possible evidence. These should emanate from different worldwide investigation projects, not only in English, which would guarantee, when implementation is compulsory, that all professionals have the best knowledge, abilities, time, and resources for implementation in a scenario of continuous evaluation for quality in assistance.[7-9]

Hence, when a pressure ulcer prevention program is to be designed, one of the first steps, and therefore one of the most important, should be the selection of a PURAS.

Since Doreen Norton[10] first published her scale in 1962, more than 30 other scales have appeared in the scientific literature, plus a large number of modifications to some of them.[11-12]

Criteria for selection and implementation of any PURAS must have scientifically based arguments. In this chapter, we shall present the tools, and the scientific evidence for the use of the PURAS, and analyze in detail the most important scales, as well as the evidence and support behind them.

Scientific Evidence for the Use of Risk Assessment Scales for Pressure Ulcers

As mentioned above, in several clinical practice guidelines (CPG), we find recommendations for the use of PURAS based on the best scientific evidence available. Nevertheless, taking into account the lack, so far, of studies that compare clinical judgment with the use of scales, we have encountered some uncertainty as to the requirement for adopting a risk assessment scale rather than relying on the clinical judgment of individual nurses.

As basic methodological support, almost all CPGs are based on the systematic reviews made by Cullum et al. in 1995[12] and McGough in 1999.[13]

These reviews, and subsequent publications, consider that there is not enough evidence to demonstrate the effectiveness of risk evaluation scales in reducing the development of pressure ulcers, even though there is some evidence that supports the use of PURAS over and above clinical judgment on it own. We should take into account the risk of a possible publication bias in these publications and CPGs, since the sources on which they are based were written in English, and any other investigations published in other languages that could reinforce or refute some of these results have not been included or considered.

In a recent systematic review of papers published in four languages (English, Spanish, French, and Portuguese) made by Pancorbo et al.,[14] well-known statements have been confirmed, but it seems that some of the knowledge disseminated in the most recent publications on the issue are still not included in clinical practice guidelines.

From the first reviews (Cullum et al.[12] and McGough[13]) we show in Tables 6.1 and 6.2 the most important risk assessment advice for the CPGs and in Table 6.3 the latest review done by Pancorbo et al. concerning works on this subject.

Table 6.1. Clinical practice guidelines on pressure ulcer prevention with graded and hierarchy defined evidence

NICE: National Institute for Clinical Excellence: Pressure ulcers risk assessment and prevention (2001)[17]	**UIGNIRC:** University of Iowa Gerontological Nursing Interventions Research Center: Research dissemination Core. Prevention of Pressure Sore (2002)[21]
EPUAP: European Pressure Ulcer Advisory Panel: Guidelines on prevention for developing pressure ulcers (1999)[18]	**RNAO:** Registered Nurses Association of Ontario: The Nursing Best practice Guideline: Risk Assessment and Prevention of Pressure Ulcers (2002)[22]
AHCPR: Agency for Health Care Policy and Research: Pressure ulcers in adults: prediction and prevention. Clinical Practice Guideline (1992)[19]	**RCN:** Pressure ulcers risk assessment and prevention. Technical Report (2000)[23]
JBI: The Joanna Briggs Institute for Evidence Based nursing and Midwifery Best Practice: Pressure Sores. Part 1: Prevention of Pressure Related Damage (1997)[20]	

All references are evidence supported and adhere to the classification of Novell and Navarro-Rubio (1997)[15] and Gálvez Toro (2001),[16] so that they can be grouped on a three-category basis of evidence: grade A = high evidence; grade B = medium evidence; grade C = low evidence.

In some aspects we find a need for adequate evidence as a result of a lack of experimental work, which provides the best evidence, and we also face an ethical

Table 6.2. Recommendations review according to evidence level and sources

Recommendation	Evidence level[a]	Sources
The use of scales in risk assessment must be used as an aid, but not to replace clinical judgment.	A	NICE,[17] AHCPR,[19] EPUAP[18]
Risk assessment is more than just using a scale for it is not a mere protocolized assessment and should be flexible according to patients' needs.	C	EPUAP[18]
Risk assessment must be performed immediately after patient admission, even though this assessment could need more time to be completed if the information is not yet available.	C	EPUAP[18]
Risk must be reassessed periodically.	A	EPUPAP,[18] AHCPR,[19] JBI[20]
To assess risk, validated scales such as Braden or Norton can be used.	Braden: B	AHCPR,[19] JBI,[20] UIGNIRC,[21] RNAO[22]
	Norton: C	AHCPR,[19] JBI[20]
Patients with a Braden scale score equal to or lower than 16 in hospitals and equal to or lower than 18 in long-term facilities must be considered at risk.	B	UIGNIRC[21]
Risk assessment must be done by professionals trained in recognizing risk factors for developing pressure ulcers.	C	RCN[23]
If a risk assessment scale is used, it should be tested on the facility that is being applied.	C	RCN[23]
All risk assessment must be documented.	C	RCN,[23] NICE,[17] AHCPR,[19] JBI,[20] UIGNIRC,[21] RNAO[22]

[a]Grade A = high evidence; grade B = medium evidence; grade C = low evidence (Novell and Navarro-Rubio[15] and Gálvez Toro[16]).

Table 6.3. Main recommendations from systematic reviews of risk assessment scales for development of pressure ulcers

	Cullum et al.[12]	McGough[13]	Pancorbo et al.[14]
Presentation date	1995	1999	2004
Period included	1962–1994	1962–1997	1962–2003
Number of studies included	15	18	33
Conclusions	• There is no evidence that the use of PURAS in scheduling care reduces the incidence of pressure ulcer • There is great variability in predictive value among different scales as well as in the same scale • No scale seems better than another • There is little evidence to demonstrate that any PURAS is better than clinical judgment or that it improves patient outcomes	• There is no evidence that PURAS are effective in reducing PU incidence or improve preventive measures • There is little evidence that demonstrates that a PURAS is better than nurses' clinical judgment • No scale is more reliable than another in identifying patients at major risk, even though the Braden scale has been more investigated than others	• There is no evidence that the use of PURAS in clinical practice reduces PU incidence in patients • There is enough evidence for the use of preventive measures adequately using as screening criteria a PURAS • There is enough evidence to determine that the use of PURAS results in better preventive methodology • Braden and Norton scales are better than nurses' clinical judgment to predict the risk of patients developing pressure ulcers • The Braden scale has the best steadiness on sensitivity/specificity, and the best predictive ability regarding patients that can develop pressure ulcers • There is no evidence that clinical judgment by itself is able to predict risk for developing pressure ulcers in all patients

Source: Pancorbo Hidalgo et al.[14]

problem in the design of studies, because the control group are at risk of being deprived of the benefits of systematic risk assessment.

This circumstance occurs in other similar situations within general nurse practice and specifically in chronic wounds, where ethically it becomes a predicament whether to switch from a low evidence type C to a higher type A. As a corollary, this implies that we should be very cautious about approaches based only on the evidence achieved from clinical trials; for low type evidence should be carefully analyzed and not disregarded, since in many cases this procedure is the only one that can ethically be chosen as an option.

Characteristics of the Ideal Scale

Several authors[8,11,19,23–28] have tried to emphasize the characteristics or requirements that the ideal scale should have, or in other words, the essential criteria of a PURAS which are, in particular, those to be considered necessary when evaluating and/or validating a scale. These aspects, listed in Table 6.4, could be:

1. High sensitivity. Defined as the ability of a test or scale to correctly identify those patients with an illness or condition among those at risk.
2. High specificity. Is the ability of the test or scale to correctly identify those patients without an illness or condition among those not at risk.

Table 6.4. Characteristics of the ideal PURAS

High sensitivity
High specificity
Good predictive value
Ease of use
Clear and definite criteria
Applicable to different healthcare settings

Source: Torra i Bou.[11]

3. Good predictive value. It may be positive: those patients with an ulcer who had been assessed as "at risk" among those who do develop an ulcer; or it may be negative: those patients without an ulcer who had been assessed as "not at risk" among those who do not develop an ulcer.
4. Ease of use, for all professionals regardless of their experience.
5. Precise definition of terms, which means that criteria must be clear and well defined in order to avoid, as much as possible, inconsistency among different nurses using the scale.
6. Applicable to the different clinical settings where ulcers appear or to those patients at risk; varying from home to residential care, hospitals or geriatric and pediatric units and intensive care.

Using these criteria we shall examine different risk assessment scales for developing pressure ulcers. It is important to consider the large number of existing scales and that new scales appear every so often (for example Fragment, Cubbin–Jackson); therefore we are only going to take into account the most important ones and the ones with valid literature.

Norton Scale

The Norton scale was the first PURAS described in the scientific literature. It was developed by Norton et al.[10] in 1962 during an investigation on geriatric patients, and has been used worldwide. The scale considers five parameters, mental status, incontinence, mobility, activity, and physical condition, and has a four-point scoring scale, 4 being the best situation for each parameter and 1 the worst (Table 6.5). This assessment scale has an inverse scoring so lower values designate higher risk. Originally a cutoff point of 14 or less implied a moderate risk of developing pressure ulcers and 12 or less indicated a high risk. Later, in 1987, Norton proposed its modification setting the cutoff point at 16.[29]

Table 6.5. The Norton scale

Physical state	Mental state	Activity	Mobility	Incontinence
4 Good	4 Alert	4 Walks	4 Complete	4 None
3 Weak	3 Apathic	3 Walks with assistance	3 Slightly limited	3 Occasional
2 Ill	2 Confused	2 Wheelchair bound	2 Very limited	2 Mainly urinary
1 Very ill	1 Stupor	1 Bed bound	1 Immobile	1 Double incontinence

Source: Norton.[29]

Table 6.6. Norton scale validation studies

Authors and publication year	Type of facility	Sample size	Sensitivity	Specificity	Positive predictive value	Negative predictive value
Norton et al., 1962[10]	Geriatric center	250	63%	70%	39%	86%
Roberts and Goldstone, 1979[30]	Hospital	64	92%	61%	37%	96%
Newman and West, 1981[30]		88	83%	63%	14%	98%
Goldstone and Roberts, 1980[32]	Hospital	64	92%	61%	—	—
Goldstone and Goldstone, 1982[33]	Hospital (traumatology)	40	89%	36%	53%	80%
Lincoln et al. 1986[34]	Hospital	50	0%	94%	—	—
Smith, 1989[35]	Hospital (traumatology)	101	60%	31%	—	—
Stotts, 1988[36]	Hospital (cardiovascular surgery and neurosurgery)	387	16%	94%	—	—
Wai-Han et al., 1997[37]	Geriatric center	185	75%	67%	9%	98%
Pang and Wong, 1998[38]	Hospital (rehabilitation)	138	81%	59%	33%	93%
García et al., 1999[39]	Hospital	3030	89%	81%	21%	99%
Schoonhoven et al., 2002[40]	Hospital	1229	46%	60%	7%	94%

Source: Created by the authors from data in Torra i Bou,[11] Cullum et al.,[12] and McGough.[13]

The Norton scale is quite easy to use[24] and has been widely validated[9,30–40] (Table 6.6). Mean values are:

- sensitivity 66% (range 0–92%);
- specificity 65% (range 31–94%);
- predictive positive value 27% (range 7–53%);
- predictive negative value 93% (range 80–99%).

As such, it displays some inconveniences that may limit its clinical effectiveness. The main deficiencies are:

1. It does not have a functional definition of the applied parameters.
2. It does not consider nutritional factors.
3. It does not take into account frictional forces on the skin surface.

Many scales have been derived from the Norton scale, adding other parameters to the five original ones. Among them are the following:

- *The Gosnell scale* (1973) includes five parameters: mental status, incontinence, activity, mobility, and nutrition (which tends to substitute the general state condition of the original scale drawn up by Doreen Norton), plus three further parameters without point scales: vital signs, skin appearance, and medication. Scoring is also inversely depicted and similar to the Norton scale.[41]
- *The Ek scale* (1987), or modified Norton scale, has seven elements, the basic Norton scale plus two nutritional parameters: food and liquid ingestion. It has been used in Scandinavia and submitted to several studies.[42]
- In Spain there are several modifications of the Norton scale, for example *the Nova-4 scale*[43,44] created by a group of nurses from the Institut Català de la Salut

Table 6.7. Validation studies of scales based on the Norton scale

Scale	Authors and publication year	Type of center	Sample size	Sensitivity	Specificity	Positive predictive value	Negative predictive value
Gosnell	Gosnell, 1973[41]	Geriatric center	30	50%	73%	—	—
Nova-4	García Fernández et al., 1999[43]	Hospital	187	84%	54%	43%	67%
EMINA	Fuentelsalz, 2001[48]	Hospital	673	77%	72%	17%	98%

(ICS—Catalan Health Institute) and the *Norton scale modified by the INSALUD* (Instituto Nacional de la Salud—Spanish National Health Institute).[45,46] The *EMINA scale* (2001) is an improvement of the Nova-4 scale in which the direction of the scale was changed so that a higher score means higher risk with an added functional definition for each parameter to assist its use.[47]

Validation data for these scales are shown in Table 6.7.

Waterlow Scale

This scale was designed by Judy Waterlow, in the UK in 1985, as an outcome from a study on pressure ulcer prevalence, where she found that the Norton scale did not classify within the "at-risk" group many patients who in time developed pressure ulcers.[48] After reviewing the factors which arise in the etiology and pathogenesis of pressure ulcers, Waterlow presented a scale with six subscales—height/weight relationship, continence, skin appearance, mobility, age/sex, appetite—and four categories of other risk factors (tissue malnutrition, neurological deficit, surgery, and medication) (Table 6.8).

Table 6.8. The Waterlow scale

Weight/size relationship:	Skin type and visual aspect of risk areas:	Sex/Age:	Special risks:
0. Standard	0. Healthy	1. Male	**Tissue malnutrition:**
1. Above standards	1. Frail	2. female	8. Terminal/cachexia
2. Obese	1. Dry	1. 14–49 years	5. Cardiac insufficiency
	2. Edematous	2. 50–64 years	6. Peripheral vascular
3. Below standards	1. Cold and humid	3. 65–74 years	insufficiency
	2. Alterations in color	4. 75–80 years	2. Anemia
	3. Wounded	5. Over 81 years	1. Smoker
Continence:	**Mobility:**	**Appetite:**	**Neurological deficit:**
0. Complete, urine catheter	0. Complete	0. Normal	5. Diabetes, paraplegic, ACV
1. Occasional incontinence	1. Restless	1. Scarce/feeding tube	
2. Urine catheter/fecal	2. Apathy	2. Liquid intravenous	**Surgery:**
incontinence	3. Restricted	3. Anorexia/Absolute diet	5. Orthopedic surgery below
3. Double incontinence	4. Inert		waist
	5. On chair		5. Over 2 hours in surgery
			Medication:
			4. Steroids, cytotoxics, anti-inflammatory drugs in elevated dosage

Scoring: Over 10 points: at risk. Over 16 points: high risk. Over 20 points: very high risk.
Source: Waterlow.[50]

Table 6.9. Waterlow scale validation studies

Authors and publication year	Type of center	Sample size	Sensitivity	Spacificity	Positive predictive value	Negative predictive value
Smith, 1989[35]	Orthopedic surgery	101	73%	38%	—	—
Edwards, 1995[49]	Primary care	31	100%	10%	7%	100%
Pang and Wong, 1998[38]	Hospital (rehabilitation)	138	95%	44%	29%	97%
Westrate et al., 1990[50]	Hospital (ICU)	594	80.9%	28.5%	8.9%	94.5%
Boyle and Green, 2001[51]	Hospital (ICU)	314	100%	13%	—	—
Schoonhoven et al., 2002[40]	Hospital	1229	89%	22%	7%	97%

Even though it is an Anglo-Saxon scale, it has an incremental positive scoring, considering a patient "at risk" with a score of 10 or higher. The validating data of this scale are shown in Table 6.9.

Mean values are:

- sensitivity 89% (range 73–100%);
- specificity 29% (range 10–44%);
- positive predictive value 14% (range 7–29%);
- negative predictive value 98% (range 97–100%).

Waterlow's scale is used in the UK, but it has not been widely implemented. Main appraisals are:

1. It tends to classify into the "at-risk" group more patients than those actually at risk.
2. It is complex to apply because of the large number of parameters that need to be evaluated.
3. It determines women with higher risk than men.

A study has been recently published of a simplified Waterlow scale with four sub-scales (appetite, continence, skin integrity, and age) and a category (cancer diagnosis) which offers an improved grading on sensitivity and specificity compared with the original scale.[52]

Braden Scale

The Braden scale was designed in 1985 in the USA, as part of a research project in residential care settings, to deal with some of the limitations of the Norton scale.[53] Barbara Braden and Nancy Bergstrom established their scale (Figure 6.1) via a conceptual scheme[54,10] (Figure 6.2) where they documented, ordered, and set relationships of facts on pressure ulcers, laying down the basis of a PURAS.[55]

The Braden scale has six subscales: sensory perception, skin exposure to humidity, physical activity, mobility, nutrition, friction and shear turning into skin damage, with a functional term definition to be checked for each of these subscales. In Figure 6.2 we can see that three subscales are measuring features related to strong and prolonged exposure to pressure, while the others are related to tissue tolerance.

The Braden scale is an inverse scoring tool, which means that the lower score implies major risk, with a range varying from 5 to 23 points. Patients "at risk" are those with scores equal to or below 16 points on this scale; 15–16 is "low risk," 13–14 "moderate risk," and between 5 and 12 "high risk." Table 6.10 shows the results of more than a dozen works for validation of the Braden scale in different care settings, varying from hospitals for acute patients to long-term facilities, including intensive care, nursing homes for the elderly, and home care.[56-67] According to these studies, mean sensitivity is 74% (range 27–100%); specificity is 69% (19–95%); positive predictive value is 43% (8–77%); and negative predictive value is 90% (71–100%).

As can be seen, this scale is the most validated by scientific literature, having the best evidence for to its usefulness, being very sensitive and specific. The main problem is its difficulty of use, for it requires more training than the Norton scale.

Patient's Name _____ Evaluator's Name _____ Date of Assessment								
SENSORY PERCEPTION ability to respond meaning-fully to pressure-related discomfort	**1. Completely Limited** Unresponsive (does not moan, flinch, or grasp) to painful stimuli, due to diminished level of consciousness or sedation OR limited ability to feel pain over most of body.	**2. Very Limited** Responds only to painful stimuli. Cannot communicate discomfort except by moaning or restlessness OR has a sensory impairment which limits the ability to feel pain or discomfort over ½ of body.	**3. Slightly Limited** Responds to verbal commands, but cannot always communicate discomfort or the need to be turned OR has some sensory impairment which limits ability to feel pain or discomfort in 1 or 2 extremities.	**4. No Impairment** Responds to verbal commands. Has no sensory deficit which would limit ability to feel or voice pain or discomfort				
MOISTURE degree to which skin is exposed to moisture	**1. Constantly Moist** Skin is kept moist almost constantly by perspiration, urine, etc. Dampness is detected every time patient is moved or turned.	**2 .Very Moist** Skin is often, but not always moist. Linen must be changed at least once a shift.	**3. Occasionally Moist:** Skin is occasionally moist, requiring an extra linen change approximately once a day.	**4. Rarely Moist** Skin is usually dry, linen only requires changing at routine intervals.				
ACTIVITY degree of physical activity	**1. Bedfast** Confined to bed.	**2 . Chairfast** Ability to walk severely limited or non-existent. Cannot bear own weight and/or must be assisted into chair or wheelchair.	**3. Walks Occasionally** Walks occasionally during day, but for very short distances, with or without assistance. Spends majority of each shift in bed or chair.	**4. Walks Frequently** Walks outside room at least twice a day and inside room at least once every two hours during waking hours.				
MOBILITY ability to change and control body position	**1. Completely Immobile** Does not make even slight changes in body or extremity position without assistance.	**2 .Very Limited** Makes occasional slight changes in body or extremity position but unable to make frequent or significant changes independently.	**3. Slightly Limited** Makes frequent though slight changes in body or extremity position independently.	**4. No Limitation** Makes major and frequent changes in position without assistance.				
NUTRITION usual food intake pattern	**1. Very Poor** Never eats a complete meal. Rarely eats more than ⅓ of any food offered. Eats 2 servings or less of protein (meat or dairy products) per day. Takes fluids poorly. Does not take a liquid dietary supplement OR is NPO and/or maintained on clear liquids or IV's for more than 5 days	**2. Probably Inadequate** Rarely eats a complete meal and generally eats only about ½ of any food offered. Protein intake incudes only 3 servings of meat or dairy products per day. Occasionally will take a dietary supplement OR receives less than optimum amount of liquid diet or tube feeding.	**3. Adequate** Eats over half of most meals. Eats a total of 4 servings of protein (meat, dairy products) per day. Occasionally will refuse a meal, but will usually take a supplement when offered OR is on a tube feeding or TPN regimen which probably meets most of nutritional needs.	**4. Excellent** Eats most of every meal. Never refuses a meal. Usually eats a total of 4 or more servings of meat and dairy products. Occasionally eats between meals. Does not require supplementation.				
FRICTION & SHEAR	**1. Problem** Requires moderate to maximum assistance in moving. Complete lifting without sliding against sheets is impossible. Frequently slides down in bed or chair, requiring frequent repositioning with maximum assistance. Spasticity, contractures or agitation leads to almost constant friction.	**2. Potential Problem** Moves feebly or requires minimum assistance. During a move skin probably slides to some extent against sheets, chair, restraints or other devices. Maintains relatively good position in chair or bed most of the time but occasionally slides down.	**3. No Apparent Problem** Moves in bed and in chair independently and has sufficient muscle strength to lift up completely during move. Maintains good position in bed or chair.					

Total Score

Figure 6.1 The Braden scale for predicting pressure sore risk.

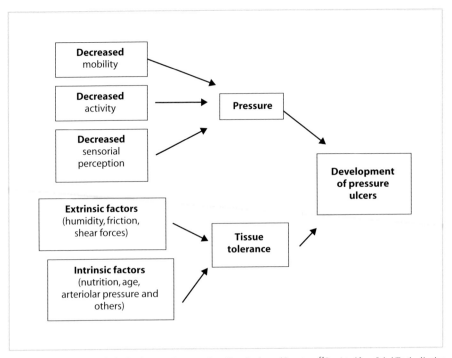

Figure 6.2 Concept diagram for the development of pressure ulcers. (From Braden and Bergstrom.[54] Reprinted from *Rehabilitation Nursing* 12:9, with permission of the Association of Rehabilitation Nurses, 4700 W. Lake Avenue, Glenview, IL 60025-1485. Copyright © 1987.)

Table 6.10. Validation of Braden scale studies

Authors and publication year	Type of center	Sample size	Sensitivity	Specificity	Positive predictive value	Negative predictive value
Bergstrom, Braden et al., 1987[55]	Hospital	99	100%	90%	70%	97%
Bergstrom, Braden et al., 1987[55]	Long-term hospital	100	100%	64%	25%	100%
Bergstrom et al., 1987[56]	Intensive care	60	83%	64%	61%	85%
Langemo et al., 1991[57]	Hospital	190	64%	87%	47%	93%
Bergstrom and Braden, 1992[58]	Nursing home	200	97%	19%	77%	71%
Salvadalena et al., 1992[59]	Hospital	99	40%	70%	23%	79%
Barnes and Payton, 1993[60]	Hospital	361	73%	91%	33%	91%
Braden and Bergstrom, 1994[61]	Nursing home	102	79%	74%	54%	90%
Ramundo, 1995[62]	Home care	48	100%	34%	21%	100%
Capobianco and McDonald, 1996[63]	Hospital	50	71%	83%	63%	88%
Halfens, 1997[64]	Hospital	320	74%	70%	30%	94%
Pang and Wong, 1998[38]	Hospital (rehabilitation)	138	91%	62%	37%	96%
Vap and Donahue, 2000[65]	Long-term hospital	555	27%	95%	53%	74%
Schoonhoven et al., 2002[40]	Hospital	1229	43%	68%	8%	95%
Seongsook et al., 2004[66]	Hospital (ICU)	125	97%	26%	37%	95%

Source: Created by the authors using data from Torra i Bou,[11] Cullum et al.,[12] and McGough.[13]

PURAS in Intensive Care Patients

The constant increase in knowledge about PURAS has led to deep and interesting debates about the need for specific tools for complex and special clinical situations, as in the case of patients in intensive care units (ICU) or pediatric patients.

For intensive care units there is wide disagreement in the literature about the use of general scales. Thus, some works stress the use of PURAS such as the Braden scale in ICU neurological patients[67,68] and cardiological surgery patients,[69,70] others propose a modification of the cutoff point for ICU traumatology patients,[71] and still others emphasize the value of the Waterlow scale,[51] while there is another group that is quite unconvinced of it.[52]

There are also PURAS specifically designed for ICU patients such as the Cubbin–Jackson scale,[51,72] which appeared in 1991 as a modification of the Norton scale; the Cornell Ulcer Risk Score,[73] the 1995 Sunderland scale,[74,75] and the Birty Pressure Risk Assessment scale.[76] Nevertheless none has validation and they are scarcely mentioned in the literature. There have been attempts to validate some such as the Decubitus Ulcer Potential Analyzer (DUPA), a modified version of the Gosnell, Norton, and Braden scales, which sensitivity wise, shows lower scores than the Braden scale on the same patients.[71]

As a further addition of specific factors on existing scales, Halfens et al.[77] underline that including variables such as blood circulation to the Braden scale does not improve its sensitivity or specificity, while Séller et al.[78] conclude that there are no specific risk factors for ICU patients that would justify the design of a PURAS exclusively for them. Therefore, many ICU professionals look at tissue damage rather than using different scales when deciding on preventive measures.[79]

PURAS in Pediatric Patients

Pressure ulcers in pediatric patients are gaining significance. Baldwin,[80] in a review on pressure ulcers in pediatric patients, found that there were 22 works published in English since 1972. Waterlow,[81] in her 1997 study of children at risk of developing pressure ulcers, considered that available PURAS were not appropriate for pediatric patients, especially babies. In 1998 Cocket published the Pediatric Pressure Sore Risk Assessment,[82] a PURAS for pediatric patients that has not yet been validated. Willock et al. later wrote an interesting review[83] about the inadequacy of using PURAS intended for adults in children, mentioning the Cocket scale and three others (Bedi A (1993), Olding L (1998) and Pickersgill J (1997)), so far not validated or at least with no published validation.

In 1996 Quigley and Curley published the Braden Q scale, which is a revised version of the Braden scale for pediatric use.[84] Recently Curley et al.[85] published a paper where they validate a modified Braden Q scale that consists of three subscales for the Braden Q scale, mobility, sensory perception, and perfusion/tissue oxygenation, with a cutoff point of 7; sensitivity was 92% and specificity 59%, values quite similar to those on the Braden scale for adults.

Summary

- Risk assessment scales for the development of pressure ulcers (PURAS) are tools that aid a nurse's clinical judgment in order to identify patients at risk and apply preventive measures.
- Risk assessment must be done soon after admittance and periodically repeated or when the clinical condition of the patient changes significantly.
- The ideal PURAS must have high sensitivity and specificity, good predictive value, clear definition of terms, and should be easy to use.
- Currently, the PURAS that offer the best validation are the Braden scale, closely followed by the Norton scale.

Acknowledgments

Our special thanks to Montserrat Robreño, assistant in the Clinical Department of the Advanced Wound Care (AWC) Division of Smith & Nephew Spain, for her help in the translation of the draft of this chapter.

References

1. Waterlow J. Pressure sore prevention manual. Taunton: Newtons; 1996.
2. Pancorbo Hidalgo PL, Garća Fernández FP. Estimación del coste económico de la prevención de úlceras por presión en una unidad hospitalaria. Gerokomos 2002; 13(3):164–171.
3. Xakellis GC, Frantz R, Lewis A. Cost of pressure ulcer prevention in long-term care. J Am Geriatr Soc 1995; 43:496–501.
4. Hodge J, Mounter J, Gardner G, et al. Clinical trial of the Norton Scale in acute care settings. Austr J Adv Nurs 1990; 8(1):39–46.
5. Bale S, Finlay I, Harding KG. Pressure sore prevention in a hospice. Wound Care 1995; 4(10):465–468.
6. Torra JE, Rueda J, Soldevilla JE, et al. 1er Estudio Nacional de Prevalencia de úlceras por presión en España. Epidemiología y variables definitorias de las lesiones y pacientes. Gerokomos 2003; 14(1):37–47.
7. Soldevilla Agreda JJ, Torra i Bou JE. Epidemiología de las UPP en España y tendencias de prevención. 2001. En, Mesa de Debate: "Las úlceras por presión, un reto para el sistema de salud y la sociedad: Repercusiones a nivel epidemiológico, ético, económico y legal." 26 and 27 II 2003. www.gneaupp.org (accessed on 25 January 2003).
8. Halfens RJG. Risk assessment scales for pressure ulcers: A theoretical methodological and clinical perspective. Ostomy Wound Manag 2000; 46(8):36–44.
9. Ayelo EA, Braden B. How and why to do pressure ulcer risk assessment. Adv Skin Wound Care 2002; 15(3):125–131.
10. Norton D, Exton-Smith AN, McLaren R. An investigation of geriatric nursing problems in hospital. London: National Corporation for the Care of Old People; 1962.
11. Torra i Bou JE. Valorar el riesgo de presentar úlceras por presión. Escala de Braden. Rev ROL Enf 1997; 224:23–30.
12. Cullum N, Deeks J, Fletcher A, et al. The prevention and treatment of pressure sores: How useful are the measures for scoring people's risk of developing a pressure sore? Eff Health Care 1995; 2(1):1–18.
13. McGough A. A systematic review of the effectiveness of risk assessment scales used in the prevention and management of pressure sore. MSc thesis. University of York, 1999.
14. Pancorbo Hidalgo PL, García-Fernández FP, López Medina I, Álvarez Nieto, C. Risk assessment scales for pressure ulcer prevention: a systematic review. In press.
15. Novell AJ, Navarro-Rubio MD. Evaluación de la Evidencia Cientćfica. Med Clin (Barc) 1995; 105: 740–743.

16. Gálvez Toro A. Enfermería Basada en la Evidencia. Granada: Fundación Index; 2001.
17. National Institute for Clinical Excellence. Pressure ulcer risk assessment and prevention. Inherited Clinical Guideline B. London: NICE; 2001.
18. European Pressure Ulcer Advisory Panel: Directrices sobre la prevención de úlceras por presión del Grupo Europeo de Úlceras por presión. Gerokomos 1999; 10(1):30–33.
19. Bergstrom N, Allman RM, Carlson CE, et al. Pressure ulcers in adults: prediction and prevention. Clinical Practice Guideline number 3. Rockville, MD: US Department of Health and Human Services. Public Health Service. Agency for Health Care Policy and Research; 1992.
20. Best Practice. Pressure sores. Part 1: Prevention of pressure related damage. The Joanna Briggs Institute for Evidence Based Nursing and Midwifery. 1997; 1(1):1–6.
21. Research Dissemination Core. Prevention of pressure sore. Iowa City: University of Iowa Gerontological Nursing Interventions Research Center; May 2002.
22. Registered Nurses Association of Ontario. The nursing best practice guideline. Risk assessment and prevention of pressure ulcers. www.rnao.org (accessed on 30 March 2003).
23. Rycroft-Malone J, MacInnes E. Pressure ulcer risk assessment and prevention. Technical Report. London: Royal College of Nursing: 2000.
24. Smith LN, Booth N, Douglas D, et al. A critique of 'at risk' pressure sore assessment tools. J Clin Nurs 1995; 4:153–159.
25. Deeks JJ. Pressure sore prediction: using and evaluating risk assessment tools. Br J Nurs 1996; 5(5):313–320.
26. Bridel J. Assessing the risk pressure sores. Nurs Stand 1993; 7(25):32–35.
27. MacDonald K. The reliability of pressure sore risk assessment tools. Prof Nurse 1995; 2(3):169–171.
28. Scott EM. The prevention of pressure ulcers through risk assessment. J Wound Care 2000; 9(2):69–70.
29. Norton D. Norton revised risk scores. Nurs Times 1987; 83(41):6.
30. Roberts BV, Goldstone LA. A survey of pressure sores in the over sixties on two orthopedic wards. Int J Nurs Stud 1979; 16(4):335–364.
31. Newman P, West J. Pressure sores 2—the value of Norton score. Nurs Times 1981; 29(21): 15–21.
32. Goldstone LA, Roberts BV. A preliminary discriminant function analysis of elderly orthopedic patients who will or will not contract a pressure sore. Int J Nurs Stud 1980; 17(1):17–23.
33. Goldstone LA, Goldstone J. The Norton score: an early warning of pressure sores? J Adv Nurs 1982; 7:419–426.
34. Lincoln R, Roberts R, Maddox A, et al. Use of Norton pressure sore risk assessment scoring system with elderly patients in acute care. J ET Nurs 1986; 13:132–138.
35. Smith I. Waterlow/Norton scoring system: a ward view. Care Sci Pract 1989; 7:93–95.
36. Stotts NA. Predicting pressure ulcer development in surgical patients. Heart Lung 1988; 17: 641–647.
37. Wai-Han C, Kit-Wai C, French P, et al. Which pressure sore risk calculator? A study of the effectiveness of the Norton scale in Hong Kong. Int J Nurs Stud 1997; 34(2):165–169.
38. Pang SM, Wong TK. Predicting pressure sore risk with the Norton, Braden and Waterlow scales in a Hong Kong rehabilitation hospital. Nurs Res 1998; 47(3):147–153.
39. Garcia AM, Rosa G de la, Garrido G, Rodriguez P. Escala de Norton: ¿es válida como método de predicción del desarrollo de úlceras por presión? Medicina Preventiva 1999; V(3):24–27.
40. Schoonhoven L, Hallboom JRE, Bousema MT, et al. Prospective cohort study of routine use of risk assessment scales for prediction of pressure ulcers. BMJ 2002; 235:797–800.
41. Gosnell DJ. An assessment tool to identify pressure sores. Nurs Res 1973; 22:55–59.
42. Berglund B, Nordström G. The use of the modified Norton scale in nursing-home patients. Scand J Caring Sci 1995; 9:165–169.
43. Garcia Fernandez FP, Bermejo J, Pérez MJ, et al. Validación de dos escalas de valoración del riesgo de úlceras por presión: Gosnell y Nova-4. Rev ROL Enf 1999; 22(10):685–687.
44. Aguado H, Aguilar M, Casado A. Protocol de prevenció i tratament de les ulceres per pressió. Institut Català de la Salut. Ciutat Sanitaria i Universitaria de Bellvitge, 1994.
45. Bermejo CJ, Beamud M, Puerta M de la, et al. Fiabilidad interobservadores de dos escalas de detección del riesgo de formación de úlceras por presión en enfermos de 65 o más años. Enf Clínica 1998; 8(6):242–247.
46. Grupo de Enfermerća del Institut Català de la Salut. Ulceras por presión: método de consenso como estrategia de mejora de la calidad asistencial. Enf Clínica 1998; 8(3):110–115.
47. Fuentelsalz C. Validación de la escala EMINA ©: un instrumento de valoración del riesgo de desarrollar úlceras por presión en pacientes hospitalizados. Enf Clćnica 2001; 11(3):97–103.
48. Waterlow J. A risk assessment card. Nurs Times 1985; 81(49):5155.

49. Edwards M. The levels of reliability and validity of the Waterlow pressure sore risk calculator. J Wound Care 1995; 4(8):373–378.
50. Weststrate JT, Hop WC, Aalbers AG. The clinical relevance of the Waterlow pressure sore risk scale in the ICU. Intensive Care Med 1998; 24(8):815–820.
51. Boyle M, Green M. Pressure sores in intensive care: defining their incidence and associated factors and assessing the utility of two pressure sore risk assessment tools. Aust Crit Care 2001; 14(1): 24–30.
52. Papanikolau P, Clark M, Lyne PA. Improving the accuracy of pressure ulcer risk calculators: some preliminary evidence. Int J Nurs Stud 2002; 39:187–194.
53. Bergstrom N, Braden B, Laguzza A, Holman V. The Braden Scale for predicting pressure sore risk: reliability studies. Nurs Res 1985; 34(6):383.
54. Braden B, Bergstrom N. A conceptual schema for the study of the aetiology of pressure sores. Rehabil Nurs 1987; 12(1):8–16.
55. Bergstrom N, Braden B, Laguzza A, Holman V. The Braden Scale for predicting pressure sore risk: reliability studies. Nurs Res 1987; 36(4):205–210.
56. Bergstrom N, Demuth PJ, Braden BJ. A clinical trial of the Braden scale for predicting pressure sore risk. Nurs Clin North Am 1987; 22(2):417–428.
57. Langemo DK, Olson B, Hunter S, et al. Incidence and prediction of pressure ulcers in five patient care settings. Decubitus 1991; 4(3):25–36.
58. Bergstrom N, Braden BJ. Prospective study of pressure risk among institutionalised elderly. J Am Geriatr Soc 1992; 40(8):747–758.
59. Salvadalena G, Snyder ML, Brogdon KE. Clinical trial of the Braden scale on an acute care medical unit. J ET Nurs 1992; 19:160–165.
60. Barnes D, Payton RG. Clinical application of the Braden scale in the acute-care setting. Dermatol Nurs 1993; 5(5):386–388.
61. Braden BJ, Bergstrom N. Predictive validity of the Braden scale for pressure sore risk in a nursing home population. Res Nurs Health 1994; 17:459–470.
62. Ramundo J. Reliability and validity of the Braden scale in the home care setting. J Wound Ostomy Continence Nurs 1995; 22(3):128–134.
63. Capobianco ML, McDonald DD. Factors affecting the predictive validity of the Braden Scale. Adv Wound Care 1996; 9(6):32–36.
64. Halfens RJ. The reliability and validity of the Braden scale. In: Harding KG, Leaper DJ, Turner TD (eds) Proceedings of the 7th European conference on advances in wound management. London: Macmillan; 1997.
65. Vap P, Donahue T. Pressure risk assessment in long-term care nursing. J Gerontol Nurs 2000; 26(6):37–45.
66. Seongsook J, Ihnsook J, Younghee L. Validity of pressure ulcer risk assessment scales; Cubbin–Jackson, Braden, and Douglas scale. Int J Nurs Stud 2004; 41(2):199–204.
67. Anonymus. Low Braden scale scores predicted the development of pressure ulcers in neurologic intensive and intermediate care units. ACP J Club 2001; 135(2):76.
68. Fife C, Otto G, Capsuto EG, et al. Incidence of pressure ulcers in a neurologic intensive care unit. Crit Care Med 2001; 29(2):283–290.
69. Lewicki LJ, Mion L, Splane KG, et al. Patient risk factors for pressure ulcers during cardiac surgery. AORN J 1997; 65(5):933–942.
70. Stordeurs S, Laurent S, d'Hoore W. The importance of repeated risk assessment of pressure sores in cardiovascular surgery. J Cardiovasc Surg (Torino) 1998; 39(3):343–349.
71. Jiricka MK, Ryan P, Carvalho MA, et al. Pressure ulcer risk factors in ICU population. Am J Crit Care 1995; 4(5):361–367.
72. Hunt J. Application of a pressure area risk calculator in an intensive care unit. Intensive Crit Care Nurs 1993; 9(4):226–231.
73. Eachempati SR, Hydo LJ, Barie PS. Factors influencing the development of decubitus ulcers in critically ill surgical patients. Crit Care Med 2001; 29(9):1678–1682.
74. Sollars A. Pressure area risk assessment in intensive care. Nurs Crit Care 1998; 3(6):267–273.
75. Lowery MT. A pressure sore risk calculator for intensive care patients: The Sunderland experience. Intensive Crit Care Nurs 1995; 11(6):344–353
76. Birtwhistle J. Pressure sore formation and risk assessment in intensive care. Care Crit Ill 1995; 11: 121–125.
77. Halfens RJ, Van Achterberg T, Bal RM. Validity and reliability of the Braden Scale and the influence of other risk factors: a multicentre prospective study. Int J Nurs Stud 2000; 37(4):313–319.
78. Séller BP, Wille J, van Ramsshort B, et al. Pressure ulcers in intensive care patients: a review of risks and prevention. Intensive Care Med 2002; 28(10):1379–1388.

79. Weststrate JT, Bruinining HA. Pressure sores in an intensive care unit and related variables: a descriptive study. Intensive Crit Care Nurs 1996; 12(5):280–284.
80. Baldwin KM. Incidence and prevalence of pressure ulcers in children. Adv Skin Wound Care 2002; 15(3):121–124.
81. Waterlow JA. Pressure sore risk assessment in children. Paediatr Nurs 1997; 9(6):21–24.
82. Cocket A. Paediatric pressure sore risk assessment. J Tissue Viability 1998; 8(1):30.
83. Willock J, Hugues J, Tickle S, et al. Pressure sores in children—the acute hospital perspective. J Tissue Viability 2000; 10(2):59–62.
84. Quigley SM, Curley MAQ. Skin integrity in the pediatric population: preventing and managing pressure ulcers. J Soc Pediatr Nurs 1996; 1:7–18.
85. Curley M, Razmus IS, Roberts KE, Wypij D. Predicting pressure ulcer risk in paediatric patients: the Braden Q Scale. Nurs Res 2003; 52(1):22–33.

7 Equipment Selection

Jacqueline Fletcher

Background Information

The European Pressure Ulcer Advisory Panel (EPUAP) guidelines for prevention of pressure ulcers[1] state that most pressure ulcers can be prevented and it is important to have prevention strategies in place that are based on the best available evidence. These strategies encompass a wide range of actions but will include the use of specialized equipment such as overlays, mattresses, and specialist beds to manage the load on the tissues.[2] Selection of the appropriate piece of equipment for any one individual is complicated as there is little good quality evidence to support the efficacy of any individual piece of equipment and indeed the tests used to determine the efficacy of these systems have been inconsistent in design and measurement techniques.[3] There is also a lack of consensus regarding the terminology used to describe the mode of action of many pieces of equipment.[2,4] Most guidelines on the prevention of pressure ulcers[2,4-7] discuss the use of equipment but are only able to give broad statements which unfortunately do not address the requirements of individual patients.

Efficacy of Equipment

There have been several published reviews of the efficacy of support surfaces[8,9] with detailed methodologies also published for clinicians wishing to replicate these reviews.[9,10]

Efficacy of individual support systems may be measured in a variety of ways including: clinical outcomes, interface pressure measurement, measurement of transcutaneous oxygen, and other measures of microcirculation. The most common method, however, appears to be the measurement of interface pressure. In order to improve comparability of published research a EPUAP working group proposed recommendations for a standardized protocol for laboratory evaluation of support surfaces.[3] It is recommended that any future research on support surfaces should follow these recommendations where possible.

Mechanisms of Action/Types of Equipment

Mattresses are defined as a piece of equipment placed directly onto the bed frame; an overlay is used in addition to the mattress and should not be placed directly onto the bed frame.

Broadly speaking equipment is described[11] as providing:

- pressure reduction—the equipment maximizes the area of skin in contact with the surface thereby reducing the pressure at an individual point; or
- pressure relief—the equipment removes pressure from a localized skin area in either a static or cyclical mechanism.

Other guidelines[9] use alternative terminology such as low-tech devices (those that use a conforming support surface to distribute body weight over a large surface area) and high-tech devices (use of alternating support surfaces where inflatable cells alternately inflate and deflate).

Pressure Reduction

Equipment that falls within this category includes static systems such as foam mattresses and overlays, fiber-filled overlays, air-filled overlays, gel-filled mattresses and overlays, and powered systems such as low-air-loss overlays and mattresses. As well as the material the mattress itself is made from, consideration must also be given to the covers of the mattress, which must be able to conform with the internal content; otherwise a hammocking effect occurs, negating the pressure-reducing properties of the mattress/overlay.[11] Consideration should also be given to the impact of the bed frame on the mattress. Solid bed frames do not allow the mattress to breathe and where condensation occurs it is possible for mold to grow between the mattress and bed frame (Figure 7.1—see color section). Mechanical bed frames that contour to improve the patient's position and reduce shearing forces may also affect the pressure-reducing properties of the mattress and care should be taken to ensure that the mattress is able to follow the contours of the frame without causing damage to the foam/gel and generating high points of pressure where the foam creases.

Pressure-Relieving Devices

Pressure-relieving devices are usually powered devices and would include, for example, alternating pressure mattresses and overlays and air fluidized systems.

Alternating systems operate by the cyclical inflation and deflation of sections of the mattress (usually known as cells). This cycle varies between products in terms of both the time taken to complete the cycle and the number of cells involved in the cycle (usually two or three). Where the cell is inflated the body is in contact and is subject to high interface pressures. However, this is for a fixed time span and as the cycle progresses the pressure is partially or totally removed and transferred to different parts of the body as the cells inflate and deflate. These devices frequently incorporate a pressure sensor and may regulate the pressure within the cells in response to the patient's weight and the distribution of the weight. For example, if the patient is in the semi-recumbent position their weight is primarily supported along the legs and buttocks as opposed to lying where the weight is distributed also along the trunk.

Air fluidized systems constantly change the points of the body supporting the weight. They operate by continually circulating warm air through fine ceramic beads covered by a permeable sheet. It is debatable whether this type of system works by redistributing the pressure through extremely close contact, or by reducing the pressure as the movement of the beads is constant and therefore the contact points are constantly changing.

Selecting Equipment

As there is such a plethora of equipment available a set of criteria need to be followed to assist in appropriate selection. These criteria usually relate to the patient's risk of developing a pressure ulcer or the grade of pressure ulcer already present, with differing criteria being available for prevention and management. It is widely acknowledged that there are limitations within the current risk assessment tools[12] and the NICE guideline[9] avoids this situation by referring to patients who are "vulnerable to" or "at elevated risk of" pressure ulcers. Their recommendations state that although there is very little evidence to suggest the high-tech devices are more effective than the low-tech equipment, professional consensus recommends use of alternating pressure or other high-tech devices:

- as a first-line prevention strategy for people at elevated risk following holistic assessment;
- when the patient has a history of previous ulceration or a clinical condition which suggests they are best cared for on a high-tech device; or
- when a low-tech device has failed.

The United Kingdom pressure ulcer benchmark statement regarding provision of equipment also clearly states that the patients should be comfortable on the equipment.[13] This is particularly important because if patients are not comfortable it is likely that they will be reluctant to use the equipment and therefore however efficacious the equipment may be they will not benefit from its allocation.

Selecting Equipment for Individual Patients

Selecting equipment for individual patients presents additional practical factors which must be considered alongside the effectiveness of the equipment. These will also determine the suitability of the equipment for use in the particular setting whether home care, hospital care, or an intermediate care setting.

These more practical considerations require in-depth knowledge of the patient and the setting in which care will be delivered. Although these are less evidence-based considerations, it is the complex interplay between these variables that may ultimately be the deciding factors in the provision of appropriate equipment for individual patients. These factors may be considered as clinical, practical, and financial.

Clinical Factors

These will include not only the current risk level but also the likely prognosis. Consideration should be given to the likelihood of the patient's condition improving or deteriorating and the level of equipment supplied should reflect this or at least plans should be made to replace the equipment as the patient's condition changes.

The overall objectives of care must also be addressed. Therefore consideration should be given to requirements for appropriate moving and handling, other wound-related factors such as management of high levels of exudate, and general clinical requirements such as control of temperature. Any factors that may contraindicate the use of a particular piece of equipment must also be considered. For example, patients with unstable spinal fractures should not be managed on alternating systems and patients with unstable cardiac conditions may also be advised to avoid this type of equipment, although a small study in the Netherlands suggests the gradual movement of these systems did not affect the patients' general medical condition.[14] Patients with bilateral amputation may also find it difficult to maintain their balance of either very soft or moving surfaces, and this will have an adverse effect on their independence. Some patients may find it difficult to sleep[14] or feel nauseated on a surface they perceive to be moving; frequently they will quickly become acclimatized to this but for some patients the movement is intolerable.

In critical care settings, where there is a higher risk of cardiac arrest, specific attention must be paid to what happens in relation to resuscitation. The surface must be suitable to resuscitate the patient on but at the same time maintain appropriate pressure redistribution while the patient has very compromised circulation. Powered systems often have a rapid deflate mechanism. However, it must be considered what happens when the mattress deflates; frequently the mattress deflates under the patient but the air remains in the edges. This results in the patient becoming enveloped in the mattress and if clinicians kneel on the edge of the mattress this can result in the patient being jerked around on the bed. When the mattress is fully deflated the patient must still be receiving some form of pressure reduction so equipment should not deflate fully onto the bed frame. In some instances a hyper-inflate facility may be preferable.

Practical Factors

Practical factors to be considered may relate to the patient, the surface, or both. Most commonly these relate to the environment in which the patient is being cared for. Patients cared for in the home setting present a much more complex scenario than those cared for in institutional settings. The shape, size, and weight of the equipment needs to be considered in terms of access to the home and sometimes into older hospital settings. Some equipment such as air fluidized beds are extremely heavy and need to be positioned carefully in any setting to avoid structural damage. The size of a mattress or overlay must be compatible with the bed frame on which it is to be used. This is a particular problem in the home, especially if the patient wishes to continue sharing a double bed with a partner (or indeed if there is nowhere else for the partner to sleep). Most standard mattress and overlays are more than half of a double bed. However, some manufacturers do supply specialist sizes designed for use on double beds which allow the partner space (Figure 7.2). There are psychological benefits to both the patient and the carer of remaining in close proximity.

Where overlays are being used, consideration must be given to the effect on the height of the mattress. Increasing the height may reduce the patient's level of inde-

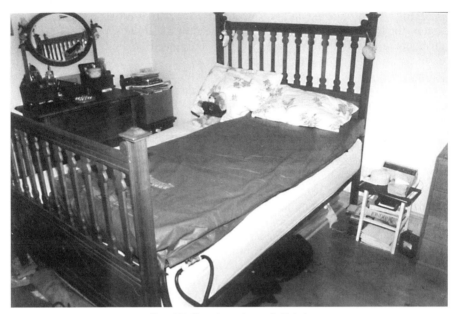

Figure 7.2 Alternating overlay on a double bed.

pendence and reduce their safety if it raises them above the level of protective cot sides. If increased height impacts on independence the use of an electronic profiling bed frame may help restore some degree of independence. However, this in itself may create additional problems as they are frequently larger than standard bed frames and also require an electrical power source. This may mean that three electrical sockets are required for a bed frame, a mattress, and seating provision. In a hospital setting where electrical supply may also be needed to power vital monitoring or drug delivery equipment this may be difficult to achieve and in a patient's own home may lead to concerns about the cost of the electricity being used when the equipment is in constant use or overloading of the system.

Most pieces of equipment including bed frames have maximum and minimum weight limits. The maximum weight limit is usually related to safety and the ability of a mattress to reach optimal performance; the minimum weight limit may also relate to optimal performance but is often a factor in patient comfort. The distribution of the patient's weight must also be considered in terms of efficacy of the equipment. Some patients, for example those with lymphedema, may have very heavy legs but the rest of their body be of "average" weight; if a pressure mat (an integral mat containing pressure sensors which identifies the weight distribution at particular points of the mattress allowing the mattress to respond to changes in weight distribution) is used within the system it may be necessary to override this to maintain patient comfort and achieve sufficient pressure reduction. Some more sophisticated systems allow zoned control of the pressure so greater support may be achieved to support the limbs.

Patients may have an individual preference for a soft or firm surface; some equipment allows small adjustments to compensate for this.

Alarm systems and the ability to rectify faults easily is a particular consideration in the home; carers must be advised what to do in the event of an alarm in the home setting. In the hospital setting the alarm needs to be sufficiently strident to be noticed above the general noise levels but not so loud that it disturbs other patients at night. Most electrical systems now have indicator panels which highlight the most common problems such as detachment of the power source.

In the home situation, particularly if the patient requires long-term care, the aesthetics of the equipment may be important. Many companies now provide electronic bed frames and other equipment designed to look as much like standard furniture as possible. This may allow the individual to feel less of a patient and more of a person.

Most equipment will need to be cleaned or even decontaminated and this needs to be considered within the selection process. If it is likely that the cover may be regularly or heavily contaminated then it may be beneficial to consider a piece of equipment with replaceable covers. Laundering of equipment such as fiber overlays may also be a factor to consider if specialist facilities are not available. Most equipment can be cleaned on site. However, some equipment, such as air fluidized beds, needs to be taken to specialist decontamination centers.

If selecting equipment for use within a healthcare setting where it may not be in permanent use, appropriate storage and transportation to and from the storage area needs to be identified.

Financial Considerations

While unit cost of equipment must always be a factor in the decision process other costs must also be taken into account. The costs of treating a patient who develops a pressure ulcer far outweigh the costs of prevention.

In terms of actual costs, differing prices are usually charged for purchase, rental or leasing of equipment and discounts are frequently available for bulk purchases or purchases of complete systems/packages such as a bed frame, mattress, and seating. More hidden costs relate to:

- the training of staff to use the equipment,
- cleaning/decontamination,
- running of the equipment, and
- service and maintenance.

Conclusion

Equipment selection is complex whether for an individual patient or for a whole service. The research and clinical evidence to support individual pieces of equipment must always be reviewed but in many instances other practical factors carry equal weight in the decision-making process. As so many types of equipment are now available many national and local guidelines[7,9] present flow charts to assist in selection. These usually commence with the patient's level of risk and then proceed through a series of clinical considerations. These are helpful in selection for the majority of patients but a thorough holistic assessment of every patient must underpin the selection process. Where patients state a dislike for a particular piece of equipment great care should be taken to determine what it is they actually dislike about it; if patients are uncomfortable on a piece of equipment it is very likely that they will not use it.

New equipment appears on the market on a regular basis. In order to make a reasoned selection the practitioner must understand the principles by which the equipment works and the clinical and practical considerations in managing patients. Care must be taken to review both the clinical effectiveness and the practical considerations of equipment usage.

References

1. EPUAP. Pressure ulcer prevention guidelines. Oxford: EPUAP; 1998.
2. EPUAP. Pressure ulcer treatment guidelines. Oxford: EPUAP; 1999.
3. Support Services Working Group. Draft guidelines for the laboratory evaluation of pressure redistributing support surfaces. EPUAP Review 2002; 4:8–12.
4. AISLeC. Council Development of consensus upon the description of patient support surfaces within Italy. EPUAP Review 2003; 5:101–102.
5. Defloor T, Vanden Bossche K, Derre B, et al. Recommandations pour la prévention des escarres. Ghent: University of Ghent; 2003.
6. CBO. Conceptrichtlijn t.b.v. richtlijnbijeenkomst Decubitus (tweede herziening). Utrecht: CBO; 2002.
7. Clinical Resource Efficiency Support Team. Guidelines for the prevention and management of pressure sores. CREST, 1998.
8. Cullum N, Nelson EA, Fleming K, Sheldon T. Systematic reviews of wound care management: (5) beds; (6) compression; (7) laser therapy, therapeutic ultrasound, electrotherapy and electromagnetic therapy. Health Technol Assess 2001; 5(9):1–221.
9. National Institute for Clinical Excellence. Clinical Guideline 7: Pressure ulcer risk assessment and prevention, including the use of pressure-relieving devices (beds, mattresses and overlays) for the prevention of pressure ulcers in primary and secondary care. London: NICE; 2003.
10. EPUAP. EPUAP and the evaluation of support surfaces. EPUAP Review 2000; 2:7–9.
11. Kenney L, Rithalia S. Technical aspects of support surfaces. J Wound Care 1999; Resource File— Mattresses and Beds Part 2:1–8.
12. Balzer K, Schrniedl C, Dassen T. Norton, Waterlow, Braden and the Care Dependency Scale: comparing their validity predicting patients' pressure sore risk. Le Mans: EPUAP 5th Open Meeting, 2001.
13. UK Department of Health. Essence of care. London: London Department of Health; 2001.
14. Grindley A, Acres J. Alternating pressure mattresses: comfort and quality of sleep. Br J Nurs 1996; 5:1303–1310.

8 Pressure Ulcer Prevention and Repositioning

Tom Defloor, Katrien Vanderwee, Doris Wilborn, and Theo Dassen

Introduction

Preventing pressure ulcers is important, but not always easy to achieve. The most effective measures decrease the level and/or the duration of the pressure and shearing force. The pressure level is reduced by means of (for example) viscoelastic mattresses or low-air-loss systems. Repositioning and (for example) alternating mattresses, by contrast, are oriented towards decreasing the duration of pressure and shearing force.

Repositioning

Repositioning is generally regarded as one of the most important and most effective measures for preventing pressure ulcers.[1] By regularly positioning patients in a different position, one modifies "the pressure points," the points on which the body is supported. If the position is modified frequently enough and the oxygen shortage in the tissues does not last too long, the chance of developing pressure ulcers is limited. Salisbury[2] demonstrated that transcutaneous oxygen levels at the level of the pressure points declined quickly in the first minutes after assuming a new body position on a standard hospital mattress. He therefore concludes that even schemes of repositioning every 2 hours will not be enough to always prevent pressure ulcers in all patients.

History

It has long been known that changing position is important in the prevention of pressure ulcers. Robert Graves (1796–1853) wrote in 1848 in his *Clinical Lectures on the Practice of Medicine* that pressure ulcers could be prevented through regular changes in position.[3]

Already in 1955 Guttman[4] recommended repositioning every 2 hours for paraplegic patients. Nevertheless, the first studies on the effect of the duration and intensity of pressure on the development of pressure ulcers date from 1961,[5] and the first pressure measurements were performed in 1965.[6]

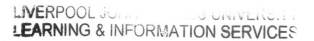

Traditional Repositioning Frequency

The frequency of changing position determines whether this preventive measure is effective, and thus leads to a decrease in the incidence of pressure ulcers. Traditionally, repositioning every 2 hours[7] or every 3 hours[8] has been recommended.

Internationally one often hears the story that the choice of a 2-hour frequency can be traced back to a nursing unit for war victims during the Second World War.[9] In this unit, two soldiers were given the task of turning all of the patients. As soon as they had finished turning them all, they immediately had to start all over again. It took 2 hours to turn all of the patients. Whether this legend has any basis in fact is uncertain, but Xakellis et al.[10] calculated that it takes an average of 3.5 minutes to change a patient's position. Thus, turning all of the patients in a 32-bed ward would take 2 hours.

Very little research has been done to determine the necessary repositioning frequency. The first study on repositioning dates from 1962. In this research Norton et al.[11] compared the pressure ulcer incidence between two groups of elderly hospitalized women. One group had their lying positions changed, while the other group did not. The pressure ulcer incidence in the repositioning group amounted to 9%, while in the other group 26% of the patients developed pressure ulcers. However, on precisely what basis the nurses decided whose position would be regularly changed, at which time(s) during their hospitalization, and how frequently, is unclear.

A PubMed search using the keywords "decubitus ulcer(s)," "pressure ulcer(s)," or "pressure sore(s)" in combination with "turning" or "repositioning" and "RCT" came up with eight references. In only two of these studies was the effect of repositioning on the development of pressure ulcers examined. Knox et al.[12] compared the effect of repositioning after 1, 1½, and 2 hours. Sixteen healthy elderly people, five whom had a dark skin type, were placed in one position for 2 hours, then in another position for 1½ hours, and finally for 1 hour in yet another position. The skin temperature had increased more after 2 hours of immobilization than after 1 or 1½ hours. No significant differences were found with respect to contact pressure and color. The test subjects found that lying in the same position for 2 hours was more uncomfortable than for 1 or 1½ hours. Due to the limited number of test subjects, the difficulty of detecting skin color changes in persons with a dark skin type, and the brief period of the study, the results are difficult to generalize.

A randomized clinical experiment with 838 geriatric patients showed that the number of pressure ulcer injuries (pressure ulcer grade 2 and higher[13]) could be reduced by changing the lying position every 2 hours and to an even greater degree by repositioning every 4 hours on a viscoelastic mattress in combination with pressure-reducing positions and seat cushions.[1,14] Changing the lying position every 3 hours did not appear to be sufficient to prevent pressure ulcers. These results have major consequences for nursing care. If patients lying on a non-pressure-reducing mattress do not have their position changed every 2 hours—both day and night, 7 days a week—it makes little sense to opt for repositioning as a preventive measure. In that case it is better to choose other measures. Changing position every 4 hours instead of every 2 hours is less labor-intensive and thus in practice much more feasible. It requires less effort on the part of the nurses and patients are less disturbed during their night's sleep. After all, changing position every 2 hours can be experienced as an unwanted intrusion by some patients.

The labor-intensive character of repositioning means that this effective prevention method is not often applied in practice, even among high-risk patients. The EPUAP prevalence study performed among 5947 patients from five European countries demonstrated that only 38.2% of the at-risk patients were having their positions changed.[15]

Combining Repositioning with Pressure-Reducing Measures

In order to make repositioning a more feasible method, its frequency can be reduced. This can be done only if repositioning is combined with pressure-reducing mattresses and cushions and adapted body positions; otherwise the preventive effect disappears, because pressure ulcers are a function of the duration and level of the pressure and shearing force. Increasing the duration can only be offset by decreasing the size of the tissue deformation.

The pressure level is determined inter alia by the position of a patient and by the hardness of the underlying layer. The contact surface is much greater in some body positions than it is in others. The greater the contact surface, the more widely the pressure can be distributed and the lower the pressure. The thickness and compressibility of the tissue on which the body is supported also differs greatly from position to position. The body position thus substantially defines the degree to which the tissue is deformed, and therefore the degree to which the oxygen supply of the tissue is impeded.

Supine Lying Position

In the flat supine lying position[16,17] and in a semi-Fowler's position of 30°,[18,19] the pressure would be lowest and thus the risk of pressure ulcers smallest. In the 30° semi-Fowler's position, the head end and the feet end are raised around 30° (Figure 8.1).

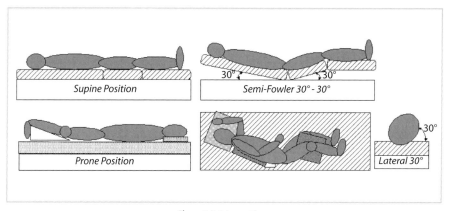

Figure 8.1 Lying positions.

Lateral Lying Position

The lowest pressure in the lateral lying position is measured in a 30° position.[20,21] In this case, the contact surface at the level of the pelvis is greater than in the classic lateral position of 90°. The tissue mass at the level of the contact surface is thicker, and so the pressure can be better absorbed and distributed. In a lateral lying position of 30° the patient is turned at a 30° angle to the mattress and is supported in the back with a cushion that has a 30° angle (Figure 8.1). The lower of the two legs is minimally bent at the level of the hip and the knee, while the upper leg is laid behind the lower one with a bend of 30° at the level of the hip and 35° at the level of the knee.[22]

Restricting Sitting Upright in Bed

The more the head end is raised, the smaller the contact surface and the more the pressure increases.[23] The pressure is greatest in a 90° upright-sitting position, because the compression area is then the smallest, which results in a high pressure and thus a greater chance of the development of pressure ulcers.

Prone Lying Position, Sometimes an Alternative

The prone lying position is sometimes used as alternative lying position (Figure 8.1). The pressure in this position is very low and roughly comparable to the pressure in the semi-Fowler's position.[18] Comfort is sometimes a problem, certainly on a harder mattress.

The prone lying position can be combined with a ventral-lateral form of the 30° lateral position. A small cushion is placed under the rib cage. The hip crest then comes to lie in a pressure-free position.

Adapted Repositioning Scheme

In a repositioning scheme the patient is placed as frequently as possible in the positions with the lowest pressure (in this case the supine lying position). In the lateral lying position the pressure is greater and the risk of pressure ulcers is also greater. A scheme which takes this into account would be: supine lying position—lateral lying position on the left—supine lying position—lateral lying position on the right.

Repositioning and Changing Sitting Position

Chair-bound patients develop pressure ulcers more frequently than bedridden patients with the same degree of helplessness.[24,25] This is because the pressure in the sitting position is much higher than in the lying position.[26] Moreover, patients often sit up for a long period.

The position must therefore also be changed while sitting, and with an even higher frequency than when lying down.[7] Changing the position of sitting patients consists of having them stand up temporarily so that the tissues can be resaturated with blood. Park[27] measured 12 test subjects in wheelchairs and found that bending forward and stretching crossways increases the pressure on one ischial protuberance and reduces it on the other.

Even in the sitting position the risk of pressure ulcers can be limited by reducing the pressure by means of adapted sitting positions and pressure-reducing cushions.

Sitting Position

The sitting position that entails the lowest pressure and thus the least risk of pressure ulcers is a backwards-sitting position with the legs supported on a small bench (Figure 8.2).[26] The contact surface is greatest and the pressure the lowest compared to other sitting positions. The disadvantage of tilting the backrest backwards is that patients have more difficulty later in standing up independently.

If the seat cannot be tilted backwards, the pressure is lowest in an upright-sitting position with the feet on the ground (Figure 8.2).[26]

Slipping down and sagging obliquely cause the pressure to increase substantially.[26,28] Using the armrests can help to stabilize the position.[29] Frequent checking of the sitting position and correction in the event of sagging to one side or slipping down should form a part of every pressure ulcer prevention policy.

Sitting upright on a chair is associated with high pressure, comparable to the pressure when sagging obliquely in an armchair.[26] The chair surface area is small and the seat of the chair is hard. While the sitting period in an armchair must already be briefer than in a lying position, the sitting period on a chair must be much shorter still.

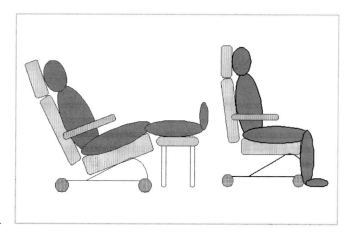

Figure 8.2 Sitting positions.

Conclusion

Repositioning is an effective way to prevent pressure ulcers, but it must be combined with sitting and lying positions in which the pressure is as low as possible. There are many opinions but little actual research on the frequency of position changes.

References

1. Defloor T. Drukreductie en wisselhouding in de preventie van decubitus [Pressure reduction and turning in the prevention of pressure ulcers]. PhD thesis, Ghent University, 2000.
2. Salisbury RE. Transcutaneous PO$_2$ monitoring in bedridden burn patients: a physiological analysis of four methods to prevent pressure sores. In: Lee BY (ed) Chronic ulcers of the skin. New York: McGraw-Hill; 1985;189–195.
3. Sebastian A. Robert Graves (1796–1853). In: Sebastian A (ed) A dictionary of the history of medicine. New York: Partenon Publishing Group; 2000.
4. Guttman L. The problem of treatment of pressure sores in spinal paraplegics. Br J Plast Surg 1955; 8:196–213.
5. Kosiak M. Etiology of decubitus ulcers. Arch Phys Med Rehabil 1961; 42:19–29.
6. Lindan O, Greenway R. Pressure distribution on the surface of the human body. Arch Phys Med Rehabil 1965; 46:378–385.
7. Panel for the Prediction and Prevention of Pressure Ulcers in Adults. Pressure ulcers in adults: prediction and prevention. Clinical practice guideline number 3. Rockville: Agency for Health Care Policy and Research, Public Health Service, US Department of Health and Human Services, AHCPR Publication No. 92–0047, 1992.
8. Bakker H. Herziening consensus decubitus [Revision of pressure ulcer consensus]. Utrecht: CBO; 1992.
9. Dealey C. Managing pressure sore prevention. Dinton: Mark Allen; 1997.
10. Xakellis GC, Frantz R, Lewis A. Cost of pressure ulcer prevention in long-term care. J Am Geriatr Soc 1995; 43:496–501.
11. Norton D, McLaren R, Exton-Smith AN. An investigation of geriatric nursing problems in hospital. New York: Churchill Livingstone; 1975.
12. Knox DM, Anderson TM, Anderson PS. Effects of different turn intervals on skin of healthy older adults. Adv Wound Care 1994; 7:48–52, 54.
13. EPUAP. Guidelines on treatment of pressure ulcers. EPUAP Review 1999; 2:31–33.
14. Defloor T. Wisselhouding, minder frequent en toch minder decubitus [Less frequent turning intervals and yet less pressure ulcers]. Tijdschr Gerontol Geriatr 2001; 32:174–177.
15. Clark M, Bours G, Defloor T. Summary report on the prevalence of pressure ulcers. EPUAP Review 2002; 4:49–57.
16. Jeneid P. Static and dynamic support systems-pressure differences on the body. In: Kenedi RM, Cowden JM, Scales JT (eds) Bedsore biomechanics. London: Macmillan; 1976: 287–299.
17. Barnett RI, Shelton FE. Measurement of support surface efficacy: pressure. Adv Wound Care 1997; 10:21–29.
18. Defloor T. The effect of position and mattress on interface pressure. Appl Nurs Res 2000; 13: 2–11.
19. Rondorf Klym LM, Langemo D. Relationship between body weight, body position, support surface, and tissue interface pressure at the sacrum. Decubitus 1993; 6:22–30.
20. Seiler WO, Allen S, Stahelin HB. Influence of the 30 degrees laterally inclined position and the "super-soft" 3-piece mattress on skin oxygen tension on areas of maximum pressure—implications for pressure sore prevention. Gerontology 1986; 32:158–166.
21. Colin D, Abraham P, Preault L, et al. Comparison of 90 degrees and 30 degrees laterally inclined positions in the prevention of pressure ulcers using transcutaneous oxygen and carbon dioxide pressures. Adv Wound Care 1996; 9:35–38.
22. Garber SL, Campion LJ, Krouskop TA. Trochanteric pressure in spinal cord injury. Arch Phys Med Rehabil 1982; 63:549–552.
23. Sideranko S, Quinn A, Burns K, Froman RD. Effects of position and mattress overlay on sacral and heel pressures in a clinical population. Res Nurs Health 1992; 15:245–251.

24. Barbenel JC, Jordan MM, Nicol SM, Clark MO. Incidence of pressure-sores in the Greater Glasgow Health Board area. Lancet 1977; ii:548–550.
25. Gebhardt K, Bliss MR. Preventing pressure sores in orthopaedic patients—is prolonged chair nursing detrimental? J Tissue Viability 1994; 4:51–54.
26. Defloor T, Grypdonck MHF. Sitting posture and prevention of pressure ulcers. Appl Nurs Res 1999; 12:136–142.
27. Park CA. Activity positioning and ischial tuberosity pressure: a pilot study. Am J Occup Ther 1992; 46:904–909.
28. Koo TK, Mak AF, Lee YL. Posture effect on seating interface biomechanics: comparison between two seating cushions. Arch Phys Med Rehabil 1996; 77:40–47.
29. Gilsdorf P, Patterson R, Fisher S. Thirty-minute continuous sitting force measurements with different support surfaces in the spinal cord injured and able-bodied. J Rehabil Res Dev 1991; 28: 33–38.

9 Skin Care

Sue Bale, Janice Cameron, and Sylvie Meaume

Introduction

The skin is the largest organ in the body and it is essential that clinicians involved in pressure area care are cognizant of the need to maintain or improve its condition. Healthy, normal skin is the first and best line of defense against the invasion of microorganisms, chemicals, and trauma. The skin is constantly exposed to potential irritants and chemicals, any of which may cause damage.[1] In addition, mechanical forces, allergy, inflammation, systemic disease, and burns also impair skin integrity, producing a range of responses. These include erosion, pressure ulceration and ulceration, erythema, papules, and vesicles.[2]

With regard to pressure ulcer prevention and management of the older person, skin care is a particular challenge, as people live for longer and are continually raising their expectations of healthcare. In addition, the developed world is experiencing increased numbers of older people within their populations. Davies[3] reports that despite differing welfare systems country policies for older people are broadly consistent in their targets. The aims of such policies are to maintain older people in their chosen environment, whilst promoting autonomy and a meaningful life.[4–6] Nolan[7] describes global initiatives that aim to prevent or delay ill health, where nurses are encouraged to be proactive in improving the health of older people, especially in the community setting.

In the UK an Audit Commission review[8] recommended that increased attention be paid to the problems of incontinence in patients cared for in the community. Incontinence has been identified as a factor that precedes skin damage and it would seem appropriate that preventing and managing incontinence should be an important aim of nursing care. As people become older, protection of the skin against the effects of incontinence is of particular importance, and as recommended by Le Lievre,[9] the development of cost-effective, evidenced-based management strategies should be a priority.

Normal Skin

Originating from the embryonic ectoderm and mesoderm, the skin is the largest organ in the human body, making up approximately 16% of total body weight (about 9 kg) and covering a surface area of $1.8 \, m^2$.[10] The skin has four main functions: protection, sensation, vitamin D manufacture, and thermal regulation.

Additional functions include acting as an energy and water reserve, excreting urea and salts in sweating.

Protection

The skin provides protection against loss of water and electrolytes, chemical and mechanical assaults, bacterial and pathogenic invasion, and ultraviolet radiation. In essence, the skin maintains a homeostatic environment and acts as a barrier.

Sensation

This is part of the body's ability to protect itself from the surrounding environment. Normal skin is sensitive to pain, touch, temperature, and pressure, through its network of nerve endings or receptors. When stimulated these receptors transmit impulses or signals to the cerebral cortex where they are interpreted.

Manufacture of Vitamin D

Vitamin D is synthesized in the presence of daylight. Epidermal cells synthesize 7-dehydrocholesterol, converting it to cholecalciferol or vitamin D when exposed to ultraviolet rays.[10]

Thermal Regulation

In health normal core body temperature is around 37°C. The skin controls this optimum temperature by the two mechanisms of sweating and blood circulation. When the body is too warm vasodilation occurs, which draws blood to the surface of the skin so cooling it down. In addition, sweat coats the skin's surface and as it evaporates, also cools the skin. When too cold vasoconstriction of blood vessels redirects heat to the body core and internal organs so preserving heat. At the same time shivering results from the arrector pili muscles attached to hair follicles contracting. This has the effect of causing the hairs to stand erect so preserving heat by forming an insular layer of air between the hair and skin.

The epidermis and the dermis are the two layers of which the skin is comprised. Supporting these main layers is a layer of subcutaneous fat as insulation and protection from physical forces, although some parts of the body including the heels, elbows, and shins do not have this protective fatty layer.

The Epidermis

The epidermis is the avascular, outer layer of the skin nourished by the diffusion of nutrients, and is thickest on the soles of the feet and palms of the hands.[11] Starting from the outside it comprises six layers:

- Horny layer—stratum corneum. The horny outer layer consisting of cells that are dead and desquamating. These cells are thin and flat and keratinized.

- Clear cell layer—stratum lucidum. The translucent layer, just below the stratum corneum and only present where the skin is thickened. The cells comprising this layer contain large amounts of keratin, and this layer is commonly found where trauma and friction are evident, leading to the development of calluses and corns.
- Granular layer—stratum granulosum. The precursor of keratin, keratohyalin a granular substance is found in this layer. Keratohyalin gradually replaces the cytoplasm of the cells in this layer.
- Prickle cell layer—stratum spinosum The cells that comprise this layer are characterized by the fine cusps or processes that resemble prickles. These hold the cells together and protect against the physical forces of shear and friction.
- Basal layer—stratum basale. The layer joins the dermis and contains cells that are rapidly dividing. Over a period of 21 to 28 days these cells migrate up to the outer layer of the epidermis.
- The epidermal/dermal junction. Here there is an undulation of dips and peaks, the rete malpighii pegs that help to give strength to the skin, protecting from physical forces such as shear and friction.

The Dermis

This vascular layer is derived from the embryonic mesoderm and is approximately 0.5 to 3 mm in thickness. Well supplied by blood vessels and nerves, it contains hair follicles, blood capillaries, sebaceous glands, and sweat glands. These structures are contained by a matrix of collagen and elastin and form support for underlying structures. Between 40 and 80% of total body water is held in the dermis.[10] The dermis includes the following structures and cells:

- Ground substance. The gel-like material in which connective tissue cells and fibers are embedded. It provides an emergency water store.
- Tissue mast cells. These cells are closely approximated to hair follicles and blood vessels, producing heparin and histamine, as part of tissue repair when injury to the skin occurs.
- Tissue macrophages. These cells are able to engulf and digest foreign bodies such as debris and bacteria and are especially active when tissues are injured. Macrophages also play a key role in regulating the healing process.
- Collagen fibers. Collagen is the major structural protein and is secreted by dermal fibroblasts as tropocollagen. Normal human dermis mainly consists of type I collagen, a fiber-forming collagen. Type I collagen accounts for between 77 and 85% of collagen.[12] Collagen is the protein that gives skin its tensile strength.
- Elastin fibers. Another dermal protein that provides skin with its elastic recoil properties. Elastin prevents skin from being permanently misshapen and these fibers form spirals or coils that allow for distraction and return to normal configuration. It contains high amounts of proline and glycine, though it accounts for less than 2% of the skin's dry weight.[12]
- Lymph vessels. Drain excess fluid and plasma proteins from the dermis[10] and connect with the body's lymphatic system.

- Nerve endings. Sensory or afferent nerves that carry information about the outside world to the brain and spinal cord, and continually monitor the environment of individuals. The sensory nerves convey the sensations of heat, cold, touch, and pain. Specialized sensory receptors are found in the dermis (and also in the basal layer of the epidermis).
- Sweat glands—sudoriferous glands. Spiral structures composed of epithelial tissue that emerge from the dermis or subcutaneous tissue, opening by a duct onto the surface of the skin. They secrete a mixture of water, sodium chloride, and small amounts of urea, lactic acid, and potassium ions. In extreme temperatures as much as 3.5 kg of body weight can be lost in a day.
- Sebaceous glands. There are thousands of these minute holocrine glands on the skin that secrete an oily, colorless, odorless fluid, sebum, through the hair follicles. Sebum is a moisturizing substance that forms a waterproof covering.

How Age Damages Skin

Aging is a normal process where humans gradually experience a degeneration of body tissues and functions. In old age the epidermis and dermis of skin gradually becomes thinner and the underlying structural support, collagen, is reported by Hunter[13] to diminish at a rate of 1% per annum.

Thinning and Loss of Elasticity

It is estimated that the paper-thin appearance of the skin in older people is due to a 20% reduction in dermal skin thickness compared to youth.[1] In the normal aging process, the epidermal junctions become flattened and dermal papillae and epidermal rete ridges or pegs are destroyed, rendering the skin vulnerable to physical damage as the epidermal layers can more easily separate from each other.[1] Skin also loses elasticity as the fibroblasts responsible for elastin and collagen synthesis decline in number, elastic fibers thicken, and the ability for elastic recoil is lost, so causing creases and wrinkles.

Reduction of Fatty Layers and Drying

At the same time the amount of subcutaneous or adipose fat lessens, so providing less of a cushion for underlying bone. This occurs primarily in areas such as the face, shins, hands, and feet. Additionally, natural moisture from sebum secretion reduces in old age, as these sweat glands become smaller, leading to increased dryness of the skin. Overall, the aging process adversely affects skin quality causing dry, thin, inelastic skin that is susceptible to damage. Potential sources of skin damage include pressure, friction, and shear, either individually or in combination. In addition, damp skin caused by exposure to excessive moisture is more vulnerable to shearing forces and at risk from loss of barrier function. Incontinence in old age renders the skin vulnerable to damage when excess or caustic moisture from urine, stool, or frequent washing reduces skin tolerance.

prevent disease, but this is not the case for patients who are experiencing incontinence. Alkaline soap reduces the thickness and number of the layers of cells in the stratum corneum and emulsifies and removes the protective lipid coating of the skin.[12] She reports that it takes 45 minutes to restore normal skin pH following washing with soap, and that prolonged exposure may need 19 hours. In addition, washing macerated, excoriated skin with soap and water will lead to dryness of the skin from a decrease in skin surface lipids.

The Evidence that Supports the Use of Specialized Skin-Care Products

Skin care of the incontinent patient consists of a regimen of skin cleansing and skin protection with a barrier preparation. Lutz and White[32] report the benefits of using specialized skin moisturizers when caring for patients with incontinence as it relieves dryness and protects against excessive moisture and irritants. These researchers report that specialized skin protectants provided better protection against washing than other protectants. Other research has demonstrated the effectiveness of implementing skin-care protocols for patients with incontinence. Lewis-Byers et al.[33] report the results of a small randomized controlled trial in which it was found that the use of soap and water together with a moisturizer was less effective and more time-consuming than using a no-rinse cleanser and a durable barrier cream. Bale et al.[30] report similar results in a study that explored the benefits of implementing a new skin-care protocol that included the introduction of specialized skin-care products. These researchers report a statistically significant reduction in the incidence of incontinence dermatitis and grade 1 pressure ulcers in combination with significant savings in staff time and product costs.

Elements of Skin Care

The US Agency for Health Care Policy and Research (ACHPR) guidelines for managing patients with urinary incontinence[28] recommend that: skin is inspected regularly, gently cleansed with a mild cleansing agent immediately after soiling, absorptive pads are used, and topical barriers are used to protect the skin from moisture.

- Skin inspections. Skin condition should be assessed regularly. For the older person with incontinence this may be daily or more frequently.
- Assess level of continence and treat incontinence appropriately. This may involve adapting patients' physical environment to include providing clothing that can be easily removed, physiotherapy, improving access to toilets, providing walking aids and assistance to access toilets, regular toileting or provision of commode, and regular cleansing and changing of soiled incontinence aids.
- Skin care. The aim here is to keep the skin clean, dry, and well moisturized to maintain the best barrier possible against skin damage. The use of specialized, pH-balanced skin cleansers, the avoidance of damaging soaps, and protecting skin with skin barriers appropriate to individual patient needs are important elements.

How Excessive Wound Exudate Damages Skin

Wound fluid has a beneficial role to play in wound repair in a normal healing acute wound. It has been shown that in the normal healing process high levels of enzyme activity, responsible for clearing the debris from the wound, decrease as the wound heals. However, research studies suggest that exudate from chronic ulceration appears to have a damaging effect on normal wound healing due to continued raised levels of tissue destructive enzymes.[34–36]

Normal skin barrier function has been shown to be compromised in peri-wound skin compared to normal skin.[37] Excessive exudate can damage the vulnerable peri-wound skin through enzymatic activity and by causing physical damage to the structure of skin. Cutting and White[38] argue that when patients have existing pressure ulcers, the exudate that drains can cause skin damage by irritating the surrounding skin. In chronic wounds, proteases (present in the exudate), particularly matrix metalloproteases, are thought to actively damage healthy skin through their enzymatic action.[36]

Excessive wound exudate can cause physical damage to the structure of the skin. Cutting[20] describes how the stratum corneum initially absorbs fluid, causing swelling. Further saturation reduces barrier function, leading to skin breakdown. As with urinary incontinence the peri-wound skin can become macerated from prolonged contact with the wound exudate.

Protection of the Peri-Wound Skin from Wound Exudate

The aim of exudate management is to achieve an optimal moisture balance within the wound environment and prevent damage to the surrounding skin. Dressing choice and peri-wound protection plays a large part in patient comfort. It is important to understand how the different dressings handle moisture and thus their suitability for the wound and the expected wear time. Dressings with adhesive borders should be avoided on patients with edematous tissue, fragile skin, wet skin, or where there is localized inflammation present around the wound.

Prolonged exposure to wound exudate on previously healthy skin may result in maceration and further loss of epithelium (Figure 9.2—see color section). The macerated skin may appear white, thickened, and hard. The use of a suitable skin protectant applied to the peri-wound skin will prevent skin damage from wound exudate and reduce the risk of further loss of epithelium. Where maceration and inflammation are present, the skin will appear erythematous and may be moist or weeping.[39] The patient may complain of burning, stinging, and itching of the affected area. Treatment of erythematous maceration may require the application of a topical corticosteroid preparation to reduce the local inflammation prior to the use of a barrier preparation. Creams are easier to apply to wet skin than ointments. A potent topical steroid should be used for 1 to 2 days only and gradually reduced over the next few days. A barrier preparation can then be applied to the peri-wound area as a skin protectant. Various skin barrier preparations are available including ointments, creams, and a barrier film that leaves a protective film on the skin surface. The barrier film comes as a spray and also in an impregnated foam on a stick. It can be applied to vulnerable skin under adhesive dressings to aid adhesion and prevent trauma on removal.

References

1. Baranoski S, Ayello EA (eds) Wound care essentials. Springhouse, PA: Lippincott, Williams & Wilkins; 2004.
2. Bryant R. Skin pathology and types of damage. In: Bryant RA (ed) Acute and chronic wounds: Nursing management. St Louis: Mosby; 2000.
3. Davies B. The reform of community and long-term care of elderly persons: an international perspective. In: Scharf T, Wenger GC (eds) International perspectives on community care for older people. Aldershot: Avebury; 1995.
4. International Association of Gerontology. Adelaide Declaration on Aging. Australas J Aging 1998; 17(1):3–4.
5. Department of Health. Modernizing social services: Promoting independence, improving protection, reviewing standards. London: The Stationery Office; 1998.
6. Hanford L, Easterbrook L, Stevenson J. Rehabilitation for older people: The emerging policy agenda. London: King's Fund; 1999.
7. Nolan J. Improving the health of older people: what do we do? Br J Nurs 2001; 10(8):524–528.
8. Audit Commission. First assessment: A review of district nursing services in England and Wales. London: Audit Commission; 1999.
9. Le Lievre S. The management and prevention of incontinence dermatitis. Br J Nurs 2001; 6:(4)180–185.
10. Docherty C, Hodgson R. Skin disorders. In: Alexander MF, Fawcett JN, Runciman PJ (eds) Nursing practice: Hospital and home, the adult. Edinburgh: Churchill Livingstone; 2000.
11. Bale S, Harding KG. Chronic wounds 3: Pressure ulcers. In: Bale S, Harding K, Leaper D (eds) An introduction to wounds. London: Emap Healthcare; 2000.
12. Wysocki AB. Anatomy and physiology of skin and soft tissue. In: Bryant RA (ed) Acute and chronic wounds: Nursing management. St Louis: Mosby; 2000.
13. Hunter JAA. Clinical dermatology, 2nd edn. Oxford: Blackwell Science; 1995.
14. Swaffield J. Continence. In: Alexander MF, Fawcett JN, Runciman PJ (eds) Nursing practice: Hospital and home, the adult. Edinburgh: Churchill Livingstone; 2000.
15. Haggar V. Strong developments. Nurs Times 2000; 91:33.
16. Willis J. Outreach for prevention. Nurs Times 1996; 92.
17. Royal College of Physicians. Incontinence: causes, management and provision. A report from the Royal College of Physicians. London: RCP; 1995.
18. Donald I, Cope B, Roberts S. Nursing care and care homes—a census view. J Community Nurs 2002; 16(8):14–15.
19. Johanson JF, Lafferty J. Epidemiology of faecal incontinence. The silent affliction. Am J Gastroenterol 1996; 91(1):33–36.
20. Cutting KF. The causes and prevention of maceration of the skin. J Wound Care 1999; 8(4): 200–201.
21. Hampton S, Collins F. SuperSkin: the management of skin susceptible to breakdown. Br J Nurs 2001; 10(11):742–746.
22. Fiers SA. Breaking the cycle: the etiology of incontinence dermatitis and evaluating and using skin care products. Ostomy/Wound Manage 1996; 2(3):33–43.
23. Leyden JJ, Katz S, Stewart R, Klingman AM. Urinary ammonia and ammonia producing microorganisms in infants with and without diaper dermatitis. Arch Dermatol 1997; 113(12):1678–1680.
24. Berg RW. Aetiology and pathophysiology of diaper dermatitis. Adv Dermatol 1986; 3:75–98.
25. Kemp MG. Protecting the skin from moisture and associated irritants. J Gerontol Nurs 1994; 20(9):8–14.
26. Andersen PH, Bucher AP, Saeed I, et al. Faecal enzymes: in vivo human skin irritant. Contact Dermatitis 1994; 30:152–158.
27. Cameron J, Powell S. Contact dermatitis: its importance in leg ulcer patients. Wound Manage 1992; 2(3):12–13.
28. Agency for Health Care Policy and Research. Urinary incontinence in adults: Acute and chronic management. Clinical Practice Guideline Number 2 (1996 Update). AHCPR Publication No. 96–0682: March 1996.
29. Gfatter R, Hackl P, Braun F. Effects of soap and detergents on skin surface pH, stratum corneum hydration and fat content in animals. Dermatology 1997; 195:258–262.
30. Bale S, Tebble N, Jones VJ, Price PE. The benefits of introducing a new Cavilon skin care protocol in patients cared for in nursing homes. J Tissue Viability 2004; 15:3.

31. Kirsner RS, Froelich CW. Soaps and detergents: understanding their composition and effect. Ostomy Wound Manage 1998; 44 (3A Suppl):62S–69S.
32. Janning B, Lutz JB. Measuring skin barrier washing-off resistance. Proceedings of the 7th European Conference on Advances in Wound Management 1997 London. EMAP Healthcare Ltd.
33. Lewis-Byers K, Thayer D, Kahl A. An evaluation of two incontinence skin care protocols in a long-term care setting. Ostomy Wound Management 2000; 48:1244–51.
34. Drinkwater SL, Smith A, Sawyer BM, Barnard KG. Effect of venous ulcer exudates on angiogenesis in vitro. Br J Surg 2002; 89(6):709–713.
35. Wysocki AB, Staiano-Coico L, Grinnell F. Wound fluid from chronic leg ulcers contains elevated levels of metalloproteinases MMP-2 and MMP-9. J Invest Dermatol 1993; 101:64–68.
36. Trengrove N, Langton SR, Stacey MC. Biochemical analysis of wound fluid from non-healing and healing chronic leg ulcers. Wound Repair Regen 1996; 4:234–239.
37. Bishop SM, Walker M, Rogers AA, Chen WYJ. Importance of moisture balance at the wound-dressing interface. J Wound Care 2003; 12(4):125–128.
38. Cutting KF, White RJ. Maceration of the skin and wound bed 1: its nature and causes. J Wound Care 2002; 11(7):275–278.
39. Newton H, Cameron J. Skin care in wound management. A clinical education in wound management booklet. Medical Communications UK; 2004.

Additional Reading

Bergstrom N, Bennett MA, Carlson CE, et al. Treatment of pressure ulcers. Clinical practice guideline, No. 15. Rockville MD: US Department of Health and Human Services. Public Health Service, Agency for Health Care Policy and Research. AHCPR Publication No 95–0652. December, 1994.
Jeter KF, Lutz JB. Skin care in the frail, elderly, dependent, incontinent patient. Adv Wound Care 1996; 9(1):29–34.
Korting HC, Kober M, Mueller et al. Influence of repeated washings with soap and synthetic detergents on PM and resident flora on the skin of forehead and forearm. Acta Derm Venereol 1987; 67:41–47.
Rottman WL, Grove G, Lutz JB, et al. Scientific basis of protecting peri-wound skin. Proceedings 3rd European Conference in Advances in Wound Management. London: Macmillan; 1994: 38–40.

10 Pressure Ulcers and Nutrition: A New European Guideline

Joseph Schols, Michael Clark, Giuseppe Benati, Pam Jackson, Meike Engfer, Gero Langer, Bernadette Kerry, and Denis Colin

Introduction

Given that the occurrence of pressure ulcers is increasingly viewed as one indicator of the quality of care delivered to patients, the development, dissemination, and implementation of appropriate guidelines and policies covering aspects of pressure ulcer prevention and treatment have been of growing interest across all healthcare sectors.[1] Despite this focused attention upon pressure ulceration these wounds remain common, with almost 20% of hospital inpatients exhibiting some form of pressure-induced damage.[2] The development of pressure ulcers is admittedly complex, depending upon a wide variety of extrinsic and intrinsic risk factors. Extrinsic risk factors such as mechanical loads on the skin and soft tissues have been frequently discussed in the literature[3] while intrinsic factors have recently been explored in a number of studies that have used logistic regression techniques to identify independent risk factors[4-7] with the following factors associated with the presence of pressure ulcers—age, sex, limitation in activity, need for assistance with the activities of daily living, bowel and/or bladder incontinence, elevated Braden scale score, anemia, infection, and nutritional status. However, the relative influence and importance of each of these factors remains unclear.

Interventions to correct many of the intrinsic risk factors are difficult. However, nutritional status is a factor that can be readily influenced by patients, their carers, and health professionals. Previous studies have indicated that poor nutritional status, a low body weight, and poor oral food intake are all independent risk factors for pressure ulcer development.[8-15] However, the exact causal relationships between nutrition and pressure ulceration remain unclear while there is also confusion regarding the precise role of various macronutrients and micronutrients in pressure ulcer prevention and healing.[10,11] Regardless of this uncertainty it is widely assumed that an adequate nutritional intake may help protect vulnerable patients from developing pressure ulcers.[16,17] Moreover, intake of oral supplements or tube feeding with a high content of protein may also improve the rate of wound healing.[18] More recently, a positive effect on wound healing was found following protein and energy supplementation, together with the use of arginine, trace elements, and vitamins with antioxidant effects.[19]

Such assumptions need to be treated with some caution for they are based on relatively small studies, typically heterogeneous with regard to type of participants and intervention.[20]

Regardless of the ambiguous nature of the evidence base implicating poor nutrition and pressure ulcers, the majority of healthcare professionals regard malnutrition as one of the main causal factors contributing to pressure ulcer development and delayed healing.[21] However, despite this conviction not only do most patients receive only limited nutritional attention; but even where this is given intervention is often started too late.[22] Perhaps one reason for the lack of intervention, or its delay, might be the relative lack of focus on nutrition within current clinical practice guidelines devoted to pressure ulcer prevention and management. A recent study on the treatment of nutrition within pressure ulcer guidelines developed across 13 countries identified a wide variation in their content related to nutrition and pressure ulcers.[23] If nutrition was mentioned at all, then the majority of guidelines focused on the need to prevent malnutrition, but were rather unspecific regarding how this was to be achieved. Most guidelines did not cover the full nutritional cycle from nutritional assessment, through nutritional intervention, to evaluation and follow-up of nutritional status; and it was also surprising how seldom referral to a dietician was recommended. Furthermore, most of the reviewed guidelines paid little attention to the possibility of providing either nutritional supplements or tube feeding, which is surprising because, in practice, many patients with pressure ulcers or at elevated vulnerability may have difficulty in obtaining sufficient nutrients entirely from their normal food intake.

In 2002 the European Pressure Ulcer Advisory Panel (EPUAP) formed a working group to develop specific clinical guidance on the role of nutrition in pressure ulcer prevention and management. This project was initially led by Professor Gerry Bennett who sadly died in 2003. The entire working group would like to pay tribute to Gerry for his enthusiasm for and support of this EPUAP initiative. The objective of the guideline development group was to prepare a clinical guideline that elaborated upon the comments about nutrition and pressure ulcers within the EPUAP's existing guidelines on pressure ulcer prevention (1998) and treatment (1999). This chapter describes the process of constructing the guideline, its content stressing the importance of nutritional assessment and intervention, and subsequent actions to enhance the practical implementation of the guideline.

Guideline Development Process

A multidisciplinary working group, with relevant healthcare professionals from six different countries, was established by Professor Bennett and subsequently facilitated by Dr Clark. This working group met in Amsterdam to agree their objectives, after which all contact was by email and telephone. Previous literature that linked nutrition and pressure ulcers was identified through a search of Medline with hand-searching of relevant conference proceedings; this identified over 400 publications. The abstracts were circulated to the working group and key papers identified for further review. In addition, the conclusions of, and studies reviewed within, a recent Cochrane Review on nutrition and pressure ulcer prevention and management were reviewed.[20]

Several drafts of the guideline were discussed within the working group with an advanced draft presented to delegates who attended the annual conference of the EPUAP held in Tampere, Finland in September 2003. Concurrently the draft was published within the *EPUAP Review*. Both the presentation and publication generated comments which were used to guide the final version of the text. The final text was published in the *EPUAP Review* early in 2003[24] and the full guideline was launched at the 2nd World Union of Wound Healing Societies Conference held in Paris in July 2004; at the time of the launch the guideline had been translated into eight languages.

The Guideline

The essentials of the guideline are summarized below. To assist the implementation of this new guideline additional work has been undertaken to draw out the essential elements of the guideline within a decision tree to aid practitioner decision-making (Figure 10.1). The view of the EPUAP is that all people vulnerable to developing pressure ulcers or with established ulcers should undergo nutritional screening and that this screening should take place within the context of all other appropriate interventions and assessments relevant for the overall management of pressure ulceration. Where the nutritional screening (which may include the outcome from a validated nutritional assessment tool) indicates that the individual may be malnourished then a comprehensive nutritional assessment should be performed by a dietician or member of a local nutritional team. Where patients are not considered to be vulnerable to malnutrition at the initial screening they should be monitored regularly, to identify any change in nutritional behavior. Where assessment of nutritional status indicates that malnutrition may be present, nutritional interventions need to be initiated, taking into account patient choice and the expected outcome of treatment. Nutritional intervention should be implemented in combination with all other appropriate interventions including load management.

The primary goal of nutritional intervention is to correct protein-energy malnutrition, ideally through oral feeding. If enhanced oral feeding is not possible, protein-energy rich oral supplements should be considered[14,15,17,19,25] and in those cases where both normal feeding and oral supplementation fail to resolve apparent malnutrition then tube feeding may be undertaken although the potential risks associated with this intervention should be considered.

Where patients already have established pressure ulcers their nutritional demands may be greater. There are a number of observational studies which suggest that protein and calorie supplementation, along with the use of arginine, vitamins and trace elements with antioxidant effects, have a positive effect on pressure ulcer healing.[14,15,17,19,25]

The nutritional plan of care, as well as the criteria for monitoring its success should be clear to the patient, caregivers, and to the healthcare professionals regardless of the care setting.[26] How is success to be monitored? The outcomes of any nutritional intervention should be reviewed within ongoing regular nutritional assessments and may be indicated by such outcome criteria as increased weight, improved functional ability, and/or enhanced health-related quality of life. Successful nutritional intervention may also be measured by a reduced incidence and/or the improved healing of established pressure ulcers, although the direct attribution of these changes in the status of pressure ulcers to the nutritional intervention alone may be problematic given the concurrent deployment of other interventions such as load management.

Where the nutritional interventions fail to meet the goals set with the patient, further diagnostic tests may be required and/or the level of nutritional

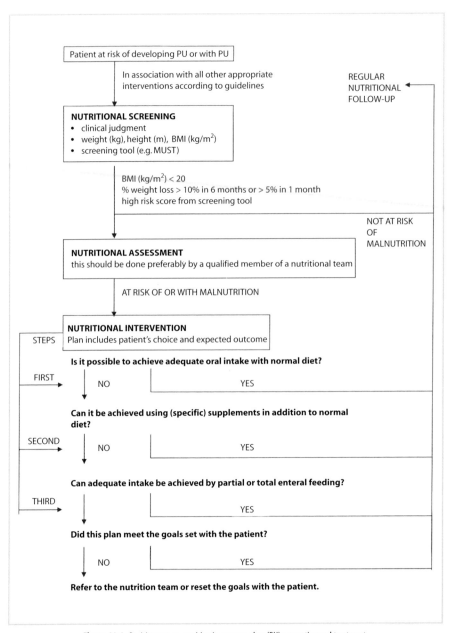

Figure 10.1 Decision tree on nutrition in pressure ulcer (PU) prevention and treatment.

intervention may need to be increased. In these cases the goals of the interventions may need to be reset with the patient.

Discussion

The nutritional guideline presented in this chapter extends the existing EPUAP guidelines on pressure ulcer prevention and treatment. The purpose of the guideline is to provide clinicians with specific guidance on nutritional screening, assessment, appropriate nutritional intervention, and follow-up within the context of pressure ulcer prevention and treatment.

The EPUAP believes that the new guideline is generally appropriate across all healthcare settings although logistical issues may prevent full compliance with all aspects of the guideline (for example access to weighing scales and dieticians may be limited). EPUAP recognizes that other clinical guidelines on nutrition exist and that the specific guidance EPUAP offers on nutrition and pressure ulcers should be considered within the context of general guidelines on nutritional management.[24] Moreover, it is also clear that the evidence base that underpins nutritional support in pressure ulcer prevention and management must be strengthened and that this process will lead to greater understanding of the relationship between one important intrinsic risk factor and pressure ulceration and so ultimately strengthen this new guideline.

Having produced a guideline there is no guarantee that its recommendations will be implemented—EPUAP now needs to consider how best all those involved in pressure area care can be made aware of such issues as the performance of nutritional screening and assessment, the preparation, presentation and delivery of attractive and appetizing meals, and the use of appropriate nutritional supplements or tube feeding, if required. Such education and training will be an important step towards establishing a nutritional culture within all care settings.

Acknowledgments

This guideline and the subsequent development of the decision tree were made possible by an unrestricted educational grant from Nutricia. The full text of the guideline can be downloaded from www.epuap.org

References

1. Clark M. Barriers to the implementation of clinical guidelines. J Tissue Viability 2003; 13(2):62–68.
2. Clark M, Defloor T, Bours G. A pilot study of the prevalence of pressure ulcers in European hospitals. In: Clark M (ed) Pressure ulcers; Recent advances in tissue viability. Salisbury: Quay Books; 2004: 8–22.
3. Bouten CV, Oomens CW, Baaijens FP, Bader DL. The etiology of pressure ulcers: skin deep or muscle bound? Arch Phys Med Rehabil 2003; 84(4):616–619.
4. Bours GJ, De Laat E, Halfens RJ, Lubbers M. Prevalence, risk factors and prevention of pressure ulcers in Dutch intensive care units. Results of a cross-sectional survey. Intensive Care Med 2001; 27(10):1599–1605.
5. Bergquist S, Frantz R. Pressure ulcers in community-based older adults receiving home health care. Prevalence, incidence and associated risk factors. Adv Wound Care 1999; 12(7):339–351.
6. Breslow R. Nutritional status and dietary intake of patients with pressure ulcers: review of research literature 1943–1989. Decubitus 1991; 4(1):16–21.

7.   Guenter P, Malyszek R, Bliss DZ, et al. Survey of nutritional status in newly hospitalized patients with stage III or stage IV pressure ulcers. Adv Skin Wound Care 2000; 13(4 Pt 1):164–168.

8.   Ek AC, Unosson M, Larsson J, et al. The development and healing of pressure ulcers related to the nutritional state. Clin Nutr 1991; 10:245–250.

9.   Green CJ. Existence, causes and consequences of disease-related malnutrition in the hospital and the community and clinical and financial benefits of nutritional intervention. Clin Nutr 1999; 18(Suppl 2):3–28.

10. Pinchcofsky-Devin GD, Kaminski MV. Correlation of pressure sores and nutritional status. J Am Geriatr Soc 1986; 34:435–440.

11. Thomas DR. The role of nutrition in prevention and healing of pressure ulcers. Clin Geriatr Med 1997; 13:497–511.

12. Berlowitz DR, Wilking SVB. Risk factors for pressure sores. A comparison of cross-sectional and cohort-derived data. J Am Geriatr Soc 1989; 37:1043–1050.

13. Green SM, Winterberg H, Franks PJ, et al. Nutritional intake in community patients with pressure ulcers. J Wound Care 1999; 8:325–330.

14. Delmi M, Rapin CH, Bengoa JM, et al. Dietary supplementation in elderly patients with fractured neck of the femur. A randomised controlled trial. Lancet 1990; 335:1013–1016.

15. Bourdel-Marchasson I, Barateau M, Rondeau V, et al. A multicenter trial of the effects of oral nutritional supplementation in critically ill older inpatients. Nutrition 2000; 16:1–5.

16. Allman RM, Walker JM, Hart MK, et al. Air-fluidized beds or conventional therapy for pressure sores. A randomized trial. Ann Intern Med 1987; 107:641–648.

17. Chernoff RS, Milton KY, Lipschitz DA. The effect of a high protein formula (Replete) on decubitus ulcer healing in long-term tube fed institutionalized patients. J Am Diet Assoc 1990; 90:A130.

18. Breslow RA, Halfrisch J, Goldberg AP. Malnutrition in tube fed nursing home patients with pressure sores. J Parenter Enteral Nutr 1992; 15:663–668.

19. Benati G, Delvecchio S, Cilla D, Pedone V. Impact on pressure ulcer healing of an arginine-enriched nutritional solution in patients with severe cognitive impairment. Arch Gerontol Geriatr 2001; 33 (Suppl 7):43–47.

20. Langer G, Schloemer G, Knerr A, et al. Nutritional interventions for preventing and treating pressure ulcers (Cochrane Review). In: The Cochrane Library, Issue 4, 2003. Chichester, UK: John Wiley; 2003.

21. Schols JMGA, Kleijer CN. Nutrition in nursing home patients with pressure ulcers; knowing is not yet doing. Tijdschr Verpleeghuisgeneeskd 2000; 24(1):9–12. (Dutch).

22. Kerstetter JE, Holthausen BA, Fitz PA. Malnutrition in the institutionalized older adult. J Am Diet Assoc 1992; 92:1109–1116.

23. Schols JMGA, de Jager-van den Ende MA. Nutritional intervention in pressure ulcer guidelines; an inventory. Nutrition 2004; 20(6):548–553.

24. Clark M (on behalf of EPUAP guideline group on nutrition). Guideline on nutrition in pressure ulcer prevention and treatment. EPUAP Review 2003; 5(3):80–82.

25. Breslow RA, Hallfrisch J, Guy DG, et al. The importance of dietary protein in healing pressure ulcers. J Am Geriatr Soc 1993; 41(4):357–362.

26. Stratton RJ, Green CJ, Elia M. Disease-related malnutrition: an evidence-based approach to treatment. Wallingford, UK: CAB International; 2003.

11 Clinical and Instrumental Assessment of Pressure Ulcers

Diego Mastronicola and Marco Romanelli

Clinical and instrumental wound assessment are essential elements in acute and chronic wound management. The main objectives of wound assessment are the identification of a proper plan of care, the quantification and monitoring of the effectiveness of several treatment modalities in an objective and reproducible way, and accurate prediction of wound healing rate. The parameters that have been included as part of general wound assessment are not only qualitative but also quantitative; they include measurements such as length, width, depth, area, volume, healing rate, as well as other wound aspects such as assessment of location, appearance of the wound bed, evaluation of wound edges, amount and type of exudates, wound odor, and monitoring of surrounding skin.

Over the past decade there has been increasing interest in the use of non-invasive assessment tools in the field of wound healing, thanks to the increasing number of measurement techniques available. The evaluation of normal wound healing processes has until now mainly been based on clinical observation.

Today non-invasive measurement techniques are able to define the stages of lesions and their evolution. The results of instrumental measurement are more sensitive, objective, reproducible, and comparable than clinical evaluation on its own. These non-invasive wound evaluations, in real time, allow significant differentiation between mild, moderate, and severe levels of tissue damage.

Clinical Assessment

The management of chronic wounds such as pressure ulcers requires an overall assessment of the general health status of the patient, together with a focus on the wound history and its characteristics. The assessment should start from a baseline recording of location, size, depth, and condition of the wound bed. These clinically assessed parameters represent a picture of the wound and serve as an evaluation tool for healing. Anatomical location is important for the definition of the healing potential of the wound and must always be recorded in the patient file.

Another essential aspect of clinical assessment is the determination of the nature of tissue involvement. In the case of pressure ulcers, a four-stage classification is used to evaluate the extent of tissue damage.

Stage 1 pressure ulcers appear as a defined area of persistent redness, which does not disappear after finger compression. Stage 2 is a superficial ulcer and clinically presents as an abrasion, blister (Figure 11.1—see color section), or shallow crater involving epidermis, dermis, or both. A stage 3 pressure ulcer presents clinically as a deeper crater involving damage or necrosis of subcutaneous tissue, with or without undermining of surrounding tissue. Stage 4 pressure ulcer involves extensive destruction of muscle, bone, joint capsule, or tendon.[1]

The amount, color, odor, and consistency of exudate should be assessed in order to exclude the presence of infection or edema. Exudate may be serous or sanguineous, reflecting a normal inflammatory process or damage to blood vessels. The presence of purulent exudate accompanied by foul odor may suggest the onset of bacterial contamination and proliferation, with progression to clinical infection.[2] Assessment of wound odor is important in the evaluation of wound parameters, being related to certain microbial species frequently found in pressure ulcers. Changes in wound condition may be suspected if there are changes in the amount and quality of odor. Contamination of the wound with specific organisms (such as *Pseudomonas aeruginosa*) or anaerobes can be detected by their characteristic odor.[3]

The amount of viable or nonviable tissue should be recorded; this procedure is commonly made by assessing the color of the wound base as a percentage of black, yellow, and red (Figure 11.2—see color section). A black wound bed reflects the presence of necrotic tissue or eschar due to local alteration of tissue perfusion or ischemia. The clinical appearance of necrotic tissue, such as color, consistency, and adherence, should be noted in order to determine the quantity and type of tissue devitalized. A yellowness in the wound bed indicates the presence of slough or fibrinous tissue. A red wound bed indicates the presence of granulation tissue, but attention must be paid to appearance and shade of red: dark red may indicate infection, while pale red with spontaneous bleeding could be a sign of ischemia or infection. Areas of hypergranulation tissue may reflect an excess of moisture in the wound bed[4] and also a malignant degeneration of the tissue into epithelial cancer, such as basal cell or squamous cell carcinoma.[5]

The presence of undermining tissue is common in pressure ulcers, reflecting a necrosis of the subcutaneous fat tissue; it is directly correlated to the severity of destruction. A careful evaluation of the location and extent of sinus tracts or undermining must be performed in full-thickness wounds that are complicated by shear forces, such as pressure ulcer.[6] A simple cotton-tipped applicator may be useful in assessing the undermining of wound edges or for documentation of the extent of sinus tracts.

Assessment of the surrounding skin and wound edges may be a source of additional information for the diagnosis and treatment of the wound. The edge should be assessed for the presence of new epithelial tissue, while surrounding skin may be characterized by the occurrence of discoloration, maceration, erythema, paleness, or erosion. Palpation of the skin may indicate the presence of an indurated area such as in lipodermatosclerosis or in stage 1 pressure ulcers.

Maceration of the wound margin may suggest an excess of exudates, possibly due to an inadequate choice of dressing or uncontrolled edema, or may be an early sign of local infection. Pressure ulcers are commonly colonized by multiple organisms even in the absence of clinical signs of infection.[7] If infection is clinically suspected, the significance of quantitative laboratory tests must be critically evaluated and drug susceptibility tests must be considered, according to the clinician's experience and the evidence from the literature.[8]

The final outcome of infected pressure ulcers depends on the balance between factors that promote further complications and those that lead to their resolution.[9] The host defense mechanisms are particularly relevant in infected pressure ulcers, because in these cases patients are generally critically ill and have already received several courses of antibiotic therapy, in addition to wound management. Because there are four different stages in pressure ulcers, according to the EPUAP scoring system,[10] it is essential to further differentiate the level of infection into superficial and deep tissue, considering also that systemic involvement may be reached after rapid progression. Superficial infection mainly affects stage 2 pressure ulcers and is characterized by the classic signs and symptoms of infection: delayed healing, change in color of the wound bed, abnormal odor, increased exudate and pain, and friable granulation tissue. In this case the use of topical antiseptics has been found to be of great benefit in controlling the bacterial burden, while at the same time avoiding systemic complications.[11] Deep infection is a frequent complication of stage 3 and stage 4 pressure ulcers and is characterized by an increase in warmth, tenderness, and pain. There may also be extended erythema, reaching to the bone, and new areas of breakdown. Osteomyelitis is a common complication in infected pressure ulcers, with *Staphylococcus aureus* the cause of approximately 60% of all cases. The diagnosis of osteomyelitis is obtained by blood culture and bone biopsy; a prolonged parenteral therapeutic regimen of 4 to 6 weeks is often required.[12]

Wound Area and Volume

Many characteristics of the wound are one-dimensional parameters. These include diameter, width, length, and circumference and can be measured by ruler devices; this procedure may, however, be problematic in terms of recognition of the wound edge or in the exact definition of perimeter in irregularly shaped wounds. Another commonly used parameter, especially for stage 3 and 4 pressure ulcers, is depth. Measurement of wound depth is done with a ruler or cotton-tipped applicator, which is inserted into the wound and marked at the deepest level. Inaccuracy in this procedure may arise if the wound bed is not uniform, and the level of inaccuracy particularly increases when measurement is performed by different people. These methods are, however, convenient, inexpensive, and very easy to perform.[13]

The area of the wound is a two-dimensional parameter and represents the best measure of wound size. Techniques include the use of rulers, acetate tracing plus manual square counting using a metric grid,[14] photogrammetry,[15] stereophotogrammetry or stereophotography,[16] image-processing methods, or the computerized planimetry of wound tracing (Figure 11.3—see color section), which is considered the gold standard.

The most popular and cost-effective indirect measurement method for wound area is sheet tracing. This method provides an inexpensive and convenient graphic reproduction of the wound shape. Furthermore, with this technique it is also possible to compare and quantify wound perimeter and area of the same lesion over time,[17] although some errors may arise in the tracing procedure itself due to problems in boundary recognition.

Another popular and inexpensive method is the electronic or computerized planimetry device, which replaces time-consuming manual counting. Digital photography and computerized planimetry techniques are very accurate and useful methods for the inspection and measurement of wound surface. Many of the photographic techniques are non-contact, non-invasive methods. They eliminate the risk of contamination of the lesion or damage to wound bed and/or surrounding skin; however, they involve expensive equipment and require proper training.

Some of these techniques can be used for wound area measurement together with color analysis.[18]

Other instruments measure wound area or volume using two digital cameras to create a three-dimensional image.[14] Pressure ulcers has also been assessed using a combined technique with full-scale photography plus transparency tracings to measure wound area.[19]

The wound volume measurement seems to be more satisfactory than two-dimensional measurement for deeper wounds with wide-scale tissue loss. There are clinical situations such as deep wounds where it is very useful to measure and assess the amount and progress of granulation tissue. Several dental impression materials, such as alginate hydrocolloid compound[20] or normal saline solution,[21] have been used to fill the ulcer and to provide an indirect estimation of tissue loss volume. These methods are very easy to perform and cost-effective, but are also time-consuming, with possible risk of infection and sensitization.

A more accurate non-invasive volume evaluation comes from the utilization of photographic methods with image processing such as structured-light technique, stereophotogrammetry, or stereophotography, but costs must be considered.

Characterization of the shape of small wounds can be achieved by using three-dimensional scanners based on active optical approaches.[22,23] Some of these systems also support the integrated acquisition of the color of the scanned region, and color plays a very important role in the analysis of the status of a skin lesion. The quality of current three-dimensional scanning devices allows accurate geometric and chromatic characterizations of the skin lesion to be achieved.

A new integrated tool has been developed at the University of Pisa to measure and assess the evolution of skin lesions over time. A laser triangulation scanner is used to acquire the wound geometry with high precision and to capture an RGB (red-green-blue) image aligned to the geometry, in order to obtain a color-based characterization of the skin lesion status. The system provides a single and uniform interface with which to manage patient data, to support three-dimensional scanning of the lesion region and to perform different kinds of geo-metric (on the three-dimensional model) and colorimetric (on the RGB image) measurements and relative comparisons. All acquired data (three-dimensional geometries and images), as well as the measures calculated, are stored in a data-base for monitoring the evolution of the skin lesion over time.[24]

Tissue Density

The assessment of tissue density in pressure ulcers is important in obtaining a wound assessment, due to the multiple anatomical structures frequently involved in patients with pressure ulcers. High frequency ultrasound imaging is often used for the assessment of inflammatory reaction and for the measurement of the echostructure, thickness, and water content of the whole dermis; for this, digital image analysis is used. Non-invasive assessment of skin structure with this tech-nique gathers further information for the understanding of fundamental patho-genic factors in wound healing.[25] This method has been shown to be an objective, valid, and reproducible instrument for the assessment of the healing process until scar formation.[26]

Using high resolution 20 MHz B-mode ultrasonography, it is possible to obtain an image of the skin and to identify physiological and pathological skin structures. This method allows the assessment of epidermal atrophy and dermal changes, providing objective quantification and the standardization of such changes.

High frequency ultrasonography, with an ultrasound velocity of about 1580 m/s, has been used for the determination of ultrastructure in chronic ulcers, hypertrophic scars, keloids, and normal surrounding skin.[27] The parameters analyzed were the depth between skin surface and the inner limit of the dermis, and the tissue density. The depth measurement, expressed in mm, can give an estimation of wound and scar thickness. The values of echogenicity are the expression of tissue density and are characterized by high echogenicity of dermis in contrast to a relative hypoechogenicity of the subcutaneous fat. The technique revealed a reduction in chronic ulcer thickness and a relatively equal echogenicity compared to normal skin. A significant increase in hypertrophic tissue thickness and an insignificant difference in echogenicity were also found. Moreover, a significant correlation between echogenicity and the duration of scars has been proven. With this technique it is also possible to make an accurate evaluation and quantification of the amount of granulation tissue, sloughy tissue, and necrotic tissue present, together with measurement of the length and width of the wound.[28]

High frequency ultrasound represents a safe, objective, non-invasive and painless method for the evaluation of the wound healing process, allowing an accurate estimation of re-epithelialization, formation of granulation tissue, and contraction of ulcers.

Tissue Perfusion

Adequate skin blood flow is fundamental to the maintenance of the normal structure and function of the skin. Different layers of local skin microcirculation can be directly detected by laser Doppler flowmetry and laser Doppler perfusion imaging. Laser Doppler techniques are non-invasive medical devices based on the Doppler effect and laser light. The movement of blood cells leads to a scattering of the laser light, inducing a Doppler shift.

Laser Doppler flowmetry is widely used because it is a non-invasive, simple, objective and fast instrumental measurement which quantifies cutaneous blood flow 1–2 mm under the skin surface and provides a continuous or near-continuous record.

The backscattered signal containing data on flux, cell concentration, and cell velocity is displayed on screens and the data may be recorded by a computer.[29]

Capillaries and dermal vessels are usually present at a depth of 1 mm and can be easily evaluated with this technique. In the healing process this measurement is able to monitor perfusion in the wound bed, adjacent normal skin, and scars. It has been shown that blood flow in all types of chronic ulcers is 170% higher than in normal skin and that a potential healing index of less than 100% is not a good prognosis. Blood flow in hypertrophic scars and keloids increases by 180% when compared to normal skin.[30] However, there are some limitations with this technique, such as the necessity for contact with the skin area evaluated, the potential for pain or sepsis when applying the probe to the skin surface, and poor accuracy in the determination of tissue volume.

Laser Doppler imaging combines laser Doppler and scanning techniques and overcomes the above limitations.[31] The instrument is equipped with a moving mirror and light collection system, instead of optical fibers. This technique displays on a computer screen a two-dimensional color-coded image of the local flux, in which each color corresponds to a different level of perfusion. It can therefore be used for evaluating tissue viability and ischemic areas[32] in patients at risk of pressure ulcer development.

With regard to colors, blue-violet is an expression of poor flux, whereas green, yellow, and red correspond to areas with higher flux. Gray areas represent regions where no flux can be detected.

These techniques have been used in the evaluation of wound healing and for definition of ischemia, inflammation, and reperfusion. They could be useful in delimiting areas that need debridement. The advantage of these methods is that they can visualize subclinical reactions through blood flow changes, at a time when clinical assessment cannot detect any modification of blood flow.[33]

Laser Doppler flowmetry is useful in the evaluation of wound healing, microangiopathy in diabetic patients, and burn depth; it has also been used to monitor flaps and replants.[34]

Laser Doppler flowmetry has been used in stage 2 and 3 pressure ulcers for the continuous evaluation of local skin microcirculation and it has been shown that the local blood flow increases at the ulcer edge at rest and after heat stress at 44°C, when compared to surrounding skin.[35]

This non-invasive instrument is not directly applicable to clinical practice, but is reliable in several fields of dermatological research, providing excellent monitoring of cutaneous microcirculation.

Wound pH

pH is defined as the negative logarithm of the activity of hydrogen ions in an aqueous solution, and is used to express the acidity and alkalinity on a scale of 0 to 14.

Normal values of pH in intact skin range from 4.8 to 6.0 due to the presence of the acid mantle, while the interstitial fluid is characterized by neutral values.[36] The acid mantle appears to play a central role as a regulating factor in stratum corneum homeostasis. Alteration in the skin pH seems to play a role in pathogenesis, prevention, and healing in several cutaneous diseases, such as irritant contact dermatitis, atopic dermatitis, ichthyosis, and also in wound healing.

Two major methods are used for measuring cutaneous pH: the colorimetric technique and the glass electrode potentiometric measurement.

The most common pH-measuring instrument, in use since 1972, is a flat glass electrode, which is connected to a meter and applied on the skin, interposing one or two drops of bi-distilled water between the electrode and the skin.[37] The measurement is non-invasive and the electrical current is low, constant and causes no skin damage.

In contrast, the colorimetric procedure with dye pH indicators is less accurate, owing to the interference of several factors. The electrode is attached to the skin for an interval of 10 seconds until stabilization of the reading. Measurements are performed at room temperature below 23°C and relative humidity less than 65%

because sweat can influence the results. Readings should be taken at least 12 hours after the application of detergents or creams to the skin.

A new instrument for pH reading makes use of pH transistor technology, in which the sensor is an ion-sensitive field effect transistor.[38] This non-invasive technique for the measurement of skin surface pH has been used in the past to assess the barrier properties of the stratum corneum and also to evaluate the relationship between changes in superficial skin microflora and the development of skin irritation. In fact, it has already been established that there is a relationship between the acidity of the skin surface and its antimicrobial activity.

There are many reports concerning the relationship between skin pH and the incidence of cutaneous diseases. Glibbery and Mani[39] used a glass electrode for the measurement of skin surface pH on ulcers and control sites, showing an association between acid medium and healing. Wound bed pH has been proven to be of fundamental importance during the healing of chronic wounds, since a prolonged acidification of the wound bed enhances the healing rate of chronic leg ulcers, while the pH of nonhealing chronic venous leg ulcers and pressure ulcers was shown to be alkaline or neutral when compared to normal perilesional skin. The same authors described a significant difference between wound pH in different stages of pressure ulcers with a progressively increasing alkalinity in the more advanced stages.

Conclusion

Wound assessment represents an essential step in wound management. The techniques involved play an important role in correct diagnosis and proper treatment of chronic, invalidating lesions such as pressure ulcers. However, what is required is a uniform, standardized, and well-established approach to wound assessment, so that non-invasive measurements may be used to identify a management strategy, determine proper standards of treatment, and appropriately reassess progress to healing together with specific modifications of intervention.

References

1. National Pressure Ulcer Advisory Panel. National Consensus Conference. Washington, DC: NPUAP: 1998.
2. Ovington LG. Dealing with drainage: the what, why and how of wound exudate. Home Healthcare Nurse 2002; 20:368–374.
3. Van Rijswijk L. Wound assessment and documentation. In: Krasner DL, Rodeheaver GT, Sibbald RG (eds) Chronic wound care: a clinical source book for healthcare professionals, 3rd edn. Wayne, PA: HMP Communications; 2001: 101–115.
4. Flanagan M. A practical framework for wound assessment 2: methods. Br J Nurs 1997; 6:6–11.
5. Harris B, Eaglstein WH, Falanga V. Basal cell carcinoma arising in venous ulcers and mimicking granulation tissue. J Dermatol Surg Oncol 1993; 19:150–152.
6. Bates-Jensen BM. Indices to include in wound healing assessment. Adv Wound Care 1995; 8(4):28.
7. Tammelin A, Lindholm C, Hambraeus A. Chronic ulcers and antibiotic treatment. J Wound Care 1998; 7(9):435–437.
8. Cooper R, Lawrence J. The isolation and identification of bacteria from wounds. J Wound Care 1996; 5(7):335–340.
9. Haalboom JR. Pressure ulcers (Letter). Lancet 1998; 352(9127):581.
10. EPUAP. Guidelines on the treatment of pressure ulcers. EPUAP Review 1999; 2:31–33.

11. Dow G, Browne A, Sibbald RG. Infection in chronic wounds: controversies in diagnosis and treatment. Ostomy/Wound Manage 1999; 45(8):23–40.
12. Darouiche RO, Landon GC, Klima M, et al. Osteomyelitis associated with pressure sores. Arch Intern Med 1994; 154:753–758.
13. Krasner D. Wound measurements: some tools of the trade. Am J Nurs 1992; 92:89–90.
14. Thawer HA, Houghton PE, Woodbury G, et al. A comparison of computer-assisted and manual wound size measurement. Ostomy Wound Manage 2002; 48:46–53.
15. Anthony D, Barnes E. Measuring pressure sores accurately. Nurs Times 1984; 80:33–35.
16. Frantz RA, Johnson DA. Stereophotography and computerized image analysis: a three-dimensional method of measuring wound healing. Wounds 1992; 4:58–64.
17. Thomas AC, Wysocki AB. The healing wound: a comparison of three clinically useful methods of measurement. Decubitus 1990; 3:18–25.
18. Williams C. The Verge Videometer wound measurement package. Br J Nurs 2000; 9:237–239.
19. Lucas C, Classen J, Harrison D, De Haan RJ. Pressure ulcer surface area measurement using instant full-scale photography and transparency tracings. Adv Skin Wound Care 2002; 15:17–23.
20. Resch CS, Kerner E, Robson MC, et al. Pressure sore volume measurement: a technique to document and record wound healing. J Am Geriatr Soc 1988; 36:444–446.
21. Berg W, Traneroth C, Gunnarsson A, Lossing C. A method for measuring pressure sores. Lancet 1990; 335:1445–1446.
22. Chen F, Brown GM, Song M. Overview of three-dimensional shape measurement using optical methods. Optical Engineering 39(10):2000.
23. Bernardini F, Rushmeier HE. The 3D model acquisition pipeline. Computer Graphics Forum 2002; 21:149.
24. Romanelli M, Gaggio G, Collugia M, et al. Technological advances in wound bed measurements. Wounds 2002; 14:58–66.
25. Whiston RJ, Melhuish J, Harding KG. High resolution ultrasound imaging in wound healing. Wounds 1993; 5:116.
26. Katz SM, Frank DH, Leopold GR, Wachtel TL. Objective measurement of hypertrophic burn scar. A preliminary study of tonometry and ultrasonography. Ann Plast Surg 1985; 14:121–127.
27. Van Den Kerckhove E, Staes F, Flour M, et al. Reproducibility of repeated measurements on post-burn scars with Dermascan C. Skin Res Technol 2003; 9:81–84.
28. Dyson M, Moodley S, Verjee L, et al. Wound healing assessment using 20 MHz ultrasound and photography. Skin Res Technol 2003; 9:116–121.
29. Nilsson GE, Tenland T, Oberg PA. Evaluation of a laser Doppler flowmeter for measurement of tissue blood flow, IEEE Trans Biomed Eng 1980; 27:597.
30. Timar-Banu O, Beauregard H, Tousignant J, et al. Development of noninvasive and quantitative methodologies for the assessment of chronic ulcers and scars in humans. Wound Repair Regen 2001; 9:123–132.
31. Wardell K, Jakobsson A, Nilsson GE. Laser Doppler perfusion imaging by dynamic light scattering, IEEE Trans Biomed Eng 1993; 40:309.
32. Gschwandtner ME, Ambrozy E, Schneider B, et al. Laser Doppler imaging and capillary microscopy in ischemic ulcers. Atherosclerosis 1999; 142:225–232.
33. Wahlberg JE. Skin irritancy evaluated by laser Doppler flowmetry. Acta Pharm Nord 1992; 4:126.
34. Olavi A, Kolari PJ, Esa A. Edema and lower leg perfusion in patients with post traumatic dysfunction. Acupunct Electrother Res 1991; 16:11.
35. Gschwandtner ME, Ambrozy E, Fasching S, et al. Microcirculation in venous ulcers and the surrounding skin: findings with capillary microscopy and a laser Doppler imager. Eur J Clin Invest 1999; 29:708–716.
36. Dikstein S, Zlotogorski A. Skin surface hydrogen ion concentration (pH). In: Levegue JL (ed) Cutaneous investigation in health and disease: Noninvasive methods and instrumentation. New York/Basel: Marcel Dekker; 1988: 59–78.
37. Peker J, Wahlbas W. Zur Methodic der pH-Messung der Hautoberflache. Dermatol Wochenschr 1972; 158:572.
38. Von Kaden H, Oelssner W, Kaden A, Schirmer E. Die Bestimmung des pH-Wertes in vivo mit Ionensensitiven Feldeffecttransistoren. Z Med Lab Diagn 1991; 32:114.
39. Glibbery AB, Mani R. pH in leg ulcers. Int J Microcirc Clin Exp 1992; 2:109.

12 Pressure Ulcers and Wound Bed Preparation

Vincent Falanga

Introduction

Over the last several years, considerable progress has been made in the field of wound healing. Clear examples are the cloning and testing of growth factors,[1,2] the evolution of better techniques for growing primary human cells in vitro,[3,4] and the development of sophisticated skin substitutes.[5,6] The process of fibrosis, too, has received great attention, and we now have a better understanding of the mechanisms that might be involved in the downregulation of scarring.[7–10] Undoubtedly, progress in our understanding of the normal wound healing process has been facilitated by increasingly complex ways of evaluating the effect of single genes in vivo, as with the use of transgenic and knockout animal models.[11]

Yet, in spite of these advances in the scientific basis for tissue repair and in the development of new and advanced therapeutic products, the improvement in our care of chronic wounds has not been as dramatic as was initially predicted. There are many reasons for this, but the most important may be our inability to properly correct the fundamental pathophysiological abnormalities present in such chronic wounds as venous, diabetic, and pressure ulcers. Recently, a new paradigm for "preparing" chronic wounds to accelerate their healing and to improve the efficacy of advanced therapeutic products has emerged. This paradigm, termed "wound bed preparation," is becoming widely accepted as a way to manage difficult-to-heal wounds. Here we will discuss the fundamental aspects of wound bed preparation in the context of pressure ulcers.

Pressure Ulcers: Basic Principles

The subject of pressure ulcers has been reviewed from the clinical standpoint in detail elsewhere.[12–19] Here we will focus on the main points as they apply to our discussion about wound bed preparation. Pressure ulcers, also called decubitus ulcers, represent the most common type of chronic wound in the western world. Figures vary as to the frequency of pressure ulcers, but they have been said to occur in up to 10% of patients in the acute care setting. The prevalence of pressure ulcers increases dramatically when patients have major predisposing factors, such as cardiovascular disease, neurological dysfunction, and orthopedic injury. The true prevalence of pressure ulcers in chronic care facilities is unknown, but a figure of approximately 20% is likely.

An important feature of pressure ulcers, one with great clinical implications, is that their apparent surface area does not correlate well with the full extent and severity of the problem. The ulcer area can appear to be quite small, but there may be extensively undermined edges and tunneling to deep structures. The classical explanation proposed for this phenomenon has been that the skin may be more resistant to pressure than subcutaneous tissue and muscle. As a result of this, the shape of the wound in pressure ulcers resembles a conical defect, with the base of the cone away from the skin. Undermining of the pressure ulcer's edges is important, because this space may provide a protected environment for bacterial overgrowth. The location of the direct pressure is also critical. For example, the amount of pressure registered over bony prominences can be as high as 2000 mmHg.

Ultimately, the actual development of ulceration is due to ischemia from pressure applied to the blood vessels. However, a number of cofactors play a fundamental role in the development, persistence, and recurrence of pressure ulcers. Malnutrition and inability to move, shearing forces, the local environment created by urinary and fecal incontinence are all important in the pathogenesis.

Full understanding of pressure ulcers has to take into account various other factors besides the direct forces of pressure alone. A number of predictors for the development of such ulcers have been proposed. Hypoalbuminemia, bone fractures, and incontinence are stated to be important, but few studies have been done to confirm these as independent predictors.

Impaired Healing and Wound Bed Preparation

It may be preferable to talk about "impaired healing" when addressing chronic wounds, although the tendency has been to use the term "failure to heal."[20] The reality is that, with ulcers due to pressure, healing should occur almost unimpeded once the pressure is removed. We will now discuss some of the pathophysiological components that lead to impaired healing, and then place them in the context of wound bed preparation. Some factors are common to all chronic wounds, while others may be more specific for pressure ulcers. Later, we will describe some of the advanced solutions for healing pressure ulcers and other types of chronic wounds. These advanced therapies rely very heavily on appropriate wound bed preparation.

Bacterial Burden and Biofilms

Colonization with bacterial and, less commonly, fungal organisms is a feature of chronic wounds. Pathophysiological factors leading to sustained bacterial colonization include absent epithelium and thus lack of barrier function, exudate conducive to bacterial growth, and poor blood flow and hypoxia.[21,22] The term "bacterial burden" has become widely used when the describing the level of bacterial colonization. Because of the lack of well-defined human experimental data, questions remain as to what constitutes an unacceptable bacterial burden that interferes with wound closure. There is evidence that, regardless of the type of bacteria present, a level greater than or equal to 10^6 organisms per gram of tissue is associated with serious healing impairment.[23-27] For pressure ulcers, governmental guidelines in the United States indicate that quantitative bacteriology, requiring a wound biopsy, may be needed in the context of continued healing impairment.

The level of bacterial burden may not be the entire story, as the configuration of bacterial growth may play a pathogenic role too. For example, there is now increasing interest in the role bacterial biofilms may play in chronic wounds, both in impaired healing as well as in ulcer recurrence. Biofilms represent bacterial colonies surrounded by a protective coat of polysaccharides; such colonies become more easily resistant to the action of antimicrobials.[28-31] Together with research aimed at a better understanding of the role of biofilms in chronic wounds, there are efforts to address therapeutic approaches, since present therapeutic measures, including antiseptic agents, do not seem to be effective. It might be that surgical debridement is important in the elimination of biofilms.

Growth Factor "Trapping"

The concept that chronic leakage of macromolecules into the wound might impair healing by "trapping" cytokines and growth factors was first developed in the context of venous ulcers, but it has applicability to a variety of chronic wounds. The idea of trapping is that, although the levels of critical cytokines might be adequate or even increased, the polypeptides are bound and unavailable to the healing process.[32] There is indirect evidence for trapping by macromolecules, and there is no question that such pathogenic events would lead to disruption of the critical processes involved in appropriate wound matrix formation and re-epithelialization. Common macromolecules that might be involved in trapping include albumin, fibrinogen, and α-2-macroglobulin.[32,33] The latter is particularly important because it is an established scavenger for growth factors. Fibrinogen can bind to fibronectin, providing a mechanism for the trapping of transforming growth factor-$\beta 1$ (TGF-$\beta 1$). Indeed, there is evidence that TGF-$\beta 1$ may be trapped and bound in the fibrin deposited in chronic wounds.[34]

Wound Fluid and Metalloproteinases

The benefits of maintaining a moist wound environment are well established. Although the notion of preventing wound desiccation is not new, it was Winter in 1962 who first proved that experimental animal wounds re-epithelialize faster when kept moist. This finding is true of human acute wounds as well.[35,36] These and other studies in acute wounds have led to the development of moisture-retentive dressings, of which there are now a very large variety.[37,38] From our perspective of wound bed preparation in pressure ulcers, we need to consider whether moist wound healing is indeed applicable. The problem has been that the best evidence for the use of moist wound healing is in acute wounds, not in chronic wounds. However, it is likely that moist wound healing does help chronic wounds in terms of the formation of granulation tissue, pain control, and debridement. Moreover, fears that moisture-retentive dressings may increase the incidence of infection are unfounded.[39-41]

The mechanisms of action by which moist wound healing contributes favorably to wound bed preparation are still unclear. The proposed mechanisms by which moisture-retentive dressings help wound healing (keeping cytokines within wound, facilitating keratinocyte migration, preventing bacterial contamination, favorable electrical gradients) remain theoretical, especially in chronic wounds. Moreover, while acute wound fluid stimulates the in vitro proliferation of fibroblasts, keratinocytes, and endothelial cells,[42–44] fluid and exudate from chronic wounds appears to have a decidedly adverse effect on cellular proliferation.[45,43] Importantly, chronic wound exudate contains excessive amounts of matrix metalloproteinases (MMPs),[46,47] which can break down wound bed proteins that are essential to keratinocyte migration, such as fibronectin and vitronectin.[48] The data regarding MMPs are mixed and, of course, they are important to the healing process.[49] Interstitial collagenase (MMP-1) is critical for keratinocyte migration.[50] However, other enzymes (MMP-2, MMP-9) may adversely affect healing.[51,52]

The above observations bring to the forefront what is sure to become a much debated issue regarding the role of exudate in chronic wounds. On one hand, the experimental evidence in acute wounds and a large clinical experience suggest that moist wound healing is clearly beneficial. On the other hand, the sheer amount of exudate in chronic wounds, particularly when they are heavily colonized with bacterial organisms and inflamed, suggests that one would not want to keep all of the wound fluid in constant contact with the wound. Therefore, modifications are needed in the way we think of moist wound healing and how much exudate should be tolerated in chronic wounds. One of the central components of wound bed preparation is to avoid excessive wound exudate, which can break down tissue, growth factors, and even bioengineered skin products. That much seems to be clear. However, we are still not certain how much and what type of exudate is tolerable. Present and evolving methods for removing fluid by vacuum-assisted devices may prove useful, but more studies are needed.[53–55]

Impaired Blood Flow and Hypoxia

Ultimately, the pathogenic step leading from pressure to tissue breakdown and necrosis is ischemia, with other contributing factors (malnutrition, bacterial colonization and infection, concomitant medical illnesses) playing an important role in impairing healing. An interesting issue is the role of low oxygen tension in wounds. There is very little question that long-term hypoxia is detrimental to the healing process. For example, and this is most evident with diabetic ulcers, low levels of transcutaneous oxygen tension ($TcPO_2$) correlate with inability to heal.[56–58] However, recent laboratory data suggest a possible role for periods of hypoxia in stimulating wound cells. This is true for fibroblast proliferation, fibroblast clonal growth, and the synthesis of certain growth factors, such as TGF-β, platelet-derived growth factor (PDGF), endothelin, and vascular endothelial growth factor (VEGF).[59–63] One might hypothesize that hypoxia may play an initial stimulatory role in the healing process. It is when the hypoxia is prolonged that healing is impaired.[64]

Phenotypic Alteration of Wound Cells

Wound bed preparation takes us beyond the clinical appearance of the wound. We need to be concerned about the cellular make-up of the wound, and what consequences that might have on impaired healing. Recently, a number of clinical and laboratory observations indicate that chronic wounds, including pressure ulcers, may be stuck in one of the phases of the repair process. Although this seems to be better worked out with pressure ulcers due to diabetic neuropathy, it is likely that similar abnormalities may be present with other types of pressure ulcers.[65] There is mounting evidence that the resident cells of chronic wounds have undergone phenotypic changes that interfere with their response to endogenous and exogenous stimuli. This might affect cellular proliferation, locomotion, and the overall capacity to heal.[66,67] Cellular senescence may also be involved in these pathogenic cellular abnormalities, and this in turn may affect the ability of cells to respond to growth factors.[68–70] Unresponsiveness to the action of TGF-β[71] and PDGF[72] has been found. Also, the signaling mechanisms, which are so critical to the action of cytokines, may be impaired.[73]

Advanced Approaches to Impaired Healing

As we approach impaired healing of pressure ulcers with a more open mind, we find opportunities in existing as well as new approaches. For example, we have now come to realize that surgical debridement may remove not only the necrotic tissue but also the excessive bacterial burden and the "cellular burden" of phenotypically abnormal cells discussed above. The concept of wound bed preparation has become a way to think more globally about chronic wounds.

Wound Bed Preparation: A New Way of Approaching Chronic Wounds

The concept of wound bed preparation is quickly gaining acceptance as a way to think about chronic wounds in a global fashion, relying not only on clinical appearance, but also on possible pathological abnormalities that need to be addressed.[74] This approach, born out of the realization that advanced therapeutic advances would not be effective unless appropriate steps are taken to maximize the status of the wound, promotes the endogenous process of wound healing. When the wound still fails to heal with standard approaches, advanced therapies can be used. Overall, there are both basic and more advanced approaches to wound bed preparation. The more basic aspects of wound bed preparation emphasize the important components we have been discussing, including debridement, decreasing the bacterial burden, and surgical correction of underlying defect when required.[75,76] There are also more advanced approaches, which may include bioengineered skin, growth factors, and other emerging therapeutic modalities, such as the use of gene therapy and stem cells.

Recently, an international advisory panel has proposed the use of the TIME concept to bring together many of the aspects of wound bed preparation. TIME is an acronym for correcting the following: T = inadequate tissue within the wound bed; I = the presence of infection and/or inflammation; M = excessive moisture control; E = lack of epithelialization. This concept can be used to further advance our discussion of what can be done to provide accelerated healing of pressure ulcers.

Growth Factors

In recent years, a number of purified recombinant growth factors have been used to accelerate the healing of impaired wounds, including venous, diabetic, and pressure ulcers. Results have been promising with such growth factors as epidermal growth factor (EGF)[77] and keratinocyte growth factor-2[78] for venous ulcers, fibroblast growth factor (FGF)[79] and platelet-derived growth factor (PDGF)[80,81] for pressure ulcers. However, at this time and based on randomized controlled clinical trials, the only commercially available growth factor in the United States is PDGF.[82–84] Some promising results have been obtained with the treatment of pressure ulcers with nerve growth factor[85,86] and basic fibroblast growth factor.[87] It remains unclear whether sequential treatment with growth factors would be more effective.[87] As mentioned at the beginning of our discussion, the use of topically applied growth factors has not resulted in dramatic outcomes for chronic wounds. Several possible explanations are applicable, including faulty dosage and mode of delivery[87–89] and, very pertinent to our discussion, inadequate preparation of the wound bed.[74] The latter may be a critical reason for the less than exciting response to growth factors. For example, a more aggressive debridement approach worked synergistically with the application of PDGF.[83]

Bioengineered Skin

While growth factors were being developed, the approach of cell and matrix therapy, mainly with the use of bioengineered skin, was being investigated in burns as well as acute and chronic wounds. As a result of numerous clinical trials, several bioengineered skin products or skin equivalents have become available. At first, an exciting development was the use of keratinocyte sheets.[4,90,91] Later, more complex constructs were developed and tested. These constructs may contain living cells, such as fibroblasts or keratinocytes or both,[6,92–94] or matrix material alone with or without other cellular components.[95,96] The results have been quite good for some allogeneic constructs consisting of living cells derived from neonatal foreskin, although the data have been best for venous and diabetic pressure ulcers.[97,98] Again, wound bed preparation has been critical to the success of these products. Bioengineered skin products may also be useful in the treatment of pressure (decubitus) ulcers.[99,100]

The mechanisms of action by which bioengineered skin works remain unknown. It has been stated that the delivery of living cells is associated with the release of growth factors and cytokines.[101,102] The available evidence indicates that the cells from these allogeneic constructs do not remain in chronic wounds.[103]

Gene Therapy

Some of the drawbacks associated with the use of topically applied recombinant growth factors (i.e. protein delivery) could possibly be corrected by the use of gene therapy methods. This often involves either the use of naked plasmid DNA or the introduction of certain growth factor-encoding genes by gene gun or biological vectors, including viruses. Therefore, a number of approaches have evolved. In ex vivo approaches cells may be manipulated before reintroduction into the wound. More direct in vivo techniques, as stated, rely on simple injection or the use of the gene gun.[104-106] This is a very active field of research.[107] It is important to realize that stable transduction may not be necessary, and that transient expression my eventually prove to be adequate and perhaps safer.[105] In addition to experimental animal wounds,[108] gene therapy has been used with promising results in human chronic wounds. This includes the use of naked plasmid DNA for such desperate situations as inoperable arterial insufficiency.[109]

Stem Cell Therapy

Cell therapy is not restricted to the use of bioengineered skin products. Indeed, it may be that the cells making up well-defined skin equivalents are simply too differentiated to greatly stimulate a nonhealing chronic wound. As a result, we are likely to see greater emphasis being placed on the use of stem or progenitor cells. These cells do not need to be embryonal, but may be derived from adult tissue.[110] Although controversy remains about the pluripotential nature (plasticity) of stem cells from different adult organs, the early results appear promising. A recent uncontrolled report suggests that direct application of autologous bone marrow and its cultured cells may accelerate the healing of nonhealing chronic wounds.[111] Since that early report, our group has worked on ways to deliver bone-marrow-derived cells using more effective delivery methods. The use of fibrin, delivered as a spray in which cells are incorporated, appears to be ideal (unpublished, V. Falanga).

Summary

Ultimately, the approach to nonhealing pressure ulcers will require a greater understanding of the clinical factors involved and the pathogenic factors leading to impaired healing. Wound bed preparation, with the TIME concept representing a crystallized form of the approach, offers hope that the endogenous process of wound healing can be accelerated. Moreover, attention to wound bed preparation can lead to greater effectiveness of advanced therapeutic products, including growth factors, gene therapy, bioengineered skin products, and stem cells.

Acknowledgment

Work supported by NIH grants AR42936 and AR46557.

References

1. Harding KG, Morris HL, Patel GK. Science, medicine and the future: healing chronic wounds. BMJ 2002; 324(7330):160–163.

2. Singer AJ, Clark RA. Cutaneous wound healing. N Engl J Med 1999; 341(10):738–746.
3. Navsaria HA, Myers SR, Leigh IM, McKay IA. Culturing skin in vitro for wound therapy. Trends Biotechnol 1995; 13(3):91–100.
4. Leigh IM, Navsaria H, Purkis PE, McKay I. Clinical practice and biological effects of keratinocyte grafting. Ann Acad Med Singapore 1991; 20(4):549–555.
5. Bell E, Ehrlich HP, Buttle DJ, Nakatsuji T. Living tissue formed in vitro and accepted as skin-equivalent tissue of full thickness. Science 1981; 211(4486):1052–1054.
6. Boyce ST. Design principles for composition and performance of cultured skin substitutes. Burns 2001; 27(5):523–533.
7. Longaker MT, Chiu ES, Adzick NS, et al. Studies in fetal wound healing. V. A prolonged presence of hyaluronic acid characterizes fetal wound fluid. Ann Surg 1991; 213(4):292–296.
8. Longaker MT, Whitby DJ, Ferguson MW, et al. Adult skin wounds in the fetal environment heal with scar formation. Ann Surg 1994; 219(1):65–72.
9. Mackool RJ, Gittes GK, Longaker MT. Scarless healing. The fetal wound. Clin Plast Surg 1998; 25(3):357–365.
10. Mast BA, Diegelmann RF, Krummel TM, Cohen IK. Scarless wound healing in the mammalian fetus. Surg Gynecol Obstet 1992; 174(5):441–451.
11. Martin P. Wound healing–aiming for perfect skin regeneration. Science 1997; 276(5309):75–81.
12. Fox GN. Management of pressure ulcers. JAMA 2003; 289(17):2210; author reply.
13. Kanj LF, Wilking SV, Phillips TJ. Pressure ulcers. J Am Acad Dermatol 1998; 38(4):517–536; quiz 537–538.
14. Kaufman JL. Management of pressure ulcers. JAMA 2003; 289(17):2210; author reply.
15. Kumar P, Bhaskara KG, Bharadwaj S. Management of pressure ulcers. Plast Reconstr Surg 2003; 111(7):2480–2481.
16. Nelson EA, Nixon J, Mason S, et al. A nurse-led randomised trial of pressure-relieving support surfaces. Prof Nurse 2003; 18(9):513–516.
17. Phillips L. Cost-effective strategy for managing pressure ulcers in critical care: a prospective, non-randomised, cohort study. J Tissue Viability 2000; 10(3 Suppl):2–6.
18. Sims A, McDonald R. An overview of paediatric pressure care. J Tissue Viability 2003; 13(4):144–146, 1488.
19. Summers JB, Kaminski JM. Management of pressure ulcers. JAMA 2003; 289(17):2210; author reply.
20. Falanga V, Grinnell F, Gilchrest B, et al. Workshop on the pathogenesis of chronic wounds. J Invest Dermatol 1994; 102(1):125–127.
21. Hunt TK, Hopf HW. Wound healing and wound infection. What surgeons and anesthesiologists can do. Surg Clin North Am 1997; 77(3):587–606.
22. Gottrup F. Prevention of surgical-wound infections. N Engl J Med 2000; 342(3):202–204.
23. Supp DM, Wilson-Landy K, Boyce ST. Human dermal microvascular endothelial cells form vascular analogs in cultured skin substitutes after grafting to athymic mice. Faseb J 2002; 16(8):797–804.
24. Robson MC. Wound infection. A failure of wound healing caused by an imbalance of bacteria. Surg Clin North Am 1997; 77(3):637–650.
25. Robson MC, Heggers JP. Bacterial quantification of open wounds. Mil Med 1969; 134(1):19–24.
26. Robson MC, Stenberg BD, Heggers JP. Wound healing alterations caused by infection. Clin Plast Surg 1990; 17(3):485–492.
27. Cooper R, Lawrence JC. Micro-organisms and wounds. J Wound Care 1996; 5(5):233–236.
28. Edwards R, Harding KG. Bacteria and wound healing. Curr Opin Infect Dis 2004; 17(2):91–96.
29. Siroky MB. Pathogenesis of bacteriuria and infection in the spinal cord injured patient. Am J Med 2002; 113(Suppl 1A):67S–79S.
30. Wysocki AB. Evaluating and managing open skin wounds: colonization versus infection. AACN Clin Issues 2002; 13(3):382–397.
31. Zegans ME, Becker HI, Budzik J, O'Toole G. The role of bacterial biofilms in ocular infections. DNA Cell Biol 2002; 21(5–6):415–420.
32. Falanga V, Eaglstein WH. The "trap" hypothesis of venous ulceration. Lancet 1993; 341(8851):1006–1008.
33. Falanga V. Chronic wounds: pathophysiologic and experimental considerations. J Invest Dermatol 1993; 100(5):721–725.
34. Higley HR, Ksander GA, Gerhardt CO, Falanga V. Extravasation of macromolecules and possible trapping of transforming growth factor-beta in venous ulceration. Br J Dermatol 1995; 132(1):79–85.

35. Winter G. Formation of scab and the rate of epithelialization of superficial wounds in the skin of the young domestic pig. Nature 1962; 193:293–294.
36. Hinman CMH. Effect of air exposure and occlusion on experimental human skin wounds. Nature 1963; 200:377–378.
37. Helfman T, Ovington L, Falanga V. Occlusive dressings and wound healing. Clin Dermatol 1994; 12(1):121–127.
38. Ovington LG. Wound care products: how to choose. Adv Skin Wound Care 2001; 14(5):259–264; quiz 265–266.
39. Hutchinson JJ. Infection under occlusion. Ostomy Wound Manage 1994; 40(3):28–30, 32–33.
40. Smith DJ, Jr, Thomson PD, Bolton LL, Hutchinson JJ. Microbiology and healing of the occluded skin-graft donor site. Plast Reconstr Surg 1993; 91(6):1094–1097.
41. Hutchinson JJ, Lawrence JC. Wound infection under occlusive dressings. J Hosp Infect 1991; 17(2):83–94.
42. Katz MH, Alvarez AF, Kirsner RS, et al. Human wound fluid from acute wounds stimulates fibroblast and endothelial cell growth. J Am Acad Dermatol 1991; 25(6 Pt 1):1054–1058.
43. Drinkwater SL, Smith A, Sawyer BM, Burnand KG. Effect of venous ulcer exudates on angiogenesis in vitro. Br J Surg 2002; 89(6):709–713.
44. Schaffer MR, Tantry U, Ahrendt GM, et al. Stimulation of fibroblast proliferation and matrix contraction by wound fluid. Int J Biochem Cell Biol 1997; 29(1):231–239.
45. Bucalo B, Falanga V. Inhibition of cell proliferation by chronic wound fluid. Wound Repair Regen 1993; 1:181–186.
46. Wysocki AB, Staiano-Coico L, Grinnell F. Wound fluid from chronic leg ulcers contains elevated levels of metalloproteinases MMP-2 and MMP-9. J Invest Dermatol 1993; 101(1):64–68.
47. Trengove NJ, Stacey MC, MacAuley S, et al. Analysis of the acute and chronic wound environments: the role of proteases and their inhibitors. Wound Repair Regen 1999; 7(6):442–452.
48. Grinnell F, Ho CH, Wysocki A. Degradation of fibronectin and vitronectin in chronic wound fluid: analysis by cell blotting, immunoblotting, and cell adhesion assays. J Invest Dermatol 1992; 98(4):410–416.
49. Madlener M, Parks WC, Werner S. Matrix metalloproteinases (MMPs) and their physiological inhibitors (TIMPs) are differentially expressed during excisional skin wound repair. Exp Cell Res 1998; 242(1):201–210.
50. Pilcher BK, Dumin JA, Sudbeck BD, et al. The activity of collagenase-1 is required for keratinocyte migration on a type I collagen matrix. J Cell Biol 1997; 137(6):1445–1457.
51. Weckroth M, Vaheri A, Lauharanta J, et al. Matrix metalloproteinases, gelatinase and collagenase, in chronic leg ulcers. J Invest Dermatol 1996; 106(5):1119–1124.
52. Yager DR, Zhang LY, Liang HX, et al. Wound fluids from human pressure ulcers contain elevated matrix metalloproteinase levels and activity compared to surgical wound fluids. J Invest Dermatol 1996; 107(5):743–748.
53. Loree S, Dompmartin A, Penven K, et al. Is vacuum assisted closure a valid technique for debriding chronic leg ulcers? J Wound Care 2004; 13(6):249–252.
54. Eldad A, Tzur T. [Vacuum—a novel method for treating chronic wounds]. Harefuah 2003; 142(12):834–836, 878, 877.
55. Ford CN, Reinhard ER, Yeh D, et al. Interim analysis of a prospective, randomized trial of vacuum-assisted closure versus the healthpoint system in the management of pressure ulcers. Ann Plast Surg 2002; 49(1):55–61; discussion.
56. McMahon JH, Grigg MJ. Predicting healing of lower limb ulcers. Aust N Z J Surg 1995; 65(3):173–176.
57. Fife CE, Buyukcakir C, Otto GH, et al. The predictive value of transcutaneous oxygen tension measurement in diabetic lower extremity ulcers treated with hyperbaric oxygen therapy: a retrospective analysis of 1,144 patients. Wound Repair Regen 2002; 10(4):198–207.
58. Kalani M, Brismar K, Fagrell B, et al. Transcutaneous oxygen tension and toe blood pressure as predictors for outcome of diabetic foot ulcers. Diabetes Care 1999; 22(1):147–151.
59. Kourembanas S, Hannan RL, Faller DV. Oxygen tension regulates the expression of the platelet-derived growth factor-B chain gene in human endothelial cells. J Clin Invest 1990; 86(2):670–674.
60. Kourembanas S, Marsden PA, McQuillan LP, Faller DV. Hypoxia induces endothelin gene expression and secretion in cultured human endothelium. J Clin Invest 1991; 88(3):1054–1057.
61. Kourembanas S. Hypoxia and carbon monoxide in the vasculature. Antioxid Redox Signal 2002; 4(2):291–299.
62. Falanga V, Qian SW, Danielpour D, et al. Hypoxia upregulates the synthesis of TGF-beta 1 by human dermal fibroblasts. J Invest Dermatol 1991; 97(4):634–637.

63. Sheikh AY, Gibson JJ, Rollins MD, et al. Effect of hyperoxia on vascular endothelial growth factor levels in a wound model. Arch Surg 2000; 135(11):1293–1297.

64. Falanga V, Zhou L, Yufit T. Low oxygen tension stimulates collagen synthesis and COL1A1 transcription through the action of TGF-beta1. J Cell Physiol 2002; 191(1):42–50.

65. Loots MA, Lamme EN, Zeegelaar J, et al. Differences in cellular infiltrate and extracellular matrix of chronic diabetic and venous ulcers versus acute wounds. J Invest Dermatol 1998; 111(5): 850–857.

66. Loot MA, Kenter SB, Au FL, et al. Fibroblasts derived from chronic diabetic ulcers differ in their response to stimulation with EGF, IGF-I, bFGF and PDGF-AB compared to controls. Eur J Cell Biol 2002; 81(3):153–160.

67. Loots MA, Lamme EN, Mekkes JR, et al. Cultured fibroblasts from chronic diabetic wounds on the lower extremity (non-insulin-dependent diabetes mellitus) show disturbed proliferation. Arch Dermatol Res 1999; 291(2–3):93–99.

68. Bruce SA, Deamond SF. Longitudinal study of in vivo wound repair and in vitro cellular senescence of dermal fibroblasts. Exp Gerontol 1991; 26(1):17–27.

69. Hehenberger K, Heilborn JD, Brismar K, Hansson A. Inhibited proliferation of fibroblasts derived from chronic diabetic wounds and normal dermal fibroblasts treated with high glucose is associated with increased formation of l-lactate. Wound Repair Regen 1998; 6(2):135–141.

70. Stanley A, Osler T. Senescence and the healing rates of venous ulcers. J Vasc Surg 2001; 33(6): 1206–1211.

71. Hasan A, Murata H, Falabella A, et al. Dermal fibroblasts from venous ulcers are unresponsive to the action of transforming growth factor-beta 1. J Dermatol Sci 1997; 16(1):59–66.

72. Agren MS, Steenfos HH, Dabelsteen S, et al. Proliferation and mitogenic response to PDGF-BB of fibroblasts isolated from chronic venous leg ulcers is ulcer-age dependent. J Invest Dermatol 1999; 112(4):463–469.

73. Kim BC, Kim HT, Park SH, et al. Fibroblasts from chronic wounds show altered TGF-beta-signaling and decreased TGF-beta type II receptor expression. J Cell Physiol 2003; 195(3):331–336.

74. Falanga V. Classifications for wound bed preparation and stimulation of chronic wounds. Wound Repair Regen 2000; 8(5):347–352.

75. Barwell JR, Taylor M, Deacon J, et al. Surgical correction of isolated superficial venous reflux reduces long-term recurrence rate in chronic venous leg ulcers. Eur J Vasc Endovasc Surg 2000; 20(4):363–368.

76. Gloviczki P, Bergan JJ, Menawat SS, et al. Safety, feasibility, and early efficacy of subfascial endoscopic perforator surgery: a preliminary report from the North American registry. J Vasc Surg 1997; 25(1):94–105.

77. Falanga V, Eaglstein WH, Bucalo B, et al. Topical use of human recombinant epidermal growth factor (h-EGF) in venous ulcers. J Dermatol Surg Oncol 1992; 18(7):604–606.

78. Robson MC, Phillips TJ, Falanga V, et al. Randomized trial of topically applied repifermin (recombinant human keratinocyte growth factor-2) to accelerate wound healing in venous ulcers. Wound Repair Regen 2001; 9(5):347–352.

79. Robson MC, Phillips LG, Lawrence WT, et al. The safety and effect of topically applied recombinant basic fibroblast growth factor on the healing of chronic pressure sores. Ann Surg 1992; 216(4):401–406; discussion 406–408.

80. Robson MC, Phillips LG, Thomason A, et al. Platelet-derived growth factor BB for the treatment of chronic pressure ulcers. Lancet 1992; 339(8784):23–25.

81. Pierce GF, Tarpley JE, Allman RM, et al. Tissue repair processes in healing chronic pressure ulcers treated with recombinant platelet-derived growth factor BB. Am J Pathol 1994; 145(6): 1399–1410.

82. Steed DL. Clinical evaluation of recombinant human platelet-derived growth factor for the treatment of lower extremity diabetic ulcers. Diabetic Ulcer Study Group. J Vasc Surg 1995; 21(1):71–78; discussion 79–81.

83. Steed DL, Donohoe D, Webster MW, Lindsley L. Effect of extensive debridement and treatment on the healing of diabetic foot ulcers. Diabetic Ulcer Study Group. J Am Coll Surg 1996; 183(1):61–64.

84. Smiell JM, Wieman TJ, Steed DL, et al. Efficacy and safety of becaplermin (recombinant human platelet-derived growth factor-BB) in patients with nonhealing, lower extremity diabetic ulcers: a combined analysis of four randomized studies. Wound Repair Regen 1999; 7(5):335–346.

85. Landi F, Aloe L, Russo A, et al. Topical treatment of pressure ulcers with nerve growth factor: a randomized clinical trial. Ann Intern Med 2003; 139(8):635–641.

86. Thomas DR. The promise of topical growth factors in healing pressure ulcers. Ann Intern Med 2003; 139(8):694–695.

87. Robson MC, Hill DP, Smith PD, et al. Sequential cytokine therapy for pressure ulcers: clinical and mechanistic response. Ann Surg 2000; 231(4):600–611.
88. Robson MC. Growth factors as wound healing agents. Curr Opin Biotechnol 1991; 2(6):863–867.
89. Cross SE, Roberts MS. Defining a model to predict the distribution of topically applied growth factors and other solutes in excisional full-thickness wounds. J Invest Dermatol 1999; 112(1): 36–41.
90. Gallico GG, 3rd. Biologic skin substitutes. Clin Plast Surg 1990; 17(3):519–526.
91. Phillips TJ, Gilchrest BA. Clinical applications of cultured epithelium. Epithelial Cell Biol 1992; 1(1):39–46.
92. Sabolinski ML, Alvarez O, Auletta M, et al. Cultured skin as a 'smart material' for healing wounds: experience in venous ulcers. Biomaterials 1996; 17(3):311–320.
93. Hansbrough JF, Dore C, Hansbrough WB. Clinical trials of a living dermal tissue replacement placed beneath meshed, split-thickness skin grafts on excised burn wounds. J Burn Care Rehabil 1992; 13(5):519–529.
94. Hansbrough JF, Mozingo DW, Kealey GP, et al. Clinical trials of a biosynthetic temporary skin replacement, Dermagraft-Transitional Covering, compared with cryopreserved human cadaver skin for temporary coverage of excised burn wounds. J Burn Care Rehabil 1997; 18(1 Pt 1):43–51.
95. Margolis DJ, Lewis VL. A literature assessment of the use of miscellaneous topical agents, growth factors, and skin equivalents for the treatment of pressure ulcers. Dermatol Surg 1995; 21(2): 145–148.
96. Phillips TJ. Biologic skin substitutes. J Dermatol Surg Oncol 1993; 19(8):794–800.
97. Gentzkow GD, Iwasaki SD, Hershon KS, et al. Use of dermagraft, a cultured human dermis, to treat diabetic foot ulcers. Diabetes Care 1996; 19(4):350–354.
98. Veves A, Falanga V, Armstrong DG, Sabolinski ML. Graftskin, a human skin equivalent, is effective in the management of noninfected neuropathic diabetic foot ulcers: a prospective randomized multicenter clinical trial. Diabetes Care 2001; 24(2):290–295.
99. Brem H, Lyder C. Protocol for the successful treatment of pressure ulcers. Am J Surg 2004; 188(1A Suppl):9–17.
100. Brem H, Tomic-Canic M, Tarnovskaya A, et al. Healing of elderly patients with diabetic foot ulcers, venous stasis ulcers, and pressure ulcers. Surg Technol Int 2003; 11:161–167.
101. Mansbridge J, Liu K, Patch R, et al. Three-dimensional fibroblast culture implant for the treatment of diabetic foot ulcers: metabolic activity and therapeutic range. Tissue Eng 1998; 4(4): 403–414.
102. Falanga V, Isaacs C, Paquette D, et al. Wounding of bioengineered skin: cellular and molecular aspects after injury. J Invest Dermatol 2002; 119(3):653–660.
103. Phillips TJ, Manzoor J, Rojas A, et al. The longevity of a bilayered skin substitute after application to venous ulcers. Arch Dermatol 2002; 138(8):1079–1081.
104. Slama J DJ, Eriksson E. Gene therapy of wounds. London: Martin Dunitz; 2001.
105. Badiavas EV, Falanga V. Gene therapy. J Dermatol 2001; 28(4):175–192.
106. Eming SA, Medalie DA, Tompkins RG, et al. Genetically modified human keratinocytes overexpressing PDGF-A enhance the performance of a composite skin graft. Hum Gene Ther 1998; 9(4):529–539.
107. Human gene marker/therapy clinical protocols. Hum Gene Ther 1999; 10:2037–2088.
108. Yao F, Eriksson E. Gene therapy in wound repair and regeneration. Wound Repair Regen 2000; 8(6):443–451.
109. Isner JM, Baumgartner I, Rauh G, et al. Treatment of thromboangiitis obliterans (Buerger's disease) by intramuscular gene transfer of vascular endothelial growth factor: preliminary clinical results. J Vasc Surg 1998; 28(6):964–973; discussion 73–75.
110. Quesenberry PJ, Colvin GA, Lambert JF, et al. The new stem cell biology. Trans Am Clin Climatol Assoc 2002; 113:182–206.
111. Badiavas E, Falanga V. Treatment of chronic wounds with bone-marrow derived cells. Arch Dermatol 2003; 139(4):510–516.

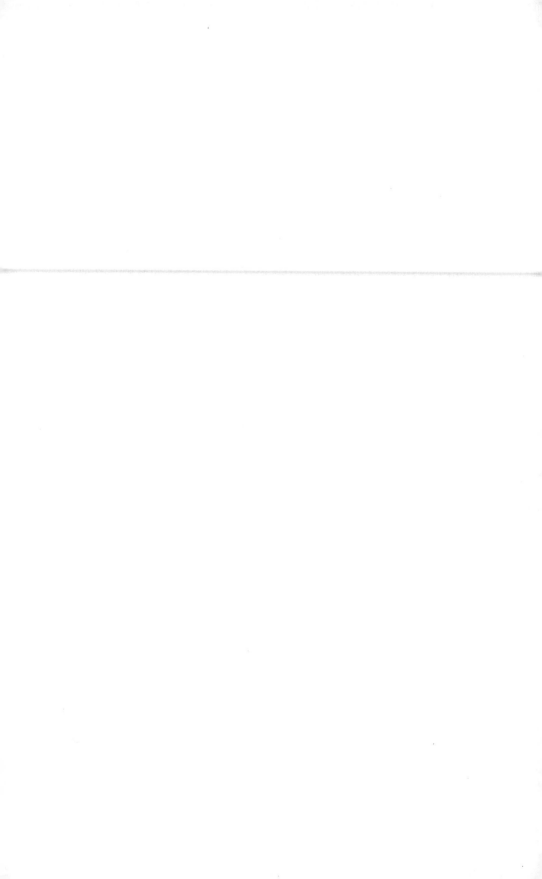

13 Conservative Management of Pressure Ulcers

Elia Ricci, Andrea Cavicchioli, and Marco Romanelli

Dressing a wound means applying local treatment, although it should be remembered that the medication of a wound in itself is only a part of the treatment and will generally help the healing process but not necessarily determine it. The objectives of medication have been established for some time now, especially in terms of microenvironment and bacterial level. There are two main theories of medication: traditional and advanced, as illustrated in Table 13.1.

Choice of Dressing

One of the problems in the choice of dressing is the wide variety of products available on the market. We have divided the dressing products into 12 groups, derived from a previous classification proposed by Ricci and Cassino,[1] with the intention of providing a general guide within the context of this vast choice.

The classification is as follows:

1. *Gauzes*: These may be simple dressings or may be impregnated with various substances (thus becoming primary medications in themselves and splitting up into various categories).

2. *Antiseptics—antibiotics*: The former are substances aimed at reducing the bacterial level and work by damaging the membrane or other cellular structures without inducing resistance. The most widely used are silver, iodine, chlorhexidine, and hypertonic solutions. They may take various forms such as solutions, creams, impregnated gauze dressings, granules, etc. Local antibiotics, long opposed by international literature, are now coming back into fashion with the discovery of products that induce a limited level of resistance and act locally (chloramphenicol, bacitracin, neomycin, etc.).

3. *Adsorbents*: These are dressings aimed at removing the exudate excess from the wound bed and take the form of granules, gel, ionic membranes (which are selective with particular regard to bacteria), alginates, and surgical fibers (which work by means of a gelling process). The latter two types of dressing have some of the typical characteristics of advanced products, but are not insulators or thermally stable. They therefore represent a link between the two categories of traditional and advanced dressings. Recently they have been used as mediums for active ingredients (e.g. silver as an antiseptic).

4. *Proteolytic enzymes*: These are enzymes aimed at breaking down necrotic tissue. They may be derived from bacteria (collagenase), vegetables (papain), or

animals (krill). They are used mainly for cleansing and, given their nature, are deactivated by drying or antiseptics. The stipulated application times should be respected.

5. *Products encouraging granulation*: The action of these products, despite much debate, is not yet fully understood. They are made from collagen or hyaluronic acid and their effect, depending on the formulation, is to provide a frame for vascular development (tablets), to control inflammation (spray, gauze), or to activate cleansing (creams).

6. *Polyurethane films*: These are very fine films of varying permeability, used to dress superficial wounds that are dry or with reduced exudate; alternatively they may be used as a secondary dressing. The permeability is rated according to the MVTR (moist vapor transmission rate), which indicates the transmission of vapor through the film. Conventionally an MVTR below 1000 indicates an occlusive dressing while above 1000 it indicates a semi-occlusive dressing.

7. *Polyurethane foams*: These are made from the same material as the film, but in a three-dimensional form, with micro cells that absorb the discharge while maintaining a moist microenvironment and controlling the excess liquid. Suitable for cleansed wounds with medium discharge, they should be replaced when they become saturated (appearance of the liquid on the surface of the dressing) or start to leak. They are sometimes covered on the outer layer by an impermeable film and can then be used on flat wounds; without such outer covering they may be used as intracavitary dressings. They may be adhesive or non-adhesive.

8. *Hydrocolloids*: These are amorphous colloids in the form of wafer, paste, or granules. They are dressings with reduced permeability and are generally occlusive. They work through absorption of the discharge and transformation of it into a fluid gel. Suitable for cleansed wounds with low to medium discharge, they have a good fibrinolytic influence and cleansing effect in the case of limited necrosis.

9. *Hydrogels*: These can be divided into two forms—fluid and on a base. Fluid hydrogels are used to induce the hydrolysis of necrotic tissue and should be used with a secondary dressing of an advanced type. Hydrogels on patches are occlusive dressings with a low-to-medium absorbency and are suitable for use in encouraging the re-epithelialization of cleansed wounds or wounds with slough.

Table 13.1. Dressing philosophy

Traditional dressing	Antisepsis
	Hemostasis
	Drying the wound
	Covering the wound
Advanced dressing	Moist environment
	Thermal stability
	Isolation from foreign environment
	Control of exudate
	Removal of necrosis and nonviable tissue
	Low cost
	Infection prevention

Table 13.2. Dressings and guidelines for their use, based on clinical examination of the wound

Wound	Dressing
Colonized/infected	Antiseptics
	Local antibiotics
	Ionic adsorbents
	Hypertonic dressings
Necrotic	Lytic enzymes
	Hydrogel
Sloughy	Lytic enzymes
	Hydrogel
	Hydrocolloids
	Hypertonic dressings
Cleansed	Products encouraging granulation
	Polyurethane film and foam
	Hydrocolloids
	Adsorbents

10. *Interactive dressings*: These include the group of biodressings, skin derivatives, metalloprotease inhibitors, engineered tissue, and growth factors. These techniques are for use by specialists only and their use is described in the section on interactive dressings below.

11. *Technical devices*: These are an evolution of dressing/debridement techniques, which combine machine-controlled functions with the action of the dressing. Although only used to a limited extent as yet, they are acquiring greater importance in daily practice. The most widespread product at the moment is the VAC system described in the section on topical negative pressure therapy below.

12. *Non-allopathic dressings*: A wide range of products held to be effective in the treatment of cutaneous lesions, often without clinical studies to support them. Although frequently based on traditions and customs that are centuries old (e.g. aloe, honey), their usage should be postponed until the effects have been scientifically proven.

With regard to guidelines for use, in a text aiming to provide quick consultation we will limit ourselves to giving some general indications. Dressing a wound means choosing the right product for the wound at its specific stage and deciding on the length of application.[2] Generally speaking we can say that the clinical status of the wound and the tissues present determine the choice of product to be used: the quantity of exudate will determine the wear time of the dressing in inverse proportion.[3] Table 13.2 shows the various clinical stages of wounds and the products suitable for dressing them.

Interactive Dressings

The next frontier in the treatment of cutaneous lesions is represented by dressings and products created by means of engineering tissues; these enable those operating in the sector to intervene directly in the healing process (Figures 13.1 and 13.2—see color section). We may say that traditional medication, based mainly on antisepsis, has turned its attention towards the outside environment and its inter-action with the wound. Advanced dressings attempt to create an environment that encourages spontaneous repair.[4] With the progressive gains in scientific knowl-edge, determined in part by increased attention to the problem, and expressed and organized according to the theories of wound bed preparation (WBP) and con-centrating in particular on the identification of corrupt and functionally limited cellular matrices in chronic cutaneous lesions, the need to interact with the healing process directly has become pressing.

We may begin by dividing these products according to method, drafting a classification as shown in Table 13.3.

This is a field that needs further exploration; not all the mechanisms behind the effects have been fully understood and the timing of their use needs to be defined; however, the initial results are promising (Figures 13.3 and 13.4— see color section). The use of single growth factors needs developing, espe-cially considering the specific language involved, which is still far from being understood.

The basic objective (which also requires developing) and the hope for this approach to dressing is to change the wound bed from a chronic to an acute state.

Therapeutic Devices

Pressure ulcers represent a major health problem, causing a considerable amount of suffering for patients and a high financial burden for healthcare systems. The percentage of the population that is geriatric, and therefore with an increased risk of chronic wound development, is rising constantly. Evidence clearly indicates that preventive measures are essential to reduce the prevalence rates of pressure ulcers; therefore healthcare professionals must be able to identify the appropriate strate-gies to adopt, in order to meet the individual patient's requirements.

The past decade has seen a rise in the number of therapeutic options available for the management of acute and chronic wounds. The introduction of advanced medical devices and new concepts of systemic treatment have led to a better under-standing of the mechanism of tissue repair in chronic wounds, which has been supported by the development of standardized guidelines for prevention and treatment.

Topical Negative Pressure Therapy

Wound management with negative pressure represents a non-invasive mechanical wound care treatment, using negative pressure to facilitate wound healing.[5] VAC® (Vacuum Assisted Closure) therapy is used to reduce wound fluid, stimulate granulation tissue formation, and reduce bacterial colonization. Negative pressure wound therapy acts by localized and controlled negative pressure, which is applied in continuous or intermittent cycles.[6,7] The equal distribution of negative pressure to every surface of the wound is ensured by a polyurethane open-cell foam dress-ing. The foam is trimmed to fit the entire surface of the lesion, placed in the wound bed, and sealed with an adhesive drape (Figure 13.5—see color section). Negative pressure is applied via an evacuation tube by means of a computerized,

Table 13.3. Interactive dressings

Group	Action	Name
Surgical		
Surgical procedures	Removal of degraded cells from the wound bed. This is an invasive, painful technique and is expensive.	Debridement
Wet to dry	Progressive removal of the bottom layer of the wound by tearing, using gauzes made to stick to the wound bed. Extremely painful.	Wet to dry
Grafting	Removal of the wound bed until healthy tissue is reached, after which the wound is covered with skin taken from elsewhere on the patient. If the skin takes, immediate healing is achieved; if not, there may in any event be a rapid resumption of the repair process and re-epithelialization.	Grafting
Skin substitutes		
Glycerol skin	This is skin taken from organ donors and treated with glycerol, which makes it non-vital and suitable for preserving. It was originally intended for use as a biological covering for patients with severe burns and has been progressively extended to chronic wounds. It is not clear how it works and a thoroughly cleansed base is required.	Skin bank
Cryopreserved skin	Skin taken from organ donors and preserved by freezing. Used as a biological covering, it may work by releasing growth factors.	Skin bank
Culture-grown skin	After a skin biopsy, the cells are placed on special mediums which make them larger and more concentrated. This is an autograft, which is capable of activating the repair process.	Apligraf®
Heterologous culture-grown skin	Skin substitute derived from the fetal prepuce. This is a heterologous graft that is capable of reactivating repair processes (growth factors?) and of taking in some cases that are not clearly defined as yet.	Dermagraft®
Metalloprotease inhibitors		
Metalloprotease inhibitors	Metalloprotease, elastase and plasmin are enzymes derived from cellular decay, which are capable of halting the healing process when present in large quantities. These products, made from oxidized and regenerated cellulose, appear to be able to deactivate the excess of such enzymes and to bind them.	Promogran®
Growth factors		
Growth factor	Proteins capable of mediating cellular functions through membrane receptors. Produced by a secretory mechanism within the body itself, they are currently being studied and are produced industrially by means of recombinant genes. The principal ones involved in the healing process are: platelet-derived growth factor (PDGF), transforming growth factor beta (TGFβ), TGFα, tumor necrosis factor (TNF), insulin-like growth factor (IGF), interleukin enhancer binding factor (ILF), interleukin-1 (IL-1), IL-2, nerve growth factor (NGF), vascular endothelial growth factor (VEGF), beta fibroblast growth factor (FGF), keratocyte growth factor (KGF).	
Platelet gel	Prepared on the spot from the patient's or donor's serum (from a blood bank) or prepared industrially, these act by releasing large quantities of growth factors, mainly PDGF.	Regranex®
Cultured cell		
Culture-grown fibroblasts	Once a sample of skin has been taken, the fibroblasts are isolated and grown so as to create a sort of "three-dimensional dressing" on a hyaluronic acid base. This is a self-graft of fibroblasts, the cells responsible for healing processes and growth factors.	Hyalograft 3D®
Culture-grown keratinocyte	As with the fibroblasts, a sample of skin is taken and once the keratinocytes have been isolated they are cultivated on a transparent sheet of hyaluronic acid. This is a very delicate product and its established use for treating acute wounds has yet to be discussed for chronic wounds.	Laser Skin® Hyalograft 3D KC®
Other		
Engineered derma	Three-dimensional structure made from cellulose and collagen or hyaluronic acid capable of providing a base mainly for neovascularization, which is considerably increased. It is covered with a coating which must be removed after 1–3 weeks.	Integra® Hyalomatrix®

programmable pump. The target pressure for wound therapies varies from 50 mmHg to 200 mmHg, based on the characteristics of the individual wound. In pressure ulcers, a negative pressure of 125 mmHg is used in a continuous cycle of 48 hours. Negative pressure therapy provides a moist wound healing environment, assists in uniformly drawing the wound border, enhances epithelial migration, reduces bacterial colonization, and reduces localized edema by increasing local blood perfusion and accelerating the rate of granulation tissue formation.[8]

Despite the successful treatment of different wound types, some limitations may occur when attempting to treat certain areas of the body that involve irregular surfaces surrounding the wounds, such as the perineum.[9] VAC® therapy is indicated in acute and traumatic wounds, dehisced incisions, neuropathic ulcers, stage 3 and 4 pressure ulcers, vascular wounds, and chronic debilitating wounds. Split-thickness mesh skin grafts also benefit from VAC® therapy.

Contraindications for negative pressure treatment include cutaneous malignant lesions, untreated osteomyelitis, necrotic tissue within the wound bed and fistula directly communicating with organs and cavities. Caution should be used when there is active bleeding, unstable local hemostasis, use of anticoagulants, or distal diabetic foot lesions.[10] The nutritional status of the patient should be stable and the patient should be continuously monitored by nurses and should be positioned on a support surface so as to redistribute his or her weight over a large area and reduce pressure. An adequate amount of intact peri-wound skin for adherent dressing should be available and the ulcer should be free of necrotic tissue or osteomyelitis.

The dressing is changed every 48h or every 12h if infection is present. The wound bed is cleansed per routine, the sponge is placed in the wound, and the evacuating tube is laid on top of the foam, linked to a collection chamber located on the pump. An adhesive clear dressing is placed over the foam and the tube. Duration of the therapy varies from 4 to 6 weeks, with continuous or intermittent cycles of treatment.[11] Continuous therapy facilitates removal of wound fluids and reduction of edema, while intermittent therapy acts as a mechanical stretch and results in the repeated release of biochemical messengers. Wound measurement, tissue and fluid characterization, odor, and surrounding skin should be monitored at each dressing change.

Negative pressure therapy should be used in pressure ulcers to achieve complete healing or to prepare the wound bed for surgical closure, especially in chronic non-healing wounds of considerable depth, rather than the traditional saline wet-to-moist dressings.

Hydrotherapy

Hydrotherapy is another treatment that is frequently used in many countries, principally in patients with leg ulcers.[12] The patient is immersed in special pools where the water, containing antiseptics, is shaken with artificial movement so as to make the removal of dead tissue easier. Hydrotherapy provides cleansing pressure-irrigation and hydromassage. The cleansing is useful either to remove secretions and bacteria or to soften necrotic wound material. This procedure is generally performed with a saline solution only or with an antiseptic solution or with other types of detergent solutions—used according to wound conditions and dressing compatibility. Pressure-irrigation uses water pressure to remove the necrotic material from the wound surface.[13] However, if the pressure used to deliver irrigation solution is too low (below 4 psi), the lavage will not clean effectively; therefore, pressure irrigation has to be in a range from 4 to 15 psi.

A simpler method uses a 35 ml syringe with a 19-gauge needle producing an 8 psi pressure action, which is able to clean a wound without causing damage to new granulation tissue.

Another method makes use of hydromassage, that is, water pressure jets generated in a whirlpool. In this case the tissue becomes soft in the whirlpool and is removed by the pressure of the jets. The massage reduces edema and inflammation and improves circulation in ischemic legs. A further refinement of this technique consists of immersing the patient for 20–30 minutes after a 30-second treatment at maximum pressure. The sessions are twice-weekly. This method is indicated in very exudative wounds, necrotic wounds, and eschars, but is contraindicated in clean and granulation wounds.

Moreover, there are now special devices available that can direct a high-pressure water jet onto lesions and then, with suction, remove the devitalized tissue before it dissolves. Among such instruments, one that deserves particular attention is a device developed in Switzerland, based on high-pressure microjet technology. The device consists of a liquid pump driven by compressed air, which generates high hydraulic pressure in a liquid directed through a nozzle installed in a hand-piece. The major advantage of this debridement technique is the reduction of the duration of treatment. The aim is to provoke a decisive healing impulse in a stagnant wound. Through the nozzle, Ringer solution, NaCl or aqua ad injectabilia are injected onto the surface of the wound in the form of a very fine jet under precisely controlled pressure. The duration of each intervention depends on the importance and degree of necrosis of the wound and varies from 10 to 30 minutes, usually at weekly intervals. Advanced dressings sustain the treatment. The three major results of this application are: shortening of the wound healing process, reduction of the scar tissue, and low stress effects for the patients, because the treatment is relatively painless. These treatments are contraindicated in patients suffering from anticoagulation, tumors, and unprotected or open blood vessels.

Warming Therapy

Most chronic wounds become hypothermic and hypothermia has been shown to impair the healing process by reducing the normal function of the immune system and promoting wound infection. A recent technology utilizing radiant heat was introduced for the treatment of chronic wounds. This warming treatment is able to maintain 100% relative humidity at the interface between dressing and wound bed and to restore both peri-wound and wound bed temperature toward normothermia. The system is provided with a temperature control unit (TCU), which operates either from an AC outlet or with a rechargeable battery pack for portability. A disposable wound cover made of a polyurethane foam provides a noncontact surface that will not disrupt the wound, will absorb the exudate, and has a transparent window which provides easy viewing for monitoring wound progress. An infrared warming card, which is connected to the TCU, slides into a sleeve in the cover and warms to a temperature of 38°C. Using warming therapy, the skin and subcutaneous tissue are returned to a temperature that is closer to normal. Warming encourages blood vessels to dilate, which increases blood flow to the wound and peri-wound area. Greater blood flow delivers more oxygen, nutrients, and growth factor to the wound. The use of warmth on fibroblasts and endothelial cells in vitro was found to reduce the inhibitory effect of chronic wound fluid upon neonatal fibroblasts.[14] In a recent study the warming therapy was compared to standard treatment in patients with stage 3 to 4 pressure ulcers.[15] Results showed a statistically significant accelerated rate of healing for patients receiving heat therapy compared to standard treatment.

References

1. Ricci E, Cassino R. Piaghe da decubito. Turin: Minerva Medica; 2004.
2. Bennet G, Moody M. Wound care for health care professionals. London: Chapman & Hall; 1995.
3. Dealey C. The care of wounds. Oxford: Blackwell; 1999.
4. Hess CT. Guida clinica alla cura delle lesioni cutanee. Milan: Masson; 1999.
5. Argenta LC, Morykwas MJ. Vacuum-assisted closure: A new method for wound control and treatment: Clinical experience. Ann Plast Surg 1997; 38(6):563–576.
6. Morykwas MJ, Argenta LC, Shelton-Brown EI, McGuirt W. Vacuum-assisted closure: A new method for wound control and treatment: Animal studies and basic foundation. Ann Plast Surg 1997; 38(6):553–562.
7. Deva AK, Buckland GH, Fisher E, et al. Topical negative pressure in wound management. Med J Aust 2000; 173(3):128–131.
8. Baynham SA, Kohlman P, Katner HP. Treating stage IV pressure ulcers with negative pressure therapy: a case report. Ostomy Wound Manage 1999; 45(4):28–32, 34–35.
9. Greer SE, Duthie E, Cartolano B, et al. Techniques for applying subatmospheric pressure to wounds in difficult regions of anatomy. J Wound Ostomy Continence Nurs 1999; 26(5):250–253.
10. Evans D, Land L. Topical negative pressure for treating chronic wounds: a systematic review. Br J Plast Surg 2001; 54:238–242.
11. Joseph E, Hamori CA, Bergman S, et al. A prospective randomized trial of vacuum-assisted closure versus standard therapy of chronic non healing wounds. Wounds 2000; 12(3):60–67.
12. Waspe J. Treating leg ulcers with high pressure irrigation devices. Nurs Stand 1996; 11(6):53–54.
13. Ho C, Burke DT, Kim HJ. Healing with hydrotherapy. Adv Directors Rehabil 1998; 7(5):45–49.
14. Park HY, Shon K, Phillips T. The effect of heat on the inhibitory effects of chronic wound fluid on fibroblasts in vitro. Wounds 1998; 10(6):189–192.
15. Price P, Bale S, Crook H, et al. The effect of a radiant heat dressing on pressure ulcers. J Wound Care 2000; 9(4):201–205.

14 Surgical Management of Pressure Ulcers

Jens Lykke Sørensen, M.J. Lubbers, and Finn Gottrup

Introduction

Most pressure ulcers do not need surgical intervention.

Candidates for surgery are a selected group of patients where debridement and conservative measures are not enough to ensure healing of a sufficient quality or speed, and where the patients will benefit from surgical intervention. In general, these patients will have grade 3 and 4 pressure ulcers.

The cornerstones of successful surgical treatment of pressure ulcers are a competent staff, correct selection of patients, correct and meticulous surgical method, and sufficient postoperative support.

No unambiguous criteria for selection of patients or methods exist, and an individual assessment is a necessity. However, guidelines are a useful tool, particularly at the initial assessment.[1–3]

The Staff

The surgeon is a link in a chain. Success in pressure ulcer treatment is dependent on a well-educated and committed multidisciplinary staff.[4]

Preceding surgery is a period of observation of the patient, either on an outpatient basis or as an inpatient, to evaluate the optimal treatment. During hospitalization the nursing staff are the most important group, since they can observe and cooperate with the patient around the clock.

Concomitant diseases must be controlled by relevant specialists preoperatively, as should the dietary intake, and pressure relief is secured as soon as possible.

Postoperatively the patient must be helped to follow restrictions to ensure total pressure relief of the operated region, and at a later stage the occupational therapist and physiotherapist participate in rehabilitating and mobilizing the patient. The hospital pharmacist is often included early in the team to prepare the discharge of the patient.

Selection of Patients

It is important to look at the whole patient and not only the ulcer. All patients with deep pressure ulcers (grade 3 or 4) should be evaluated for surgical treatment. Pressure ulcer patients, however, tend to have other diseases as well as the pressure ulcer, and this must be taken into account before deciding whether to operate. As mentioned, concurrent diseases must be dealt with preoperatively. The patient's ability to cooperate and to tolerate operation and the postoperative regimes must be evaluated. The patient's activities of daily living should be compatible with postoperative pressure relief and general care, and education of the patient is necessary.

Debilitated patients without the capacity for cooperation or patients expected to make a full recovery might be sufficiently treated by revision alone. Terminal patients are not candidates for reconstructive procedures. Spinal cord injured patients usually are. Special attention must be paid to patients with advanced disseminated sclerosis and other diseases influencing their intellect, since these patients will often have difficulties in cooperating because of the impact of the disease on their behavior.

In patients likely to make a total recovery, such as some multitrauma patients, even large pressure ulcers may eventually heal and these could be left for spontaneous healing. However, other factors such as time and the restrictions caused by the pressure ulcer can be an indication for surgery.

Surgical Methods

The initial step in surgical treatment of pressure ulcer is always a thorough debridement including removal of not only necrotic tissue but also inferior, scarified tissue, extra-osseous calcifications, and infected bone. This is dealt with in Chapter 15. Denuded bone should always be smoothed out to create an even pressure-distributing surface beneath the soft tissue used in the reconstruction.[2]

When the pressure ulcer cavity is clean and vital, the decision is whether to leave the cavity to a time-consuming spontaneous healing or to perform a fast but more or less complicated reconstruction.

Small and superficial pressure ulcers should be left for secondary healing. Correct wound care and sufficient pressure relief are prerequisites for success. Large superficial pressure ulcers should usually be operated on. Small but deep pressure ulcers will often benefit from reconstructive procedures.

One-stage procedures with revision and immediate reconstruction are usually recommended.[1,5,6] A number of reconstructive alternatives exist, and the least demanding method suitable for the purpose should be chosen.

Split-Thickness Skin Grafts

From a surgical point of view split-thickness skin grafting is a simple and fast procedure. Donor sites are abundant in pressure ulcer patients. The recipient site must be clean and well vascularized. The skin graft consists of the epidermis and a fraction of the dermis. Split-thickness skin grafts are harvested with a dermatome adjusted to a thickness of about 0.3–0.4 mm. The graft is meshed to allow fluid to escape since this will hamper healing if it is trapped beneath the graft. The graft sticks to the graft bed, where granulation tissue will turn into scar tissue after healing, covering the area with a thin non-pliable surface making the split skin graft prone to erosion.[7] The graft is covered with a bandage, which allows diffusion of superfluous liquid away from the graft without desiccation. One of the few indications for use of local antibiotics is in the dressing covering the graft to prevent infection. If a tie-over dressing or an ordinary bandage is not suitable, a VAC® (Vacuum Assisted Closure) sponge can secure the graft.[8] The bandage is removed after 2–6 days depending on the method, the risk of complications, and the surgeon's preference. Healing is completed in about 10 days, but the skin graft should not be submitted to mechanical loading for about 3 weeks. The donor site is covered with a bandage for moist healing. After 7–10 days the donor site should be healed and the bandage removed.[9]

Split-thickness skin grafting is indicated for well-granulating, large, shallow ulcers, where future mechanical loading will be limited. The sacral area and the back are the typical locations where split-thickness skin grafting may be indicated.

Full-Thickness Skin Grafts

Full-thickness skin grafts contain all the dermis. This makes the full-thickness graft thicker and more resistant to mechanical wear and tear, but the demand for vascularization of the recipient bed is bigger. When a full-thickness skin graft is considered, a skin flap will often be indicated as well. Full-thickness skin grafts can usually only be harvested when skin is loose enough to allow direct suture of the donor site, since no epithelial elements are left to allow healing from the donor bed. The recipient bed must have a good blood supply, and the graft must be firmly immobilized. Full-thickness skin grafts are not meshed.

Full-thickness skin grafts are indicated for small superficial pressure ulcers with well-granulating, even surfaces on locations where friction is to be expected or cosmetic outcome is to be taken into consideration. Grafting does not alter the character of the skin.[9] The heel, the plantar, and the head can sometimes be treated with a full-thickness skin graft.

Direct Closure

Direct closure is the simplest surgical method for eliminating a defect, but in pressure ulcer surgery it is only exceptionally indicated. If it is indicated, closure is performed in layers over suction drainage. An underlying cavity must be avoided. A pressure ulcer develops when tissue is too scanty. With direct suture even less tissue is available, increasing the risk for recurrence of the pressure ulcer.[5,10]

Skin Flaps

Skin flaps, or cutaneous flaps if no subcutaneous tissue is incorporated in the flap, can literally be raised anywhere on the body. As with other types of flaps, their blood supply can be random, or an axial vessel can be incorporated in the flap. An axial vessel makes the planning more pliable, since the blood supply to the flap is independent of the supply from the base of the flap. Skin flaps are elevated by cutting the skin and subcutaneous tissue to the desired depth according to the drawing on the patients from the preoperative planning. The underside of the flap is cut to its base, the surroundings are mobilized as necessary, the flap is moved to the defect, and the donor site and the flap are sutured in layers. Suction drainage is compulsory.

In pressure ulcer surgery, no tightness of the flaps or the surroundings can be accepted, reducing the availability of these flaps. The donor site must be without scarification or other consequences of being close to a pressure ulcer.

Cutaneous flaps are indicated anywhere where a skin graft is insufficient and a myocutaneous flap is too much. Pressure ulcers of moderate size, not too deep, and without underlying bony disorders or exposure are potential candidates for cutaneous flaps.[2,9,11]

Fasciocutaneous Flaps

Adding an underlying fascia to a skin flap improves the blood supply. The extra padding probably adds little to the pressure-distributing abilities of the flap.

Fasciocutaneous flaps are managed in the same way as skin flaps but with incorporation of the underlying fascia in the flap. The fascia in the donor site can usually not be sutured.

Fasciocutaneous flaps are indicated in reconstruction of pressure ulcer defects without too deep a tissue defect, preferably without a history of osteomyelitis, and without a big demand for pressure distribution in the region.[12,13]

The scrotal flap[9] is a well-known fasciocutaneous flap. This flap is not often used by the authors. The distal part of the tensor fasciae latae flap (the central part is actually a myocutaneous flap) is a more recommendable type of fasciocutaneous flap.[5,9,14]

Myocutaneous Flaps

Myocutaneous flaps are axial flaps. They possess muscle tissue with an excellent blood supply and provide full-thickness skin coverage; a large amount of tissue can be incorporated in the flap to supply it with sufficient bulk to fill even large defects. The excellent blood supply makes these flaps well suited for fighting infection and promoting healing. The intact skin and subcutaneous tissue have the potential for effective pressure and shear distribution, and the bulk adds to the ability to distribute pressure and fill a large defect. These physiological and mechanical properties make myocutaneous flaps the treatment of choice for deep pressure ulcers.[1,10,15]

In general the pressure points on the human body are not padded with muscle. Yet, experiments indicate that muscle tissue beneath pressure-loaded skin is advantageous.[16]

Some muscles are indispensable for normal muscle function, for example gluteus maximus in normal gait. This fact must be considered when the selection of a myocutaneous flap is carried out in an ambulatory patient. In spinal cord injured patients, a group constituting the majority of patients with myocutaneous flap surgery, these considerations are usually irrelevant.

The myocutaneous flap is advanced into the defect by cutting its cutaneous, subcutaneous, and fascial borders according to a drawing from the planning on the patient. The muscles are then freed from their bony connections or tendons, and the areolar tissue around the vessels is loosened enough to mobilize the flap into the defect. Usually the vessels do not need to be totally freed, not with the primary use of the flap, anyhow. The whole mass of tissue is then advanced into the defect, and over suction drainage in both the donor and the recipient site the flap and donor site are sutured in layers. The drains in the pressure ulcer cavity can be left for a couple of weeks, if formation of a cavity beneath the flap is feared.[5]

Myocutaneous flaps are indicated anywhere on the body where deep pressure ulcers are treated for osteomyelitis or optimal pressure-distributing abilities are requested. The pelvic region is the region most often treated with myocutaneous flaps, since many of the pressure ulcers needing a myocutaneous flap are situated here.[5,17]

In the pelvic region the ischial region is most often the site of pressure ulcers. Several flaps are available for the repair.[1,2,9,18–20] The primary choice of the authors is a flap based on the hamstrings (Figure 14.1—see color section). This is a versatile and safe flap, which can be readvanced in case of recurrence[18]—if it is raised in its full length. The muscle content of the flap can be varied, making it usable for both spinal cord injured and ambulatory patients. The gluteus maximus or the tensor fasciae latae are alternative solutions.[2,9]

The sacral pressure ulcer is often treated using a flap based on the gluteus maximus muscle.[5,13,21] Several variations in creating myocutaneous flaps based on the muscle exist, making the flap very versatile.[5,9,21] By splitting the muscle, which has a dual blood supply, ambulatory patients can benefit from this flap too.[9]

A trochanteric pressure ulcer invites the use of a tensor fasciae latae flap, which is just at the edge of the ulcer (Figure 14.2—see color section). The flap is safe, and the muscle is expendable. Often the donor site can be closed primarily; otherwise a split skin graft can be used for the donor defect.[10,14,22,23] Alternatives are the vastus lateralis muscle, the rectus femoris muscle, or the inferiorly based gluteus maximus muscle.[2,5,9]

Flaps Without Skin Coverage

In selected cases—or merely by need—a muscle flap can be indicated. If too much bulk from subcutaneous tissue is to be avoided (not a frequent problem in pressure ulcer surgery!) or if the survival of the cutaneous part of a myocutaneous flap is hampered, a muscle flap can be used to supply bulk and blood supply, and the flap can be covered by a split-thickness skin graft. If possible a myocutaneous flap should be preferred.

In flaps without skin coverage the tissue is isolated and transposed to the recipient site using the same dissection technique as in raising other flaps.

Isolated fascial flaps are hardly ever indicated in pressure ulcer surgery except if they are the only way to get a vital ulcer bed.

Special Types of Flaps or Surgical Procedures

Sensate myocutaneous flaps in some spinal cord injured patients can be elevated to transfer sensate skin to an insensate region with a pressure ulcer.[15,24,25] Recurrence rates might be reduced by making the skin sensitive to pain from pressure and ischemia, but the new sensation might be unpleasant, making the patient move support to an insensitive area, where a new pressure ulcer can develop.[10,24]

Complicated procedures to gain sensitivity in pressure ulcer risk areas exist, but the more simple tensor fasciae latae flap is probably the most popular with a lesion below L3.[15,24]

Free flaps are an option in selected cases of pressure ulcers.[26,27] The procedures are demanding and time-consuming and are infrequently indicated. An example is a free latissimus dorsi myocutaneous flap to a pelvic pressure ulcer. Temporary casting or external fixation of the region might be indicated to avoid lesion of the microvascular anastomosis.

Muscle-sparing perforator flaps are attracting increasing interest in pressure ulcer surgery.[12,28]

Tissue expansion has been used in both skin and other tissue to gain coverage of pressure ulcer defects.[10,29,30] Implantation of foreign material to reinforce tissue covering former or threatening pressure ulcers[31] has not been widely reported. The authors have no experience with the latter two methods.

Multiple or Recurrent Pressure Ulcers

Extensive or multiple pressure ulcers should be treated in as few sessions as possible to reduce time, the use of resources, and, probably, the risk of cross-infection from an untreated to a treated pressure ulcer.[5,17] When reconstruction becomes an option, the extensive ulcers are situated in the pelvic region. A total thigh flap gives good soft tissue covering even for huge pressure ulcers on the ipsilateral pelvis.[5,32] A smaller amount of tissue can be provided by a rectus abdominis myocutaneous flap.[33]

Recurrence is unfortunately a quite common problem in pressure ulcer surgery.[5,15,17,21,34] There is no major difference in treating primary or recurrent pressure ulcers. The same reconstructive methods are used. In the primary planning it is important to design the reconstruction so that the future use of flaps is not hampered. The flaps should, if possible, be designed large enough for reuse in case of recurrence. With an intelligent design it is usually possible to close the donor site without grafting.[5]

Postoperative Care

Postoperatively the pressure ulcer is dealt with, but the risk factors might still be present and will need continuous monitoring. The patient will still need optimal pressure relief, diet, and treatment of concomitant diseases. If this is forgotten, recurrence is almost inevitable.

Postoperative Pressure Ulcer Prevention

Immediately after the operation impairment to the circulation in the region must be avoided, otherwise healing might be hampered. Skin grafts tolerate some pressure. Actually a certain amount of pressure is an advantage to immobilize the graft to the recipient bed and to avoid oozing of liquid beneath the graft. Flaps must not be loaded in the initial postoperative period.

The operated region can be pressure relieved in two ways: The patient can be positioned to totally relieve the region; for example, a reconstruction on the back of the pelvis can be relieved by the prone position. Some patients, such as tetraplegics, may be unable to stay in the prone position, since their respiration might be obstructed. Other complications can also occur as a result of lying in the prone position for long periods.[10] An alternative to positioning the patient is a pressure-relieving mattress. Turning regimes are necessary with some types of mattresses. Loading or straining the flap during the turning must absolutely be avoided. Social isolation of the patient during the postoperative restrictions should also be avoided.[5]

A number of mattresses and special beds are available (see Chapter 7). Air-fluidized beds and some of the low-air-loss beds and mattresses are recommended for relieving flaps.[5,15,35] The recommended period for postoperative pressure relief varies. Usually 2–3 weeks are recommended.[5,10]

After total pressure relief the flap is conditioned to loading[5] In ambulant patients normal behavior can be resumed. In high-risk patients restrictions on loading the risk areas should continue, since the risk factors are permanent. As a general principle, risk areas should not be loaded for more than 2 hours.[10] The authors advocate fixed planes for mobilization and regular postoperative control, naturally with individually based variations.

Postoperative Patient Care

The operation field is observed according to normal surgical procedures. Fluid accumulation, infection, and tissue necrosis are particularly observed for, and intervention should generally be swift.[5]

In the postoperative period the protein and caloric intake should be increased after estimation of need by a dietician.

The operation wound, as well as being protected from load and strain, should be kept clean. Indwelling catheters, fluid or low fiber diet for a few days preceded by preoperative enema and constipating medicine can be used.[10,15] Medication to treat spasm is sometimes necessary.[36]

Physical training for all patients is a prerequisite. Mobilization is performed to a degree compatible with the individual patient's ability. All of the staff are responsible for participating in teaching patients to take responsibility for their own training and pressure sore prevention. Prevention and educational programs are used to help with training and reduce recurrence.[4,10,37,38]

Pressure prevention is modified according to alterations in the patient's condition. If the pressure ulcer risk is permanent, the prevention measures should be permanent.

References

1. Foster RD, Anthony JP, Mathes SJ, Hoffman WY. Ischial pressure sore coverage: a rationale for flap selection. Br J Plast Surg 1997; 50:374–379.
2. Linder RM, Morris D. The surgical management of pressure ulcers: a systematic approach based on staging. Decubitus 1990; 81:32–38.

3. Pressure Ulcer Advisory Panel. Pressure ulcer treatment. Am Fam Physician 1995; 51:1207–1222.
4. Sinclair L, Berwiczonek H, Thurston N, et al. Evaluation of an evidence-based education program for pressure ulcer prevention. J Wound Ostomy Continence Nurs 2004; 31:43–50.
5. Sørensen JL, Jørgensen B, Gottrup F. Wound management: Surgical intervention. In: Morison MJ (eds) The prevention and treatment of pressure ulcers. London: Mosby; 2001: 155–175.
6. Rubayi S, Burnett CC. The efficacy of a single-stage surgical management of multiple pressure sores in spinal cord injured patients. Ann Plast Surg 1999; 42:533–539.
7. Place MJ, Herber SC, Hardesty RA. Basic technique and principles in plastic surgery. In: Aston SJ, Beasley RW, Thorne CNM (eds) Grabb and Smith's Plastic surgery, 4th edn. London: Little, Brown and Company; 1997: 13–26.
8. Genecov DG, Schneider AM, Morykwas MJ, et al. A controlled subatmospheric pressure dressing increases the rate of skin graft donor site reepithelialization. Ann Plast Surg 1998; 40:219–225.
9. Bergström N, Bennett MA, Carlson CE, et al. Treatment of pressure ulcers. Clinical Practice Guideline no. 15. Rockville, MD: US Department of Health and Human Services, Public Health Service, Agency for Health Care Policy and Research; December 1994.
10. Strauch B, Vasconez LO, Hall-Findlay EJ (eds) Grabb's encyclopedia of flaps. London: Little, Brown and Company; 1990: 1529–1800.
11. Mithat Akan I, Sungur N, Ozdemir R, et al. "Pac Man" flap for closure of pressure sores. Ann Plast Surg 2001; 46:421–425.
12. Yu P, Sanger JR, Matloub HS, et al. Anterolateral thigh fasciocutaneous island flap in perineoscrotal reconstruction. Plast Reconstr Surg 2002; 109:610–616.
13. Borman H, Maral T. The gluteus fasciocutaneous rotation-advancement flap with V-Y closure in the management of sacral pressure sores. Plast Reconstr Surg 2002; 109:2325–2329.
14. Dermiseren ME, Gökrem S, Özedemir OM, et al. Hatchet-shaped tensor fascia lata musculocutaneous flap for coverage of trochanteric pressure sores: A new modification. Ann Plast Surg 2003; 51:419–422.
15. Niazi ZBM, Salzberg CA. Surgical treatment of pressure ulcers. Ostomy/Wound Manage 1997; 43: 44–52.
16. Naito M, Ogata K. Vulnerability of the skin circulation without underlying muscle. An experimental study. 33rd Annual Meeting of the ISOP, Kobe, 1994; MT V-1.
17. Schryvers OI, Stranc MF, Nance PW. Surgical treatment of pressure ulcers: 20-years experience. Arch Phys Med Rehabil 2000; 81:1556–1562.
18. Kroll SS, Hamilton S. Multiple and repetitive use of the extended hamstring V-Y myocutaneous flap. Plast Reconstr Surg 1989; 84:296–302.
19. Angrigiani C, Grill D, Siebert J, Thorne C. A new musculocutaneous island flap from the distal thigh for recurrent ischial and perineal pressure sores. Plast Reconstr Surg 1995; 96:935–940.
20. Josvay J, Donath A. Modified hamstring musculocutaneous flap for coverage of ischial pressure sores. Plast Reconstr Surg 1999; 103:1715–1718.
21. Aggrawal A, Sangwan SS, Siwach RC, Batra KM. Gluteus island flap for repair of sacral pressure ulcers. Spinal Cord 1996; 34:346–350.
22. Siddique A, Wiedrich T, Lewis VL. Tensor fascia latae V-Y retroposition myocutaneous flap: clinical experience. Ann Plast Surg 1993; 31:313–317.
23. Ercöen AR, Apaydin I, Emiroglu M, et al. Island V-Y tensor fasciae latae fasciocutaneous flap for coverage of trochanteric pressure sores. Plast Reconstr Surg 1998; 102:1524–1530.
24. Kuhn BA, Lüscher NJ, de Roche R, et al. The neurosensory musculocutaneous tensor fasciae latae flap: long term results. Paraplegia 1992; 30:396–400.
25. Thomson HG, Azhar AM, Healy H. The recurrent neurotrophic buttock ulcer in the myelomeningocele paraplegic: a sensate flap solution. Plast Reconstr Surg 2001; 108:1192–1196.
26. Park S, Koh KS. Superior gluteal vessel as a recipient for free flap reconstruction of lumbosacral defects. Plast Reconstr Surg 1998; 101:1842–1849.
27. Hung SJ, Chen HC, Wei FC. Free flap for reconstruction of the lower back and sacral area. Microsurgery 2000; 20:72–76.
28. Blondeel PN, Van Landuyt K, Hamdi M, Monstrey SJ. Soft tissue reconstruction with the superior gluteal artery perforator flap. Clin Plast Surg 2003; 30:371–382.
29. Espositio GE, Ziccardi P, Di Caprio G, Scuderi N. Reconstruction of ischial pressure ulcers by skin expansion. Scand J Plast Reconstr Surg 1993; 27:133–136.
30. Gray BC, Salzberg CA, Petro JA, Salisbury RE. The expanded myocutaneous flap for reconstruction of the difficult pressure sore. Decubitus 1990; 3:17–20.
31. Minns RM, Sutton RA. Carbon fibre pad insertion as a method of achieving soft tissue augmentation in order to reduce the liability to pressure sore development in the spinal injury patient. Br J Plast Surg 1991; 44:615–618.

32. Peters JW, Johnson GE. Proximal femurectomi for decubitus ulceration in the spinal cord injury patient. Paraplegia 1990; 28:55–61.
33. Kierney PC, Cardenas DD, Engrav LH, et al. Limb-salvage in reconstruction of recalcitrant pressure sores using the inferiorly based rectus abdominis myocutaneous flap. Plast Reconstr Surg 1998; 102:111–116.
34. Evans GRD, Dufresne CR, Manson PN. Surgical correction of pressure ulcers in an urban centre: is it efficacious? Adv Wound Care 1994; 7:40–45.
35. Allen V, Ryan DW, Murray A. Air-fluidized beds and their ability to distribute interface pressures generated between the subject and the bed surface. Physiol Measure 1993; 14:359–364.
36. Mess S-A, Kim S, Davison S, Heckler F. Implantable Baclofen pump adjuvant in treatment of pressure sores. Ann Plast Surg 2003; 51:465–467.
37. US Department of Health and Human Services. Preventing pressure ulcers. A patient's guide. Decubitus 1992; 5:34–40.
38. Maklebust HA, Magnan MA. Approaches to patient and family education for pressure ulcer management. Decubitus 1988; 5:18–28.

15 Debridement of Pressure Ulcers

Andrea Bellingeri and Deborah Hofman

Debridement is an accepted principle of good wound care, especially when debris is acting as a focus for infection. (NICE Guidelines, UK, 2001)

Introduction

The term debridement was first used by a French surgeon in the eighteenth century to describe surgical removal of debris from open wounds.[1] Debris may consist of foreign bodies in a wound, for example following trauma, but in chronic wounds such as pressure ulcers it is more likely to be devitalized tissue. This may manifest itself as: slough (soft and ill-defined yellow-brownish hydrated tissue), necrotic tissue (black or brown), or eschar (well-circumscribed black adherent slough).[2] Such devitalized tissue may be distributed over the entire surface of the wound, separated from the wound edges, or patchy over the wound surface. Chronic wounds and in particular pressure ulcers are particularly prone to accumulate devitalized necrotic tissue, which reduces the possibility of nutrients reaching the wound and damages new epithelial and granulation cells. The removal of this type of tissue or debridement is therefore essential to facilitate healing.

Why Necrotic Tissue Is Present in Chronic Wounds

Tissue ischemia resulting from poor circulation, from unrelieved pressure or from a combination of both of these factors deprives the tissue of oxygen and causes tissue death. Devitalized tissue deprived of blood tends to become dehydrated and to contract, forming an eschar. Classically the eschar is dry, black, and rigid and with the passage of time tends to separate at the margins from the surrounding tissue. When the tissue becomes hydrated either as a result of occlusive dressings, edema, or exudate the eschar softens and the color changes, becoming first brown and then yellow. In the final stages of degeneration the eschar becomes slough, a yellowish fibrous tissue which adheres to the wound bed. This is part of the natural healing process (autolysis) in which the endogenous proteolytic enzymes digest the devitalized tissue.

129

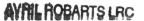

Reasons for Debridement

Removal of dead tissue from the wound is necessary to promote the proliferation of new cells. The presence of necrotic tissue in the wound bed will result in:

- a heightened risk of infection (since devitalized tissue is a medium for bacterial growth);
- increased odor;
- cellular dysfunction—necrotic tissue gives a persistent pro-inflammatory stimulus resulting in impaired cell migration and connective tissue deposition and inhibition of growth factors;[3]
- inability of the wound to contract because the eschar forms a "plug" within the wound.

The presence of necrotic tissue will also prevent assessment of the depth and extent of the wound.

As in many other aspects of wound management, debridement must be carried out following a detailed clinical and nursing assessment taking into account the patient's objectives and expectations as well as those of the clinicians. There are many criteria which should be taken into account before deciding whether or not to debride. Sibbald et al.[4] suggested that the choice of method should depend on:

- the speed of debridement required;
- how selective it needs to be;
- level of wound-related pain;
- the presence or absence of infection;
- cost.

In addition, the site and extent of the lesion, the general condition of the patient, availability of resources and the environment in which debridement is to take place, for example community or hospital, should be factors influencing choice. Selection of the debridement procedure should be made after discussion with the patient.

When Not to Debride

It is often the nurse who is attending to the patient on a daily basis who makes the decision as to whether the wound should be debrided and by what means. Sometimes it is in the patient's best interests for the wound(s) to be left with the necrotic tissue in place.

1. A patient who is terminally ill should have as few interventions as possible, and unless the necrosis is causing unacceptable odor, debridement should not be undertaken. An eschar is at least a covering requiring infrequent dressing compared to a wound from which the eschar has been removed.

2. There is debate as to whether black heels should be debrided. The European Pressure Ulcer Advisory Panel's guidelines[5] recommend that black eschar should be left until it shows signs of separation.

3. It is rarely beneficial to perform limited debridement in the presence of obliterative arterial disease as amputation through vital tissue is preferred. It is

generally advisable not to attempt any form of debridement on an ischemic limb and to keep the necrosed area as dry as possible, avoiding the use of moist occlusive dressings.

4. There are certain conditions, such as pyoderma gangrenosum, where removal of necrotic tissue is contraindicated in the acute phase of the disease as there is a risk that debridement will extend the wound necrosis.[6]

It should always be borne in mind that the presence of devitalized tissue in a wound bed is due to poor local perfusion. Unless the blood flow is improved, necrotic tissue will rapidly reappear following its removal. If there is no possibility of improving local perfusion debridement should only be carried out to reduce bacterial burden and odor.

Nurses attempting wound debridement should have an adequate knowledge of local anatomy and be able to distinguish between different abnormal wound coverings and tissue within the wound, for example yellow slough, fibrin, tendon, ligament, cartilage, and fatty tissue (Figure 15.1—see color section).

Black necrotic tissue may also pose some problems in correct identification. For example, it may be confused with heavy anaerobic contamination which is best treated with appropriate antibacterial therapy, or with dried blood where a product to dissolve the blood such as a dilute hydrogen peroxide preparation is the most effective tool. On close examination the differences become apparent. Contamination with anaerobic bacteria gives rise to a slimy appearance to the wound, whereas eschar is black and dry. Dried blood in a wound will have a reddish hue.

Debridement is complete when 100% of the wound bed consists of healthy granulation tissue.[7] To achieve complete clearance of devitalized tissue consecutive treatments and use of a combination of methods may be necessary.

In discussing the various methods of wound debridement it should be remembered that there are limitations in availability among different countries. For example, enzymatic debridement is not available in the UK, apart from a streptokinase preparation that is now rarely used. Larval debridement is not yet available in some European countries. Some countries allow nurse practitioners to perform sharp debridement whereas others do not.

Practitioners should be aware of the limits of their expertise and be able to decline intervention if they feel unsure of their competence. This is of course of particular importance when undertaking sharp debridement.[8]

Sharp Debridement

There is often confusion between the terms sharp and surgical debridement. Surgical debridement involves wide excision of necrotic tissue often removing viable tissue from the wound margins. This procedure is normally carried out by a surgeon in theater. Sharp debridement can be defined as the removal of loose necrotic tissue or dead material to just above the level of viable tissue. However, podiatrists and surgeons will often sharp debride to bleeding tissue. The procedure is carried out with the assistance of instruments such as scalpel or scissors. If nurses are to undertake sharp debridement they must do so in line with hospital policy and only accept the responsibility if they are confident that the appropriate level of knowledge and understanding of the procedure has been achieved. They should be aware of the underlying structures likely to be encountered during

Table 15.1. Contraindications and cautions for nurses carrying out sharp debridement

Contraindications for nurses attempting sharp debridement
Ischemic digits
Blood clotting disorders
Fungating/malignant wounds
Necrotic tissue near/involving vascular structures, Dacron grafts, prosthesis
Dialysis fistula
Debridement of the foot (excluding heel region)
Hands and face
Cautions
Ischemia of the lower limbs
Patients on long-term anticoagulant therapy
Achilles tendon area

Source: Fairbairn et al.[9] (p. 372).

debridement and stop if they become uncertain at any time during the procedure. The following recommendations for nurses carrying out a sharp debridement procedure were devised by a group of tissue viability nurses in the UK and are laid out in Table 15.1.[9]

In the UK it is now recommended that the nurse should have undertaken an accredited education course in wound management and attended a minimum of one study day on the subject. They should also have gained practical supervised practice, completed a competency document, and subsequently been assessed by a competent practitioner.

Prior to carrying out the procedure, informed consent should be obtained from the patient. Complications of sharp debridement include pain, damage to underlying structures, and bleeding. Removal of dead tissue is normally painless, but if the procedure involves approaching viable tissue, then pain may occur. Pain can be minimized during debridement with the application of EMLA cream half an hour prior to the procedure.[10] If damage to underlying tissues is suspected then the practitioner must immediately stop the procedure, document the occurrence in the patient notes, and inform the patient's doctor. If substantial bleeding occurs then the procedure should be stopped and appropriate action taken, for example applying pressure on the bleeding point, suturing the vessel, and/or hemostatic dressings.

Maggot Debridement Therapy/Biosurgery

The literature provides evidence on the use of maggot debridement therapy (MDT) dating back to the 1930s but its use fell into decline with the introduction of antibiotics in the 1940s. It remained a medical curiosity until Dr Ron Sherman from the University of California used larvae to treat pressure ulcers and other chronic wounds.[11] MDT was reintroduced in the UK in 1995 by Mr John Church, orthopedic surgeon, when maggots of the common greenbottle *Lucilia sericata* were introduced into necrotic wounds. Sterile maggots were then produced in a fly culture laboratory in Bridgend, Wales, and their use has grown steadily throughout the UK. Similar production facilities have now been developed elsewhere in the world including Germany, Hungary, Sweden, Belgium, Israel, Ukraine, and Tanzania. Studies have shown that the treatment is efficient and cost effective.[12] The great advantage of larval therapy over sharp debridement is that the larvae are highly selective and will only attack dead tissue and are therefore less likely than a clinical practitioner to damage healthy tissue during the debridement procedure. It has even been observed that they appear to leave small capillary vessels intact while consuming adjacent necrotic tissue. They are also able to access sinuses and cavities which would not be possible without laying the wound open with extensive surgery. They are, however, air breathing and this limits the depth to which they can penetrate wounds.

Maggots, when introduced into a wound containing devitalized tissue, produce secretions containing proteolytic enzymes, which break down necrotic tissue into a semiliquid form that they subsequently ingest. In addition, research indicates that larvae have an antibacterial effect.[13] They ingest and destroy bacteria including methicillin-resistant *Staphylococcus aureus*. Further, maggot secretions have been shown to stimulate the growth of fibroblast cells, which may explain the regularly observed finding that granulation tissue formation is enhanced after successful MDT. When using MDT it is important to ensure that any secondary dressings permit the ingress of oxygen and free drainage of excess fluid. Although the development of maggots is unaffected by commonly prescribed antibiotics, their development can be adversely affected by the presence of residues of hydrogel dressings containing propylene glycol.[14] All traces of such dressings should therefore be thoroughly removed before the application.

Figures 15.2 to 15.5 (see color section) show a pressure ulcer on the calf being treated with maggot debridement.

There are no reported significant adverse reactions to maggot therapy. As with any debriding agent, care must be taken to protect the surrounding skin from secretions. Some patients, especially those with ischemic or vasculitic ulcers, report increased levels of pain during treatment. However, in general, patient acceptance of the technique is very high. Recently larvae bags have been introduced which contain the larvae and yet allow them to feed through the pores of the bag. Such bags make the treatment much more acceptable for patient and practitioner, but may be less effective at cleansing wound sinuses and wound crevices.

Enzymatic Debridement

In many cases when autolytic debridement is not sufficiently rapid and invasive methods such as surgical or sharp debridement need to be avoided, enzymatic debridement is the treatment of choice. There are several different pharmaceutical enzyme preparations. One of the most widely used is *collagenase*, which is a purified product derived from the bacterium *Clostridium histolyticum* and acts best with a pH of between 6 and 8,[15] which is the pH of normal skin. It is a hydrosoluble proteinase favoring the removal of the necrotic "plug." It is sensitive to temperature[16] and is naturally found in wounds as a metalloprotease matrix.[4] In cultivated cells collagenase accelerates keratinocyte migration threefold and the individual cellular mobility tenfold.[15] Antiseptics with metallic ions (e.g. silver or mercury) will inactivate the product. It is therefore necessary to avoid using products containing silver concurrently with collagenase.[15] Some patients suffer skin irritation when the collagenase cream comes into contact with the skin surrounding the wound.[4,15] Collagenase acts most effectively on fibers of collagen and elastin fibers in the center of the eschar, so that its activity is at the base of the wound rather than on the surface.[18-22] Clinically collagenase may seem the slowest of the enzymatic debriding agents since its activity is at the base of the wound where it is less visible. To enhance its activity it is advised that the eschar should be scored so that the enzyme can penetrate to where it is most effective, i.e. the base of the eschar.

Papaina is derived from the vegetable product papaya, blended with a chemical agent, urea, which enhances the enzymatic action of papaya.[21] Papaina can be inactivated by hydrogen peroxide as well as by products containing silver and mercury. It appears to be most effective on the superficial areas of necrotic tissue where there is the greatest concentration of fibrin and fibronectin so that clinically its action appears more rapid than collagenase. Papaina/urea causes the wound to produce more exudates,[22] which can cause skin irritation and necessitates more frequent dressing change. Papaina/urea is of greatest use when there is extensive eschar which needs to be rapidly removed.

The third group of enzymatic debriding agents discussed here are *fibrinolysin* and *deoxyribonuclease*. These enzymes are obtained from bovine pancreas, and promote wound debridement by the lysis of deoxyribonucleic acid and deoxyribonucleoproteins present in necrotic tissue. The product is insoluble in water and soluble in saline solution. During the debridement process the product releases enzymes within 6–8 hours and the products that result from the fibrinolysis are not reabsorbed so that it is necessary to clean the wound bed after use, to avoid irritation.[23] In a recent study which compared this enzyme with collagenase on 134 patients with pressure ulcers there were no significant statistical differences between the two agents.[24]

Autolytic Debridement

Any dressing that maintains a moist wound environment will exploit the natural properties of the wound to dissolve necrotic tissue with its own enzymes. *Hydrocolloids, hydrogels*, and *polyacrylates* are particularly useful in the management of dry eschar as they rehydrate the wound and hence promote enzymatic activity and the subsequent degradation of necrotic tissue.[15,25,26] The advantage of this type of debridement is that it is painless but it may take several days and sometimes weeks to effect. If after the application of this type of dressing there is no sign of autolysis within 72 hours, then other methods of debridement should be considered. In the workplace there is still ignorance about the mode of action of occlusive dressings, despite extensive literature on the subject. There is sometimes concern about the risk of infection under such dressings. However, clinical trials have provided evidence that there is a lower risk of infection under these dressings compared with conventional dressings.[23,27,28] This can be explained by the relative impermeability of the dressings to external pathogens, and by the accumulation of neutrophils in the wound fluid which inhibits the growth of bacteria and reduces the amount of necrotic tissue in the wound bed.[23,29]

Occlusive dressings are contraindicated in the presence of infection as an infected wound should be inspected daily and occlusive dressings should remain in place for several days undisturbed.

Hydrogels are amorphous gels in a base of water or glycerin used for rehydrating a dry/necrotic wound. They should not be used on a moderate or heavily exuding wound. Some hydrogels also contain hydrocolloid or alginates. They should be used as a primary dressing and used with either a hydrocolloid dressing polyurethane film or non-adherent dressing and pad. Hydrogels have also been combined with gauze to form a cavity dressing or a dressing that can be laid in the wound bed. Rehydration of a necrotic wound will inevitably produce more exudate and care must be taken to protect the surrounding skin from maceration.

Superabsorbent polyacrylate surrounded by a covering layer of polypropylene is a new type of dressing introduced into the market in recent years. The dressing must be activated by Ringer's solution prior to application, which is then continuously delivered to the wound. At the same time the exudate is absorbed by the dressing. The continual supply of the solution to the wound facilitates softening and debridement of necrotic tissue.[30,31] This dressing must be renewed at least once every 24 hours.

Alginate or *cellulose* dressings maintain a moist environment in a heavily exuding wound and will hence encourage autolysis but are not effective in a dry environment.

Antiseptic Dressings

Hypochlorite solutions were at one time the only dressing available in the management of sloughy/contaminated wounds. Following Leaper's animal studies in 1985[29] to illustrate the inhibition of angiogenesis when applied to healthy tissue, its use was largely discredited. It is now generally accepted that hypochlorites can damage granulation tissue and can act an irritant to surrounding skin. However, hypochlorites are cheap and effective antiseptics. If surrounding skin is protected while a hypochlorite dressing is being used and if its use is discontinued as soon as the wound bed is showing vital tissue there would seem to be some indication for re-evaluating its use, especially now when there is a problem of increased antibiotic resistance. Recently there has developed an increased interest in *honey*, an even older remedy, and research supports its therapeutic effectiveness. Honey is reported to resolve infections, promote debridement, and stimulate tissue regeneration. The debriding effect of honey may be due to the activation of proteases in wound tissues by hydrogen peroxide generated by oxidation.[27] *Cadexomer iodine* dressings have been on the market for over 20 years. Cadexomer iodine is distinguished from dextranomer iodine by its greater absorptive capacity. The product absorbs wound exudate while simultaneously releasing iodine into the wound bed, thus providing a prolonged antibacterial action. Studies have shown that it is effective at removing debris from the wound bed.[28] Some patients find iodine treatment very painful and some patients may have an iodine sensitivity; its use should therefore be avoided in such patients. Recently dressings containing *silver* have been marketed and are designed to release free silver ion into the wound site. Silver dressings are indicated primarily for the treatment of soft tissue infections having a broad spectrum of activity and are rarely associated with resistance and depend on the ability of low concentrations of silver ions to kill a broad spectrum of microorganisms.[32]

It is known that removal of devitalized tissue from the wound surface reduces the bacterial load on the wound but clinical observation would also suggest that the reverse is also true and that the reduction of the bacterial load reduces the continuing production of devitalized tissue in the wound; thus dressings with an antibacterial action play a vital role in the management of pressure ulcers containing devitalized tissue.

Conclusion

"Devitalized material is an integral part of pressure ulcer pathology and is a major barrier to healing."[2] The problem for the practitioner when healing is the desired outcome is how best to achieve debridement. The Cochrane report on debriding agents concluded that there were no trials which suggested that any dressing was more effective than any other in the removal of devitalized tissue from a wound.[33] Clinical experience is necessary in making the correct choice for each individual patient.

References

1. Dolynchuk K. Debridement. In: Krasner D, Rodeheaver GT, Sibbald G (eds) Chronic wound care. Wayne, PA: HMP Communications; 2001; 385–389.
2. Romanelli M, Mastronicola D. The role of wound bed preparation in managing chronic pressure ulcers. J Wound Care 2002; 11(8):305–310.
3. Mast BA, Schultz GS. Interactions of cytokines, growth factors and proteases in acute wounds. Wound Repair Regen 1996; 4:411–420.
4. Sibbald RG, Williamson D, Orsted HL, et al. Preparing the wound bed: debridement, bacterial balance and moisture balance. Ostomy Wound Manage 2000; 46(11):14–35.
5. European Pressure Ulcer Advisory Panel. Guidelines on treatment of pressure ulcers. EPUAP Review 1999; 1(2):31–33.
6. Coady K. The diagnosis and treatment of pyoderma gangrenosum. J Wound Care 2000; 9:282–285.
7. Vowden K, Vowden P. Wound debridement: 2 Sharp techniques. J Wound Care 1999; 8(6):291–294.
8. Ashworth J, Chivers, M. Conservative sharp debridement: the professional and legal issues. Prof Nurse 2002; 17(10):585–588.
9. Fairbairn K, Gier J, Hunter C, Preece J. A sharp debridement procedure devised by specialist nurses. J Wound Care 2002; 11(10):371–375.
10. Hansson C, Holm J, Lillieborg S, Syren A. Repeated treatment with lidocaine/prilocaine cream (EMLA) as a topical anaesthesic for the cleansing of venous leg ulcers. Acta Derm Venereal (Stockh) 1993; 73:231–233.
11. Sherman RS, Wyle F, Vulpe M. Maggot therapy for treating pressure ulcers in spinal cord injury patients. J Spinal Cord Med 1995; 18(2):71–74.
12. Thomas S, Jones M, Wynn K, Fowler T. The current status of maggot therapy in wound healing. Br J Nurs 2001; 10(22 Suppl):5–8.
13. Thomas S, Andrews A, Nigel P, et al. The antimicrobial activity of maggot secretions, a result of a previous study. J Tissue Viability 1999; 9:127–133.
14. Thomas S, Andrews A. The effect of hydrogel dressings on maggot development. J Wound Care 1999; 8(2):75–77.
15. Ayello EA, Cuddingan JE. Debridement: controlling the necrotic/cellular burden. Adv Skin Wound Care 2004; 17(2):66–75.
16. Dolynchuk K, Keast D, Campbell K, et al. Best practices for the prevention and treatment of pressure ulcers. Ostomy Wound Manage 2000; 46(11):38–52.
17. Rao CN, Ladin DA, Liu YY, et al. Alpha 1 antitrypsin is degraded and non-functional in chronic wounds but intact and functional in acute wounds: the inhibitor protects fibronectin from degradation by chronic wound fluid enzymes. J Invest Dermatol 1995; 105:572–578.
18. Herman I. Stimulation of human keratinocyte migration and proliferation in vitro: insights into the cellular responses to injury and wound healing. Wounds 1996; 8(2):33–41.
19. Herman I. Extracellular matrix–cytoskeletal interactions in vascular cells. Tissue Cell 1987; 19(1):1–19.
20. Kreig T. Collagen in the healing wound. Wounds 1995; 7(Suppl):5A–12A.
21. Hebda PA, Lo C. The effects of active ingredients of standards debriding agents—papain and collagenase—on digestion of native and denatured collagenous substrates, fibrin and elastin. Wounds 2001; 13(5):190–194.
22. Hebda PA, Flynn KJ, Dohar JE. Evaluation of efficacy of enzymatic debriding agents for removal of necrotic tissue and promotion of healing in porcine skin wounds. Wounds 1998; 10:83–86.
23. Falabella A. Debridement of wounds. Wounds 1998; 10(Suppl C):1C–9C.

24. Pullen R, Popp R, Volkers P, et al. Prospective randomized double-blind study of the wound-debriding effects of collagenase and fibrinolysin/deoxyribonuclease in pressure ulcers. Age Ageing 2002; 31:126–130.

25. O'Brien M. Method of debridement and patient focused care. JCN online 2003; 17, 11.

26. Zacus H, Kirsner S. Debridement: rationale and therapeutic options. Wounds 2002; 14(7, Suppl):2S–6S.

27. Molan PC. The role of honey in the management of wounds. J Wound Care 1999; 8(8):415–418.

28. Hillstrom L. Iodosorb compared to standard treatment in chronic venous leg ulcers—a multi-center study. Acta Chir Scand Suppl 1988; 544:53–56.

29. Cameron S, Leaper D. Antiseptic toxicity in open wounds. Nurs Times 1988; 25:77–78.

30. Scholz S, Rompel R, Petres J. A new approach to wet therapy of chronic leg ulcers. Arzt & Praxis 1999; 816:517–522.

31. Mosti G, Mattaliano V, Iabichella ML, Picerni P. Uso del tenderwet nella detersione delle ulcere degli arti inferiori ad eziologia vascolare. Acta Vulnologia (in press).

32. Lansdown ABG. Silver 1: Its antibacterial properties and mechanism of action. J Wound Care 2002; 11(4):125–130.

33. Bradley M, Cullum N, Sheldon T. The debridement of chronic wounds: a systematic review. Health Technol Assess 1999; 3:(17 Pt 1).

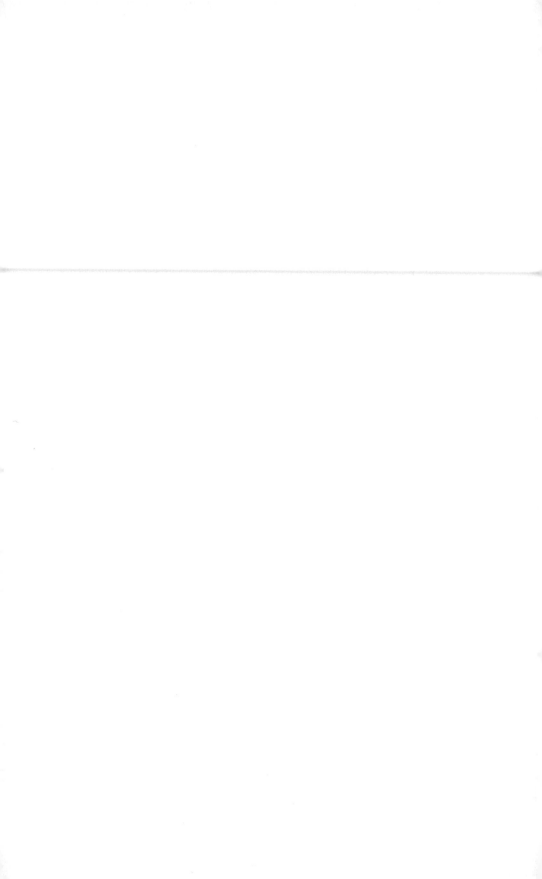

16 The Role of Bacteria in Pressure Ulcers

R. Gary Sibbald, Paul Chapman, and Jose Contreras-Ruiz

Introduction

The approach to a person with a pressure ulcer must start with treating the cause and patient-centered concerns before the bacteria–host relationship can be adequately assessed and treated (Table 16.1). The role of bacteria in pressure ulcers is complex. There is no longer a straightforward clinical distinction between contamination, colonization, and infection. A number of factors must be examined to determine the effect of bacterial burden on chronic pressure ulcer healing. For healing to occur the patient must be assessed holistically with the cause treated and the local wound care optimized. An ulcer that is not healing at the expected rate may be the result of a nonhealable or uncorrected cause. Alternatively, bacteria can damage local tissue and delay healing (critical colonization) with or without the classical features of infection.

The bacterial burden can be assessed in pressure ulcers using a compartmental model that delineates multiple levels of bacterial involvement (above the wound, surface and deep wound compartments, surrounding skin, and systemic sepsis). A clinical approach to management and assessment of bacterial burden can then be outlined depending on the level of invasion. Most bacterial contamination originates from external sources requiring infection control measures. The level of damage caused by bacteria will then determine the choice of topical and/or systemic treatment.

The effect of bacteria on pressure ulcer healing is dependent on organism numbers and virulence, but the most important factor is host resistance. The relationship can be expressed as:

$$\text{Infection} = (\text{Organism number} \times \text{Virulence})/(\text{Host resistance})$$

The approach to infection in a person with pressure ulcers is illustrated in Figure 16.1.[1] We must look at the whole patient before treating the hole in the patient.

Table 16.1. The approach to a person with pressure ulcers and increased bacterial burden / infection

Patient as a whole
1. *Assess the cause* of the ulcer and determine the ability for healing (healability).
2. *The patient and the caregivers* should be part of the decision-making process to improve adherence to treatment plans and to optimize pain control and quality of life.

Regional treatment
3. *The diagnosis of infection is made clinically* with the choice of topical and/or systemic antimicrobial therapy guided by investigative testing (bacterial swab, X-rays, and laboratory tests including CRP and ESR).
   Do not use swab cultures to diagnose infection.
4. Diagnose and treat deep infection with appropriate systemic antimicrobial agents (deep compartment, surrounding skin, systemic infection). Determine clinical and investigative parameters to monitor treatment and wound healing.

Local wound care
5. *Cleanse or compress the local wound* with saline or water.
6. *Topical antiseptics* may be appropriate in patients with *nonhealable ulcers* or where the reduction of bacterial burden is more important than toxicity to granulation tissue.
   (a) In general, choose agents with broad spectrum antimicrobial activity and low tissue toxicity.
7. *Debride devitalized tissue* to decrease bacterial burden and control pro-inflammatory stimulus.
   (a) Choose most appropriate method (surgical, mechanical, biotherapy, enzymatic, autolytic).
   (b) Use systemic antibiotics prior to deep surgical debridement procedures, especially in the compromised host.
   (c) In wounds without the ability to heal, aggressive sharp surgical debridement to bleeding base is contraindicated.
8. *Consider a 2-week trial of topical antimicrobials* if wound is not healing despite optimal care (increased bacterial burden or covert infection suspected).
   (a) Use agents with low tissue toxicity that can also promote moisture balance.
   (b) Avoid agents that can cause allergic sensitization or frequent bacterial resistance.
9. *Perform semiquantitative bacterial cultures* and re-evaluate for infection or osteomyelitis if wound fails to improve.
10. *Reassess outcomes* of therapy at appropriate time intervals by monitoring clinical, laboratory, and investigative parameters.

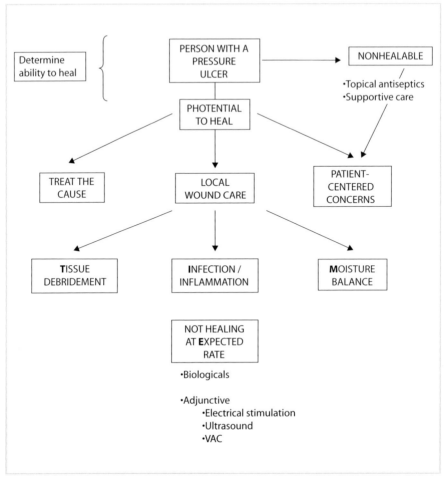

Figure 16.1 Holistic approach to pressure ulcer management. VAC, Vacuum Assisted Closure.

Assessment and Diagnosis of Patients with Pressure Ulcers

Case one scenario

Ms S is a 57-year-old woman with a nontreatable brain tumor (anaplastic astrocytoma). She has been semi-comatose for the past month and developed four pressure ulcers located in the occiput, sacrum, and both heels. The family advocated for palliative care and you were called by the treating physician to address the nonhealing skin ulcers because the odor is disturbing both the family and other patients.

Can this individual make new granulation tissue and heal? Is healing the ulcer part of the patient- or caregiver-centered plan? How much more should be done to treat or heal the pressure ulcers?

Many factors are involved in this assessment. The patient and caregiver must be involved in the decisions. The general health and fitness of the patient must be determined including: ability to perfuse tissue, vital organ function (brain, heart, lungs, kidney, liver), and drugs that will inhibit healing (e.g. chemotherapeutic agents, corticosteroids).

Although the diagnosis of pressure ulcers is usually obvious, there are some cases where other diagnoses are confused with pressure ulcers. An early stage (1 or 2) pressure ulcer in the gluteal fold region of the buttocks can be confused with candidial intertrigo or a contact dermatitis. Deeper lesions mistakenly labeled as pressure ulcers may in fact be perianal bacterial abscesses or ruptured pilonidal sinuses. Once the diagnosis is established, specific pressure ulcer contributing factors must also be corrected (e.g. nutritional deficiencies, friction and shear, incontinence) and patient/caregiver cooperation with the treatment plan is vital.[2] In some settings availability of resources can be a limiting factor. All these factors must be considered as part of the holistic assessment of the patient's healing potential.

Patient/Caregiver-Centered Concerns

Patient-centered concerns often revolve around issues of quality of life and pain. Ulcer healing may be less important than other issues facing a patient including the control of odor, sleep, and pain.[3] Particularly in persons with nonhealable pressure ulcers, sepsis prevention and minimizing dressing changes become very important considerations of the care plan. It is senseless to concentrate only on healing an ulcer and not take into account previous social activities. It is very demoralizing to put a person with a pressure ulcer to bed for long periods of time for maximum healing only for them to resume normal activities and have a recurrence.[4]

Treat the Cause

Host resistance can only be maximized if the pressure ulcer cause has been effectively corrected. One of the most important aspects is to optimize the systemic environment in which healing will occur. Underlying conditions such as anemia, organ failure, and medications that impair healing should be evaluated, corrected, or changed to optimize the wound healing environment. Attention must be directed to local factors including pressure relief and reduction as well as minimizing shearing forces, friction, and local moisture.[5] Some additional risk factors include prolonged immobilization, sensory deficit, circulatory disturbances, and poor nutrition.[5] Vasille et al. suggested that the patient's mobility level may be more important than many factors including bacteriology.[6]

Pressure Ulcers Without the Potential to Heal

If the ulcer is deemed nonhealable, then topical antiseptics may be perfectly legitimate as a primary treatment to decrease local bacterial burden. Lower surface bacterial counts will help prevent bacterial invasion with the risk of adjacent and systemic sepsis that may lead to increased morbidity and mortality. Antiseptic agents with low tissue toxicity and appropriate antibacterial coverage should be chosen (Table 16.2). Paradoxically these agents may even result in healing of the ulcers[7] since toxicity in vitro has not been clearly demonstrated in well-controlled in vivo studies.[8] In ulcers that have the ability to heal, topical antiseptics may be useful to decrease surface bacterial counts and discourage granulation tissue until systemic agents can treat the deeper infection.

Table 16.2. Antiseptics most commonly used in wound care

Class and agent	Action	Effect in healing	Effect on bacteria	Comments
Alcohols				
Ethyl alcohol Isopropyl alcohol	Dehydrates, denatures proteins, and dissolves lipids	Cytotoxic May cause dryness and irritation on intact skin	Bactericidal and viricidal	Used as a disinfectant on intact skin Stings and burns if used on open skin
Biguanides				
0.02–0.05% Chlorhexidine	Acts by damaging the cell membranes	Relatively safe. Little effect on wound healing. Toxicity—small effect on tissue	Highly bactericidal against Gram-positive and -negative organisms	Highly effective as hand washing agent and for surgical scrub Binds to stratum corneum and has residual effect
Halogen compounds				
Sodium hypochlorite (e.g. Hygeol, Eusol, Dakins)	Lyses cell walls	Acts as a chemical debrider and should be discontinued with healing tissue	Dakins solution and Eusol (buffered preparation) can select out Gram-negative microorganisms.	High pH causes irritation to skin

Table 16.2. *(Continued)*

Class and agent	Action	Effect in healing	Effect on bacteria	Comments
1% Iodine (povidone) (e.g. Betadine)	Oxidizes cell constituents, especially proteins at –SH groups; iodinates proteins and inactivates them	Povidone iodine Cytotoxicity depends on dilution. Potential toxicity in vivo related to concentration and exposure	Prevents and controls bacterial growth in wounds Resistance has not been reported Broad spectrum of activity, although decreased in the presence of pus or exudate	Toxicity is of concern with prolonged use or application over large areas Potential for thyroid toxicity
Organic acids Acetic acid (0.25–1%)	Lowers surface pH	Cytotoxicity in vitro; in vivo is concentration-dependent	Effective against *Pseudomonas*. May be useful for other Gram-negative rods and *Staphylococcus aureus*	Often burns and stings on application
Peroxides 3% Hydrogen peroxide	May induce cell death by oxidative damage	Can harm healthy granulation tissue and may form air emboli if packed in deep sinuses	Very little to absent antimicrobial activity	Acts more like a chemical debriding agent by dissolving blood clots and softening slough. Safety concerns— deep wounds due to reports of air embolisms
Tinctures Gentian violet	Very weak antiseptic	Carcinogenic and cytotoxic. May cause erosions, ulcers or areas of necrosis especially on mucous membranes	Kills Gram-positive organisms and some yeasts such as *Candida*, more effective at higher pH but can select out overgrowth of Gram-negative organisms	High irritancy potential and occasional allergies
Mercurochrome	A very weak antiseptic with action inhibited in the presence of organic debris	Epidermal cell toxicity	Not enough data available	Contact allergen and irritant; systemic toxicity and rare death through topical application, possible aplastic anemia
Cetrimide (quaternary ammonium)	Disrupts membranes, may inactivate some proteins	High toxicity to tissues	Gram-positive and -negative organisms	Good detergent but very irritating to open wounds

Source: From Lineaweaver et al.,[9] Rodeheaver,[10] White et al.,[11] Drosou,[8] Lawrence.[12]
© Dr. R. G. Sibbald.

Case One Completion

Returning to our patient with the nontreatable brain tumor, the cause cannot be treated and the patient's family is advocating palliative treatment. There was no deep infection requiring systemic agents. The patient had excellent pain control, with long-acting narcotic agents for normal nerve function pain, a short-acting narcotic for breakthrough, and a tricyclic agent high in norepinephrine (noradrenaline) for the neuropathic component of chronic wound pain. The odor was derived from nonviable slough and *Pseudomonas*. The debris was removed with surgical debridement and acetic acid compresses to acidify the local wounds and discourage *Pseudomonas* growth. A new modern dressing combining ionized silver with calcium alginate was then applied every second day for bacterial balance and moisture balance and autolytic debridement. The wounds were monitored every second day for deep infection and size. Non-viable slough that accumulated on the wound surface was removed with dressing changes. The patient died 3 weeks later with no further extension of the wounds, no significant local pain even at dressing changes (short-acting breakthrough narcotic was administered 30 minutes prior to the procedure).

Pressure Ulcers with Potential to Heal

Local Wound Care

Local wound care includes three components: tissue debridement, control of increased bacterial burden or prolonged inflammation (infection/inflammation), and moisture balance. If these three components are controlled and the wound is still not healing, we need to reassess the cause, patient-centered concerns, and the local wound care to be sure that treatment has been optimized. If the wound is not healing at the expected rate, the edge effect of the TIME (Tissue debridement, Infection/Inflammation, Moisture Balance, Edge Effect) paradigm[13,14] reminds us of the appropriate use of advanced therapies in our toolkit: biological agents (growth factors, living skin equivalents), adjunctive therapies (ultrasound, electrical stimulation, negative pressure therapy), and skin grafts or flaps. Advanced therapies are expensive and will only work when patient care has been optimized as outlined in Figure 16.1. These advanced therapies are not a substitute for best wound care practices.

Debridement

Debridement is necessary to remove devitalized tissue and to reduce bacterial contamination. There are five methods to consider for debridement: sharp surgical, autolytic, enzymatic, biological, and mechanical.[13] Devitalized tissue serves as a good culture medium for bacteria to grow within a chronic wound. This dead tissue

also acts as a foreign body that may induce a pro-inflammatory response. Persistent inflammation as well as infection can delay healing (Figure 16.2—see color section). The presence of foreign material such as necrotic debris, retained packing materials, or small fragments of gauze dressing will significantly decrease host resistance and lower the number of bacteria necessary to cause wound infection or damage to the granulation tissue in the ulcer base. Universal precautions are necessary to prevent wound contamination. The surface compartment may have an increased bacterial burden and this area of the wound can be treated topically with newer antibacterial dressings that will also control moisture balance and on occasion have additional autolytic debridement functions. The deep compartment of the wound requires systemic antimicrobial therapy and is defined as the area that is not accessible by topical treatments. This compartment can have bacterial invasion of the underlying bone or localized infections in the form of an abscess. In individuals with pressure ulcers, abscesses below the surface must be sought and this deep compartment infection drained (Figure 16.3—see color section).[15]

The choice of debridement depends on the availability of healthcare providers with skill in performing sharp surgical debridement or local preference for autolytic methods with dressings (calcium alginates, hydrogels, or hydrocolloids), topical enzymatic agents, biological methods with maggots, or mechanical irrigation with saline wet to dry dressings.

Deep surgical debridement has been associated with transient bacteremia in patients with pressure ulcers.[16] Positive blood cultures were obtained during five out of eight active surgical debridement procedures in a study by Glenchur et al.[16] A majority of these included anaerobes so the recommendation is that the significant incidence of bacteremia occurring during surgical debridement indicates the need for broad spectrum antibiotic coverage during and after deep surgical procedures.[17] This is important when large and/or deep ulcers are debrided, especially in the compromised host.[16]

Bacteremia is a common complication of pressure ulcers and may lead to morbidity and mortality. Galpin et al.[18] documented bacteremia in 16/21 patients with pressure ulcers. The most commonly isolated bacteria were anaerobes. In patients with spinal cord injury, a mortality of 7–8% is frequently associated with secondary wound infection.[19] In a study of 21 patients with systemic bacteremia (frequently polymicrobial) and sepsis, 76% of the isolated bacteria originated from a pressure ulcer. Overall, mortality was 48% and all patients over 60 died despite empiric antibiotic treatment. Five patients had bacteremia that persisted with antibiotic treatment and resolved only after local debridement. The mortality rate among patients with pressure ulcers and bacteremia is close to 50%.[18] Another grave and often fatal complication of pressure ulcers is necrotizing soft tissue infection.[20,21]

Bacterial Balance/Chronic Inflammation

Assessment of Infection

The diagnosis of infection is made based on clinical criteria, with bacterial swabs or deep cultures, laboratory and radiological tests used as adjuncts for diagnosis and treatment. Pressure ulcers are prone to infection.[13] All wounds contain

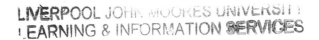

bacteria at levels ranging from contamination, through colonization, critical colonization (also known as increased bacterial burden, occult or covert infection) to infection. The increased bacterial burden may be confined to the superficial wound bed or may be present in the deep compartment and surrounding tissue of the wound margin. Therefore, it becomes very important to diagnose both the bacterial imbalance and level of invasion in order to diagnose and treat infection properly. Increased bacterial burden in pressure ulcers has been demonstrated to delay healing in patients with chronic ulceration.[22]

Clinical Assessment

In this discussion, we identify contamination as the presence of bacteria on the wound surface. Colonization is the presence of replicating bacteria attached to the wound tissue but not causing injury to the host. Infection is the presence of replicating microorganisms in a wound with associated host injury. The borders between these concepts are not clearly established. The clinician must assess the patient's symptoms and signs present in the wound to distinguish contamination, colonization, and healing from critical colonized or infected wounds that are not healing, or even endangering the life of the patient. Critical colonization occurs when bacteria delays or stops healing of the wound without the classical symptoms and signs of infection being present. The wound care specialist needs to carefully identify the clinical signs and symptoms of infection to make an accurate diagnosis. In patients with pressure ulcers some of these signs may be obscured[23] by factors such as malnutrition, anemia, drugs, or immunosuppression including chronic illness such as diabetes.

The classical signs of infection are: pain, erythema, edema, purulent discharge, and increased warmth. These are related to the inflammatory process occurring in the wound. Increased blood flow produces a rise in temperature, and fluid leaking from intravascular spaces accumulates in the tissue, causing visible swelling. Vasoactive mediators such as histamine produce the characteristic erythema, and pain is caused through activation of biochemical mediators secreted near unmyelinated nerve fiber endings.

In chronic wounds other signs should be added: delayed healing or new areas of breakdown, increased discharge (often it is initially serous or clear and watery before it becomes pustular), bright red discoloration of granulation tissue, friable and exuberant granulation, new areas of slough on the wound surface, undermining, and a foul odor (Figure 16.4—see color section).[24] Serous exudate may be increased in a chronic wound with increased bacterial burden before purulence is noted with the clinical signs usually recognized in infections. It has been suggested that chronic wounds should show some evidence of healing within 4 weeks to progress to healing by week 12. If this time limit is exceeded then increased bacterial burden or infection should be suspected as one of the causes of delayed healing.[25]

Discoloration of granulation tissue arises from loose, poorly formed granulation tissue, while friable granulation tissue that bleeds easily occurs from excessive angiogenesis stimulated by bacterial pathogens (Figure 16.5—see color section). Healthy granulation tissue is pink-red and firm with a moist translucent appearance. When infected, it will appear dull and may have patches of greenish or yellow discoloration. Certain anaerobic species such as *Bacteroides fragilis* and streptococci can produce a dullish, dark-red hue, while *Pseudomonas* will produce green or blue patches which may fluoresce at 365 nm (Wood's) light. Undermining results from atrophic granulation tissue inhibited or digested by bacteria. Foul odor is usually produced by Gram-negative bacilli especially *Pseudomonas* species or anaerobes digesting granulation tissue.[26]

Deep infection will often cause erythema and warmth extending 2 cm or more beyond the wound margin when the surrounding skin becomes involved (Figure 16.6—see color section). This bacterially stimulated increased inflammatory response is painful and will cause the wound to increase in size or lead to satellite areas of tissue breakdown resulting in adjacent tissue ulceration. Deep infections, especially in ulcers of long duration, can often lead to underlying osteomyelitis. Probing to bone is a simple clinical test that may indicate osteomyelitis, especially in patients with neuropathic foot ulcers often associated with diabetes.[27]

These symptoms and signs of wound infection are summarized in Table 16.3.

Gardner et al.[29,30] examined the reliability and validity of clinical signs of infection in two recent papers. These studies identified various symptoms and signs of infection and compared diagnoses made using these signs with the results of quantitative cultures from tissue biopsies to correlate each sign or symptom with the stated criteria of infection. Increasing pain, friable granulation tissue, foul odor, and wound breakdown all demonstrated validity for a diagnosis of infection based on discriminatory power and positive predictive values. A checklist was then constructed to test the ability of different observers to distinguish these signs (reliability). There was a very high level of agreement between observers but it is also important to assess the discriminatory power of the sign or symptom when infection is present compared to when it is absent. A kappa test was performed to quantify the usefulness of each criterion. High kappa values (above 0.7) indicate a high reliability associated with a diagnosis of infection and the values for the symptoms and signs were:

- increasing pain (1.0),
- edema (0.93),
- wound breakdown (0.89),
- delayed healing (0.87),
- friable granulation (0.8),
- purulent exudate (0.78),
- serous exudate (0.74).

Table 16.3. Clinical signs of wound infection

Superficial increased bacterial burden	Deep or surrounding wound infection	Systemic infection
Nonhealing	Pain	Fever
Bright red granulation tissue	Swelling, induration	Rigors
Friable and exuberant granulation	Erythema	Chills
New areas of breakdown or necrosis on the wound surface (yellow, brown, or black slough)	Increased temperature Wound breakdown	Hypotension Multiple organ failure
Increased exudate that may be translucent or clear before becoming purulent	Increased size or satellite areas Undermining	
Foul odor	Probing to bone	

Source: Adapted from Sibbald et al.[28]

The sample size was small with only 31 patients and there were five different types of wounds including pressure ulcers. Although these observations must be considered preliminary, these characteristics (especially when more than one is present) will assist clinicians to more accurately identify bacterial damage and infection in chronic wounds. These studies need to be expanded to larger numbers of patients and separate analysis of each wound type including pressure ulcers must be determined.

The classical signs of overt infection are generally easy to identify but it is more difficult to make a judgment about wounds that display abnormal or persistent inflammation. Wounds may display signs of covert infection, where the host is harmed enough to impede healing but not enough to cause typical inflammatory symptoms. Covert infection is difficult to diagnose as many of the signs listed above may be absent. The most obvious sign is the failure of the pressure ulcer to heal or initial progress to healing is stalled. Disorganization (hypertrophy or atrophy) of previously healthy granulation tissue, discoloration of granulation tissue to pale gray or deep red, and increased friability and bleeding are also likely to be detectable. The exudate may increase in quantity and can be serous or watery in consistency. Some clinicians utilize infrared thermometry as an aid in the diagnosis of infection or inflammation, as validated by Armstrong and colleagues for the active inflammatory process associated with a Charcot foot in people with diabetes.[31,32] This technique has not been properly validated in pressure ulcer patients but it may be a useful tool to discriminate the increase in temperature in the surrounding skin compared to mirror image locations. In general, the clinician should assess for swelling, warmth, tenderness, pain, and erythema extending more than 2 cm beyond the ulcer margin to diagnose surrounding skin cellulitis and probable deep tissue compartment infection in the ulcer base.

Bacterial Tests

Bacterial swabs and cultures are not used to diagnose infection but to guide antimicrobial therapy choices and screen patients for multiresistant bacterial organisms such as methicillin-resistant *Staphylococcus aureus* (MRSA). There is no need to culture a pressure ulcer that is healing at an expected rate and does not display any signs or symptoms of infection. As all wounds are contaminated and potentially colonized, a culture will simply confirm that microorganisms are present without providing any information as to whether they are having a detrimental effect on the host.

Bacterial swabs can provide information on the predominant flora on the surface of a nonprogressing, deteriorating, or heavily exuding wound. Microbiological tests can also screen for multiresistant bacteria such as MRSA and vancomycin-resistant enterococcus (VRE). The degree of the inflammatory response is measured by the presence and number of neutrophils per high power field in the Gram stain. The relationship between increased local infiltration of neutrophils and chronicity of wounds is extremely important. A granulation tissue biopsy study of pressure ulcers by Diegelmann[33] demonstrated delayed healing when the biopsies included an increased number of neutrophils. The numbers of neutrophils correlated well with an increase in myeloperoxidase activity and metalloproteinases. The elevated number of neutrophils and their destructive enzymes may be the cause of the matrix dysfunction and perpetuation of the ulcer. Sibbald et al.[34] demonstrated an association between increased bacterial burden and an increased number of neutrophils in nonhealing venous stasis ulcers. Both the bacteria and neutrophilic infiltrate delayed healing. Once bacterial load reaches 10^6 colony-forming units (CFU) per gram of tissue, wound healing is usually impaired.[35] In 1964 Bendy et al.[36] reported that healing in pressure ulcers was inhibited if the bacterial load was greater than 1×10^6 CFU/ml of wound fluid. Superficial wound swabs were used in this study, but other studies using the gold standard (tissue biopsy specimens) reported similar results for pressure ulcers and surgical wounds.[37–41] In quantitative biopsies from 17 patients Vande Berg et al.[42] determined that fibroblast growth inhibition was not related to the type of bacteria but to the bacterial load (greater than 1×10^5 CFU/g).

Quantitative microbiology has a role to play in predicting the risk of infection as many studies have shown that bacterial load correlates with risk.[43] Nevertheless, these findings need to be viewed in perspective. At least 20% of wounds colonized with more than 10^5 CFU/g of bacteria will still heal.[44] If host resistance is high, normal skin flora present in very high quantities have the potential in some clinical situations to enhance wound healing.[45] On the other hand, reduced host resistance, or the presence of foreign objects in the wound, can significantly reduce the bacterial load that is required to trigger infection. Some microorganisms such as streptococcus may cause tissue damage at very low concentrations.[15,46] Thus quantitative microbiology does not necessarily provide an unambiguous diagnosis of infection. Under certain circumstances, quantitative biopsies may also have poor sensitivity and low reliability. Woolfrey et al.[47] showed that there was a 25% chance of missing an organism using biopsy probably due to uneven distribution of organisms within the wound bed and the techniques used to clean the specimen. Results varied by 2 logarithms (logs) in 27% of paired isolates. Ehrenkranz et al.[48] demonstrated that an irrigation-aspiration technique could produce similar results to qualitative biopsy in pressure ulcers.[49] It is not always necessary in everyday clinical practice to quantify the bacterial load through tissue biopsy or alternative invasive techniques that require expertise and timely processing in the microbiology laboratory.

Evidence for the Clinical Use of the Bacterial Swab

Evidence from comparative studies confirms that microbiology obtained by a swab may adequately correlate with qualitative findings obtained through tissue biopsy.[50,51] When plated in the laboratory bacteria are streaked in four quadrants on blood agar in a Petri dish. Growth in the fourth quadrant (the most dilute bacterial swab specimen streaking of the Petri dish) corresponds to a growth of 105 CFU/g of tissue as determined by quantitative biopsy.[46,50] In most cases the colonizing bacteria come from exogenous sources, and would be present in the superficial compartment before reaching the deep tissues.[15] Sapico et al.[26] compared pressure ulcer bacterial swab results with quantitative biopsy cultures and demonstrated a 75% concordance. In a similar comparison of diabetic foot ulcer infections Wheat et al.[52] obtained comparable bacterial culture results with swabs and tissue biopsy. There was a fairly high rate of false positive and negative results using the swab but most of the false positives were commensal organisms that did not require antimicrobial therapy. The authors concluded that 92% of antibiotic therapy choices would have been adequate based on the swab alone. Rudensky et al.,[49] on the other hand, concluded that blood samples or deep tissue biopsies are more clinically significant than bacterial swabs due to the high number of false positive isolations in the latter.

Taking a Bacterial Swab

The appropriate use of bacterial swabs is for antibacterial therapy selection and to identify the specific organisms in a chronic wound such as multiresistant bacteria.

A bacterial swab result is only as good as the technique used to obtain the specimen and the processing in the laboratory. There is much discussion about the type of swab to use and the procedure for taking a specimen. Some clinicians have recommended alginate or rayon-tipped swabs in the belief that the fatty acids contained in cotton swabs might inhibit growth in certain bacteria. However, the organisms commonly encountered in infection are likely to withstand the environment of a cotton swab. Pre-moistening a swab in the transport media is useful if the surface of the wound is dry as it can improve the yield. This is not necessary if the wound is already very moist. There are two swab culture techniques commonly used in clinical practice. In the first technique, the tip of the swab should be rolled on its side for one full rotation over the part of the wound granulation tissue with the most obvious signs of infection, avoiding slough and surface purulent discharge. A zigzag pattern can be used for sample collection on the swab surface for wounds larger than $5\,cm^2$. This technique is likely to increase the yield of nonsignificant colonizers and it may be preferable to take more than one regional swab from the upper and lower areas of the wound. An alternative technique involves pressing the swab on the surface at a single point of the granulation to express wound fluid and then rotating the swab 360° to obtain the bacterial specimen. The wound bed must first be cleaned with saline or water and superficially debrided so that the cultures from the surface of the wound more closely resemble those in the tissue. There will undoubtedly be more colonizing organisms than pathogens on the surface of the wound but there is a correlation between the pathogens found on the surface and in the deep compartments. Culture results by themselves, even results of bone culture or culture of other deep-tissue biopsy specimens, should not be used as the sole criteria for infection without clinical or histopathological evidence of infection.

Infected Wounds: Causative Species

The microbial flora in a chronic wound changes over time in a predictable fashion.[46] Clinicians often need to treat infected wounds before the results of bacterial cultures are available. In wounds of less than one month's duration there is usually a high percentage of Gram-positive organisms. In wounds of longer than one month's duration, the wound is likely to acquire multiple organisms including Gram-negatives and anaerobes in addition to the Gram-positive bacterial flora.[46] In combination with clinical signs it may be possible to attempt identification of the invading pathogens while waiting for culture results (Table 16.4).

It is widely believed that aerobic or facultative pathogens such as *Staphylococcus aureus*, *Pseudomonas aeruginosa*, and the beta-hemolytic streptococci are primarily responsible for delayed healing and infection in all types of wounds, but this has largely been based on studies in which the culture and isolation of anaerobic bacteria was minimal or omitted.[43] However, anaerobes can be highly viru-

Table 16.4. Microbial flora in a chronic wound over time

Time	Type of microorganism	Clinical and laboratory findings
First few days	Cutaneous flora	
1 to 4 weeks	Cutaneous flora accompanied by Gram-positive aerobic cocci, often streptococci, *Staphylococcus aureus*	Suppurating, Gram-positive, single species
4 weeks onwards	Cutaneous flora accompanied by Gram-negative facultative anaerobic bacteria, particularly coliforms followed by anaerobic bacteria and *Pseudomonas* spp.	Polymicrobial mixture of aerobic and anaerobic pathogens, tissue necrosis, undermining, deep involvement

lent and may be the cause of postoperative infections when routine culture fails to yield bacterial growth.[53] Traditional culture methods have underestimated the presence of anaerobic bacteria in chronic wounds. In their review, Bowler et al.[43] summarized the studies published in this area and conclude that anaerobic bacteria are found in 48% of infected wounds (compared with 38% in noninfected wounds). They conclude that there is a definite role of anaerobes in wound infection. Two studies involving pressure ulcers within the scope of this review are summarized in Table 16.5.

Is the Causative Organism Relevant?

Some studies have identified specific microorganisms responsible for delayed wound healing or wound infection, but Bowler and colleagues comment in their review that no particular colonizing species is more likely associated with infection.[43] Based on the collective evidence, the role of specific microorganisms in many kinds of infected wound is still debatable and it may be that the presence of a number of different types of organisms is the key factor. Virulence is also important: beta-hemolytic streptococci produce a number of exotoxins and spreading factors which enable them to cause infection at lower concentrations than many other organisms.[46] Most chronic wounds contain more than three species of microorganisms but not all of these organisms are pathogens.[15,56] The risk of infection may increase if more than one species are present as they may develop synergies with each other. The combined effects of aerobes and anaerobes in wounds may be synergistic, producing effects that are not seen with just one type of microorganism. Oxygen consumption by aerobic bacteria brings about tissue hypoxia, which favors the growth of anaerobic bacteria; one bacterium may produce specific nutrients that are required by other microorganisms; and some anaerobes are able to impair the host immune cell functions, providing a competitive advantage to themselves and other microorganisms.[43] Ulcers containing four or more pathogens are more likely to be associated with clinical infection.[26,57–60] In

Table 16.5. Predominant isolates in people with pressure ulcers

Study	Isolation technique, type and number of wounds	Predominant isolates
Heym et al.[54]	Swabs, deep tissue, and liquids from 101 pressure ulcers	Enterobacteria (*Enterococcus faecalis*, *Escherichia coli* and *Proteus* sp.) *Staphylococcus aureus* (MRSA > non-MRSA)
Vande Berg et al.[42]	Quantitative biopsies from 17 pressure ulcers	*Pseudomonas aeruginosa* *Staphylococcus aureus* *Acinetobacter calcoaceticus*

Infected pressure ulcer bacterial flora is polymicrobial and is often similar to that seen in some acute necrotizing soft tissue infections.[55]

a study of chronic leg ulcers, Trengove et al.[61] reported that no single microorganism or group of bacteria were more detrimental to healing than any other but that there was a significantly lower probability of healing if there were four or more bacterial groups present in the ulcer. Bowler and Davies[62] also reported that there were more species isolated in infected than in noninfected leg ulcers. A similar trend may be found in pressure ulcers but the data have not been analyzed to date. In wounds that are infected with a number of species it is often impossible to detect the specific causative role of each organism.

In conclusion, bacterial swabs or wound cultures do not diagnose infection but they can be used as guidance for antimicrobial therapy: The diagnosis of infection is based on clinical symptoms and signs.

Osteomyelitis

Deep infection, especially in ulcers of long duration, can often be complicated by underlying osteomyelitis. Osteomyelitis is caused by an infecting organism creating an inflammatory process and resulting in bone destruction.[63–68] The diagnosis of osteomyelitis under pressure ulcers is important, but is also challenging because deep signs of infection can be obscured in patients with pressure ulcers. A study of clinical signs of a single criterion for the diagnosis of osteomyelitis found a 53% accuracy rate, with sensitivity of 33% and specificity of 60%.[69] The use of a sterile probe to determine if any sinuses or deeper pocketing or undermining is present can often alert clinicians to potential deeper tissue and bony involvement. The diagnosis of bone infection in pressure ulcers should be considered in deep ulcers whenever the ulcer fails to improve with proper conventional local treatment or after removal of pressure.[69–71] Sugarman et al.[72] discovered osteomyelitis in 32% of pressure ulcers that did not respond promptly to local therapy (as early as 2 weeks). These ulcers often had surrounding erythema and drainage. Three studies detected osteomyelitis in 17 to 32% of patients with long-standing pressure ulcers,[69,70,72] with one study noting a less frequent occurrence.[73] The presence of a nonhealing wound or exposed bone did not always indicate osteomyelitis;[69] nevertheless probing to bone is a simple clinical test that may indicate osteomyelitis, especially in those with diabetic foot ulcers (Figure 16.7—see color section).[27]

The role of surface bacterial swabs to help in antibiotic selection is controversial. Some authors[15,46,50] support the idea that bacteria on the surface may eventually penetrate the deeper tissue and potentially infect bone; therefore, a swab may isolate the responsible bacteria. Other authors believe that organisms in bone cannot be accurately detected with a swab. This belief stems from evidence that sinus tract cultures do not usually correlate with those cultures obtained from the bone biopsy, except when *Staphylococcus aureus* is isolated from the sinus (it is likely to be the cause of the underlying osteomyelitis).[17,54,74] These authors conclude that bone biopsies are superior to swabs at picking infecting organisms from the bone rather than surface colonizers.

Bone biopsies remain the gold standard for diagnosing osteomyelitis in patients with pressure ulcers. If a bone biopsy is performed, one sample should be sent for culture and another for histological examination. Cultures should be performed for both aerobes and anaerobes. The most common organism isolated in any type of osteomyelitis is *Staphylococcus aureus*. Other microorganisms associated with osteomyelitis secondary to pressure ulcers are streptococci, Gram-negative bacilli, and anaerobes.[64,64] The histopathology is very important since high neutrophil counts are associated with the inflammatory response that is a marker for bone infection as distinguished from bacterial colonization. More than 5 neutrophils per high power field indicates infection with sensitivity of 43–84% and specificity of 93–97%.[75] Sugarman et al.[70] concluded that cultures of bone biopsy specimens are difficult to interpret because of bacterial colonization or infection overlying pressure sores, and with few exceptions should not be relied on unless a histological examination of bone is also performed. These observations were confirmed in a study of 36 patients where 73% of cultures from bone biopsies grew bacteria even when osteomyelitis was not considered to be present. These authors used pathological examination of bone tissue as the standard criterion for diagnosing osteomyelitis. Blood culture isolation of osteomyelitis-associated organisms occurs intermittently in a minority of cases and is less reliable than direct biopsies from the involved bone.[76,77]

Imaging studies for osteomyelitis are only helpful if combined with a proper clinical assessment of the patient as a whole. Ultrasound is helpful for detecting purulent collections in chronic osteomyelitis and in the diagnosis of acute osteomyelitis. Conventional X-rays are necessary at both presentation and follow-up, with bone destruction apparent after 10–21 days.[78-80] Computed tomography (CT) and magnetic resonance imaging (MRI) are excellent for detecting osteomyelitis. MRI has the added advantage of better soft tissue visualization and early detection. Bone scintigraphy (scanning) is generally useful because of its high negative predictive value (>90%), although the positive predictive value is only 80%.[81,82] Scintigraphy depends on the method used. Methylene diphosphonate is a good test for acute osteomyelitis. Radiolabeled leukocytes or antibody labeling scanning techniques have reported high sensitivities and even higher specificities, but they are expensive and not widely used.[81-83] Fluorodeoxyglucose-positron emission tomography (FDG-PET) combined with CT appears promising for the research setting, but is costly and unavailable to most clinicians.[63,64,84,85]

Laboratory tests commonly used in the diagnosis of osteomyelitis include total leukocyte count, erythrocyte sedimentation rate (ESR), and C-reactive protein (CRP).[86,87] For the diagnosis of osteomyelitis an elevated white blood cell count is not a reliable indicator. ESR is elevated in more than 90% (especially values over 40 mm/h) of the cases, but although it is helpful for diagnosis, its kinetics are too slow for it to be used for follow-up. CRP elevations returning to normal levels may be more reliable for follow-up of the response to treatment. It is always important to remember that ESR and CRP may be elevated for reasons other than osteomyelitis. Calcium, phosphorus, and alkaline phosphatase are elevated in metastatic bone disease.[63,64]

Treatment of Infection

Methicillin-resistant *Staphylococcus aureus* (MRSA) may be present in as many as 50–71% of all pressure ulcer inpatients in some long-term care facilities.[88] Using molecular characterization of subspecies, it has been found that patients are often infected from acute hospitals; the MRSA is then carried into the nursing home and transferred to other patients and staff. Previous studies and reviews have evalu-

Table 16.6. Infection-control recommendations

1. Reduce contamination of pressure ulcers by: sterilizing instruments for debridement applying clean dressings (except sterile dressings in immune compromised patients)

2. Healthcare workers should: use alcohol cleansers or wash hands between contacts with different patients treat the most contaminated ulcer last (patients with multiple ulcers) use sterile gloves with newly debrided or deeper pressure ulcers

3. Ulcers should be protected from sources of contamination such as feces

4. To prevent spread of pathogenic organisms from pressure ulcers: wear gloves change gloves and wash hands between patients and after any type of patient contact use additional barriers such as gowns, masks, goggles to avoid contact with clothing or skin

5. Place soiled or reusable items in securely sealed containers

6. Place needles in designated sharps containers

Source: Modified from US Department of Health and Human Services Clinical Practice Guideline No. 1594, National Pressure Ulcer Advisory Panel Recommendations.
© Dr. R. G. Sibbald.

ated the most effective methods of controlling MRSA. The results demonstrate that alcohol hand rinses are more effective for healthcare providers in preventing MRSA contamination of pressure ulcers compared to hand washing with antiseptic (chlorhexidine) soap.[89–91] The alcohol hand rinses decreased the number of bacteria on healthcare providers' and patients' hands by a number of logarithms. Another study assessing the best hand rinses found that chlorhexidine 0.5% in alcohol-based hand-rubs was the most effective agent tested.[92] Infection-control recommendations[25] from the Agency for Health Care Policy and Research for residents of long-term care facilities illustrate these principles (Table 16.6).

Superficial Bacterial Imbalance (Colonization/Critical Colonization)

Topical Antimicrobials

The aim of a topical antimicrobial is to reduce bioburden; therefore, the choice of agent is often broad spectrum or related to the identity of the causative organisms, assessed either through bacteriological culture or clinical judgment. The choice of topical agent should also include an awareness of their potential to induce sensitization. Neomycin is a well-known allergen, along with perfumes contained in the delivery vehicles.

Tables 16.7 and 16.8 list the properties of available topical antimicrobials.

Iodine

Iodine is a potent broad spectrum antiseptic agent but its role in wound management is controversial because some traditional iodine formulations (povidone iodine) have been shown in vitro to impair the functioning of cells involved in wound healing. However, in vivo this cellular toxicity was not observed, when concentrations used were below 1%.[93] Povidone iodine can significantly decrease the microbial load without accelerating healing.[94]

Improved formulations are now available which release low levels of iodine over longer periods of time (cadexomer iodine) and this low concentration of iodine has been shown to be effective against wound pathogens, without impairing wound healing.[94] The sustained release of iodine overcomes the neutralizing effect of organic material in the wound and a literature review concludes that cadexomer iodine is safe, effective, and economical in the treatment of many chronic wounds.[95] This formulation of iodine into an absorbent hydrogel dressing also acts as a debriding agent, removing pus and debris from chronic wounds.[8] Cadexomer iodine has also been shown to inhibit proliferation of MRSA in experimental wounds[94] and expert opinion now supports the role of this form of iodine in healable chronic wounds that have an increased bacterial burden in the superficial wound compartment.[96] Cadexomer iodine significantly reduces pus, debris, and pain in pressure ulcers and accelerates the healing rate. In one study, roughly 80% of the cadexomer-treated ulcers healed compared with 60% of the control ulcers.[97]

Silver

The antimicrobial properties of silver have been known about and exploited for thousands of years, even though the mechanism of action was unknown. The first documented silver preparation to be used in medicine was a 1% silver nitrate solution which was used to prevent neonatal ocular infections.[98] In 1887, Von Behring documented that 0.25% and 0.01% silver nitrate solutions were effective against typhoid and anthrax bacilli respectively.[98] In the early 1900s, hammered foil and colloidal silver were used to treat nonhealing wounds and it was noted that they brought about a decrease in erythema (rubor). In the 1920s the US Food and Drug Administration acknowledged that colloidal silver was an effective wound treatment.[99] Research into antibiotics in the 1940s shifted the emphasis away from silver and it was 30 years before Fox[100] introduced 1% silver sulfadiazine cream for the treatment of burn wounds.

Table 16.7. Topical antimicrobials used in wounds with overt/covert infection

Agent	S. aureus	MRSA	Streptococcus	Pseudomonas	Anaerobes	Comments	Summary
Cadexomer iodine	+	+	+	+	+	Also debrides Low potential for resistance Caution with thyroid disease	Safe and effective
Polymyxin B sulfate/ bacitracin zinc	+	+	+	+	+	Bacitracin in the ointment is an allergen: the cream formulation contains the less-sensitizing gramicidin	
Mupirocin	+	+				Reserve for MRSA and other resistant Gram+ spp.	
Metronidazole					+	Reserve for anaerobes and odor control. Low or no resistance of anaerobes despite systemic use	
Benzoyl peroxide	Weak	Weak	Weak		Weak	Large wounds. Can cause irritation and allergy	Use selectively
Gentamicin	+		+	+		Reserve for oral/intravenous use—topical use may encourage resistance	
Fusidin ointment	+		+			Contains lanolin (not in cream)	
Polymyxin B sulfate/ bacitracin zinc neomycin	+	+	+	+	+	Neomycin component causes allergies, and in 40% of cases cross-sensitizes to aminogycosides	Use with caution

Table 16.8. Silver preparations used in wound management

Preparation	Current use	Product name	Benefits	Disadvantages
Silver salts				
Silver nitrate	0.5% solutions in burn wounds	Silver nitrate solution	Easy to use Host cytotoxicity[105–108]	Staining Eschar formation may delay healing
Silver sulfadiazine	1% in cream for burns/wounds	Flamazine, Silvadene, SSD Cream	Low cytotoxicity in vivo[109]	Cytotoxic (in vitro);[110] broad spectrum
Silver-calcium-sodium phosphates	Co-extruded in polymer matrix; for superficial wounds with limited exudate	Arglaes	Residual antimicrobial activity lasts from 24 hours to 4 days	Limited absorption of fluid
Silver-sodium carboxy-methylcellulose dressing	Hydrofiber dressing +1.2% ionic silver (released via ion exchange)	Aquacel-AG	Provides fluid lock to prevent excess wound fluid from macerating surrounding skin	Low concentration of silver released Hydrofiber may trap bacteria
Silver coated foam	Highly exudating chronic wounds	Contreet Foam	Provides bacterial balance in a foam dressing with partial fluid trapping	Low concentration of silver released with high absorption
Silver combined with hydrocolloid	Chronic wounds with increased bacterial burden	Contreet-HC	Provides odor control under hydrocolloid dressing	Moderate fluid absorption Autolytic debridement Low concentration of silver release
Adsorbed silver				
Silver charcoal	Silver adsorbed onto charcoal for odor control	Actisorb	Silver kills organisms which are adsorbed onto the charcoal	No release of silver into the wound
Nanocrystalline silver				
Silver coating and absorptive core	Burns Chronic wounds	Acticoat Burn	Equivalent to silver nitrate in burns with less frequent dressing changes	Release of high concentration of ionized silver + absorptive of fluid
Silver coating—3 layers with two absorptive cores	Leg ulcers and other chronic wounds for up to 7 days wear time	Acticoat 7	Sustained release of bactericidal concentrations of silver over 7 days	Useful for weekly compression therapy in venous ulcers
Silver coated calcium alginate	Moderately exudating chronic wounds	Acticoat Absorbent	Provides absorption and hemostasis	Bio-absorbable controlling bacteria, fluid, and hemorrhage

Silver was first incorporated into modern dressings adsorbed onto charcoal. The silver kills bacterial organisms that are adsorbed into the dressing and the charcoal provides a wound deodorizer. Film dressings were then the backbone for a calcium sodium phosphate polymer matrix that releases most silver over the first few hours with some delayed release over the next few days, but this dressing has limited fluid handling capabilities. Several newer delayed release vehicles for silver have been developed that incorporate longer dressing wear time with moisture balance, and in some products autolytic debridement may also be available.

Silver is effective against a broad range of aerobic, anaerobic, Gram-negative and Gram-positive bacteria as well as yeast, fungi, and viruses.[101–103] Silver has an effect on bacterial DNA, enzymes, and membranes, requiring several bacterial mutations for resistant organisms to appear. It has very low mammalian cell toxicity, low sensitization potential and is not used systemically so that it is an ideal agent for superficial compartment infection treatment.

In vitro concentrations of silver as low as 10 μg/l can control bacteria. Higher concentrations are delivered in some topical wound dressings. The minimum inhibitory concentration (MIC) in wounds in one study was estimated to be between 20 and 40 μg/l.[104] A study on common wound pathogens using a complex organic growth medium found that the MIC in vitro ranged between 5 and 12.5 μg/ml.[103]

In a study of 29 chronic wound patients not healing at the expected rate, Sibbald et al.[28] applied nanocrystalline silver dressings after baseline superficial bacterial swabs and quantitative biopsies. Improved healing was related to improvement in the semiquantitative surface swabs but the deep quantitative bacterial biopsies were often unchanged. If the deep compartment was out of bacterial balance and this was delaying healing, topical silver dressings did not reverse the impaired healing response or the increased bacteria in the deep compartment requiring systemic therapy.

Uncommon or rare silver allergic sensitization has been reported but there have been no other significant adverse effects despite the large amounts of silver used in burn wound treatment. On the other hand, the nitrate molecule in silver nitrate may be pro-inflammatory while the cream base in silver sulfadiazine reacts with serious exudate to produce a pseudo-eschar which must be removed before reapplication.[105] In both of these preparations, a large excess of silver has to be supplied to the wound to compensate for inactivation; new technologies have therefore been developed to improve the controlled release of silver ions. The silver ions can provide antibacterial and anti-inflammatory properties topically as well as providing moisture balance with absorptive dressing cores as outlined in Table 16.8.

Nanocrystalline Silver

Nanocrystalline silver is composed of very small crystals of less than 20 nm where the silver may exist in a new lattice solid state.[111] In amorphous matter, atoms and molecules interact only with their nearest neighbor, whereas in crystals each component interacts with immediate and distant neighbors through the crystal lattice. During dissolution, the silver reaches a steady state where the concentration in solution is between 70 and 100 μg/ml and antimicrobial levels can be maintained in the dressing for at least 7 days. Nanocrystalline silver is effective against a broad range of bacteria, including MRSA and VRE.[28]

For over a century the anti-inflammatory effects of silver have been observed and documented but the mechanism by which silver exerted this effect was not understood. The anti-inflammatory effect was largely masked or even countered by the silver preparations available in the twentieth century (silver nitrate, silver sulfadiazine) whereas the development of nanocrystalline silver may shed some light on this mechanism. Wright et al.[112] studied matrix metalloproteinases (MMP), cell apoptosis, and healing in a porcine wound model where wounds were dressed with nanocrystalline silver, silver nitrate, and saline soaks. They suggest that the nanocrystalline silver may modulate the actions of the MMPs. Another pilot study examined the wound fluid of ten patients treated with either a nanocrystalline dressing or a control. Those patients with the active dressing had lower MMP-9 and tumor necrosis factor α (TNFα) levels relative to the controls.[112] Newer topical silver products offer variable levels of silver release with moisture balance and may have autolytic debridement properties for optimal wound bed preparation.

The European Pressure Ulcer Advisory Panel recommends that systemic antibiotics are not required for pressure ulcers that have clinical signs of local infection (or increased bacterial burden) only.[113] A period of 2 weeks would be a reasonable trial with these agents before considering systemic treatments or re-examining the treatment of the cause or the ability of the ulcer to heal. This paradigm in Figure 16.1 will now be used to illustrate the steps in the diagnosis and treatment of the role of bacteria in chronic pressure ulcers.

Case Two

Mr CP, a 45-year-old man, has been paraplegic since a motor vehicle accident 18 years ago. He developed a deep pressure ulcer over the buttocks 18 months ago and a satellite area opened up 12 cm from the original opening (Figure 16.3—see color section).

Patient as a whole:

1. Assess case. The patient's ulcer is caused by sliding from the bed to the wheelchair with friction and shearing during transfers. The problem can be corrected.

2. The patient and caregivers decided to install an automatic ceiling lift for self-transfers from the bed and to use a transfer board at other times.

Regional treatment:

3. Clinically there were increased exudates and bright red granulation tissue that was friable, with undermining and a communication between the two ulcer beds. A bacterial swab grew *S. aureus* (not MRSA) and *Pseudomonas*. The ESR was elevated at 45 (NI.20) and CRP high at 25.0. An X-ray of the pelvis was normal with no evidence of osteomyelitis.

4. The deep infection was treated with oral ciprofloxacin 500 mg twice daily and clindamycin 300 mg four times daily by mouth for 6 weeks.

5. The wounds were cleansed with saline.

6. Topical antiseptic treatment with Betadine-soaked gauze ribbon was changed daily until surgical debridement was scheduled.

7. Surgical debridement was performed to remove the bridge of tissue over the undermined wound edge.

8. Topical ionized silver impregnated foam was applied to the wound to perform autolytic debridement, surface bacterial balance, and moisture balance three times per week.

9. The wound was 25% of its initial size at week 12. Swabs showed scant *S. aureus* and ESR was 15; C-reactive protein was normal at 7.

10. The wound completely healed at 20 weeks and Mr CP adhered to his new transferring technique.

References

1. Schultz GS, Sibbald RG, Falanga V, et al. Wound bed preparation: a systematic approach to wound management. Wound Repair Regen 2003; 11(Suppl 1):S1–S28.
2. Von Renteln-Kruse W, Krause T, Anders J, et al. [High-grade pressure sores in frail older high-risk persons. A retrospective postmortem case-control-study]. Z Gerontol Geriatr 2004; 37:81–85.
3. Reddy M, Keast D, Fowler E, Sibbald RG. Pain in pressure ulcers. Ostomy Wound Manage 2003; 49:30–35.
4. Norton L, Sibbald RG. Is bed rest an effective treatment modality for pressure ulcers? Ostomy Wound Manage 2004; 50(10):44–52.
5. Kanj LF, Wilking SV, Phillips TJ. Pressure ulcers. J Am Acad Dermatol 1998; 38:517–536.
6. Vasile J, Chaitin H. Prognostic factors in decubitus ulcers of the aged. Geriatrics 1972; 27:126–129.
7. Lee BY, Trainor FS, Thoden WR. Topical application of povidone-iodine in the management of decubitus and stasis ulcers. J Am Geriatr Soc 1979; 27:302–306.
8. Drosou A, Falabella A, Kirsner RS. Antiseptics on wounds: an area of controversy. Wounds 2003; 15(5):149–166.
9. Lineaweaver W, Howard R, Soucy D, et al. Topical antimicrobial toxicity. Arch Surg 1985; 120: 267–270.
10. Rodeheaver G. Wound cleansing, wound irrigation, wound disinfection. In: Krasner DL, Rodeheaver GT, Sibbald RG (eds) Chronic wound care: a clinical source book for healthcare professionals, 3rd edn. Wayne, PA: HMP Communications; 2001: 369–383.
11. White RJ, Cooper R, Kingsley A. Wound colonization and infection: the role of topical antimicrobials. Br J Nurs 2001; 10:563–578.
12. Lawrence JC. The use of iodine as an antiseptic agent. J Wound Care 1998; 7:421–425.
13. Ayello EA, Dowsett C, Schultz GS, et al. TIME heals all wounds. Nursing. 2004; 34:36–41.
14. Sibbald RG, Orsted H, Schultz GS, et al. Preparing the wound bed 2003: focus on infection and inflammation. Ostomy Wound Manage 2003; 49:23–51.
15. Bowler PG. The 10(5) bacterial growth guideline: reassessing its clinical relevance in wound healing. Ostomy Wound Manage 2003; 49:44–53.
16. Glenchur H, Patel BS, Pathmarajah C. Transient bacteremia associated with debridement of decubitus ulcers. Mil Med 1981; 146:432–433.
17. Brem H, Lyder C. Protocol for the successful treatment of pressure ulcers. Am J Surg 2004; 188:9–17.
18. Galpin JE, Chow AW, Bayer AS, Guze LB. Sepsis associated with decubitus ulcers. Am J Med 1976; 61:346–350.
19. Reuler JB, Cooney TG. The pressure sore: pathophysiology and principles of management. Ann Intern Med 1981; 94:661–666.
20. Cunningham SC, Napolitano LM. Necrotizing soft tissue infection from decubitus ulcer after spinal cord injury. Spine 2004; 29:E172–E174.
21. Chan JW, Virgo KS, Johnson FE. Hemipelvectomy for severe decubitus ulcers in patients with previous spinal cord injury. Am J Surg 2003; 185:69–73.
22. Heggers JP. Defining infection in chronic wounds: does it matter? J Wound Care 1998; 7:389–392.
23. Parish LC, Witkowski JA. The infected decubitus ulcer. Int J Dermatol 1989; 28:643–647.
24. Cutting KF, Harding KG. Criteria for identifying wound infection. J Wound Care 1994; 5(4): 198–201.
25. Bergstrom N, Bennett MA, Carlson CE, et al. Clinical practice guideline number 15: Treatment of pressure ulcers. AHCPR Publication 95-0652. Rockville, MD: Agency for Healthcare Policy and Research (AHCPR); 1994.
26. Sapico FL, Ginunas VJ, Thornhill-Joynes M, et al. Quantitative microbiology of pressure sores in different stages of healing. Diagn Microbiol Infect Dis 1986; 5:31–38.
27. Grayson ML, Gibbons GW, Balogh K, et al. Probing to bone in infected pedal ulcers. A clinical sign of underlying osteomyelitis in diabetic patients. JAMA 1995; 273:721–723.
28. Sibbald RG, Browne AC, Coutts P, Queen D. Screening evaluation of an ionized nanocrystalline silver dressing in chronic wound care. Ostomy Wound Manage 2001; 47:38–43.
29. Gardner SE, Frantz RA, Doebbeling BN. The validity of the clinical signs and symptoms used to identify localized chronic wound infection. Wound Repair Regen 2001; 9:178–186.
30. Gardner SE, Frantz RA, Troia C, et al. A tool to assess clinical signs and symptoms of localized infection in chronic wounds: development and reliability. Ostomy Wound Manage 2001; 47:40–47.
31. Armstrong DG. Infrared dermal thermometry: the foot and ankle stethoscope. J Foot Ankle Surg 1998; 37:75–76.

32. Murff RT, Armstrong DG, Lanctot D, et al. How effective is manual palpation in detecting subtle temperature differences? Clin Podiatr Med Surg 1998; 15:151–154.

33. Diegelmann RF. Excessive neutrophils characterize chronic pressure ulcers. Wound Repair Regen 2003; 11:490–495.

34. Sibbald RG, Coutts P, Freiheller M, et al. Use of nanocrystalline silver dressing in the treatment of non-healing venous ulcers. In preparation. 2004.

35. Dow, G. Infection in chronic wounds. In: Krasner DL, Rodeheaver GT, Sibbald RG (eds) Chronic wound care: A clinical source book for healthcare professionals, 3rd edn. Wayne, PA: HMP Communications; 2001: 343–356.

36. Bendy RH, Jr, Nuccio PA, Wolfe E, et al. Relationship of quantitative wound bacterial counts to healing of decubiti: effect of topical gentamicin. Antimicrob Agents Chemother 1964; 10:147–155.

37. Robson MC, Lea CE, Dalton JB, Heggers JP. Quantitative bacteriology and delayed wound closure. Surg Forum 1968; 19:501–502.

38. Robson MC, Heggers JP. Bacterial quantification of open wounds. Mil Med 1969; 134:19–24.

39. Robson MC, Heggers JP. Delayed wound closure based on bacterial counts. J Surg Oncol 1970; 2:379–383.

40. Vande Berg JS, Rudolph R. Cultured myofibroblasts: a useful model to study wound contraction and pathological contracture. Ann Plast Surg 1985; 14:111–120.

41. Vande Berg JS, Rudolph R. Pressure (decubitus) ulcer: variation in histopathology—a light and electron microscope study. Hum Pathol 1995; 26:195–200.

42. Vande Berg JS, Rudolph R, Hollan C, Haywood-Reid PL. Fibroblast senescence in pressure ulcers. Wound Repair Regen 1998; 6:38–49.

43. Bowler PG, Duerden BI, Armstrong DG. Wound microbiology and associated approaches to wound management. Clin Microbiol Rev 2001; 14:244–269.

44. Robson MC, Duke WF, Krizek TJ. Rapid bacterial screening in the treatment of civilian wounds. J Surg Res 1973; 14:426–430.

45. Tenorio A, Jindrak K, Weiner M, et al. Accelerated healing in infected wounds. Surg Gynecol Obstet 1976; 142:537–543.

46. Dow G, Browne A, Sibbald RG. Infection in chronic wounds: controversies in diagnosis and treatment. Ostomy Wound Manage 1999; 45:23–40.

47. Woolfrey BF, Fox JM, Quall CO. An evaluation of burn wound quantitative microbiology. I. Quantitative eschar cultures. Am J Clin Pathol 1981; 75:532–537.

48. Ehrenkranz NJ, Alfonso B, Nerenberg D. Irrigation-aspiration for culturing draining decubitus ulcers: correlation of bacteriological findings with a clinical inflammatory scoring index. J Clin Microbiol 1990; 28:2389–2393.

49. Rudensky B, Lipschits M, Isaacsohn M, Sonnenblick M. Infected pressure sores: comparison of methods for bacterial identification. South Med J 1992; 85:901–903.

50. Dow G. Bacterial swabs and the chronic wound: when, how, and what do they mean? Ostomy Wound Manage 2003; 49:8–13.

51. Hill KE, Davies CE, Wilson MJ, et al. Molecular analysis of the microflora in chronic venous leg ulceration. J Med Microbiol 2003; 52:365–369.

52. Wheat LJ, Allen SD, Henry M, et al. Diabetic foot infections. Bacteriologic analysis. Arch Intern Med 1986; 146:1935–1940.

53. Nichols RL, Smith JW. Anaerobes from a surgical perspective. Clin Infect Dis 1994; 18(Suppl 4): S280–S286.

54. Heym B, Rimareix F, Lortat-Jacob A, Nicolas-Chanoine MH. Bacteriological investigation of infected pressure ulcers in spinal cord-injured patients and impact on antibiotic therapy. Spinal Cord 2004; 42:230–234.

55. Kingston D, Seal DV. Current hypotheses on synergistic microbial gangrene. Br J Surg 1990; 77:260–264.

56. Bucknall TE. The effect of local infection upon wound healing: an experimental study. Br J Surg 1980; 67:851–855.

57. Eriksson G, Eklund AE, Kallings LO. The clinical significance of bacterial growth in venous leg ulcers. Scand J Infect Dis 1984; 16:175–180.

58. Gilchrist B, Reed C. The bacteriology of chronic venous ulcers treated with occlusive hydrocolloid dressings. Br J Dermatol 1989; 121:337–344.

59. Annoni F, Rosina M, Chiurazzi D, Ceva M. The effects of a hydrocolloid dressing on bacterial growth and the healing process of leg ulcers. Int Angiol 1989; 8:224–228.

60. Handfield-Jones SE, Grattan CE, Simpson RA, Kennedy CT. Comparison of a hydrocolloid dressing and paraffin gauze in the treatment of venous ulcers. Br J Dermatol 1988; 118:425–427.

61. Trengove NJ, Stacey MC, McGechie DF, Mata S. Qualitative bacteriology and leg ulcer healing. J Wound Care 1996; 5:277–280.
62. Bowler PG, Davies BJ. The microbiology of infected and noninfected leg ulcers. Int J Dermatol 1999; 38:573–578.
63. Lew DP, Waldvogel FA. Osteomyelitis. N Engl J Med. 1997; 336:999–1007.
64. Lew DP, Waldvogel FA. Osteomyelitis. Lancet 2004; 364:369–379.
65. Waldvogel FA, Medoff G, Swartz MN. Treatment of osteomyelitis. N Engl J Med 1970; 283: 822.
66. Waldvogel FA, Medoff G, Swartz MN. Osteomyelitis: a review of clinical features, therapeutic considerations and unusual aspects. N Engl J Med 1970; 282:198–206.
67. Waldvogel FA, Medoff G, Swartz MN. Osteomyelitis: a review of clinical features, therapeutic considerations and unusual aspects. 3. Osteomyelitis associated with vascular insufficiency. N Engl J Med 1970; 282:316–322.
68. Waldvogel FA, Papageorgiou PS. Osteomyelitis: the past decade. N Engl J Med 1980; 303:360–370.
69. Darouiche RO, Landon GC, Klima M, et al. Osteomyelitis associated with pressure sores. Arch Intern Med 1994; 154:753–758.
70. Sugarman B. Pressure sores and underlying bone infection. Arch Intern Med 1987; 147:553–555.
71. Thornhill-Joynes M, Gonzales F, Stewart CA, et al. Osteomyelitis associated with pressure ulcers. Arch Phys Med Rehabil 1986; 67:314–318.
72. Sugarman B, Hawes S, Musher DM, et al. Osteomyelitis beneath pressure sores. Arch Intern Med 1983; 143:683–688.
73. Brandeis GH, Morris JN, Nash DJ, Lipsitz LA. The epidemiology and natural history of pressure ulcers in elderly nursing home residents. JAMA 1990; 264:2905–2909.
74. Mackowiak PA, Jones SR, Smith JW. Diagnostic value of sinus-tract cultures in chronic osteomyelitis. JAMA 1978; 239:2772–2775.
75. Abdul-Karim FW, McGinnis MG, Kraay M, et al. Frozen section biopsy assessment for the presence of polymorphonuclear leukocytes in patients undergoing revision of arthroplasties. Mod Pathol 1998; 11:427–431.
76. Howard CB, Einhorn M, Dagan R, et al. Fine-needle bone biopsy to diagnose osteomyelitis. J Bone Joint Surg Br 1994; 76:311–314.
77. Jacobson IV, Sieling WL. Microbiology of secondary osteomyelitis. Value of bone biopsy. S Afr Med J 1987; 72:476–477.
78. Gold RH, Hawkins RA, Katz RD. Bacterial osteomyelitis: findings on plain radiography, CT, MR, and scintigraphy. AJR Am J Roentgenol 1991; 157:365–370.
79. Kaim AH, Gross T, von Schulthess GK. Imaging of chronic posttraumatic osteomyelitis. Eur Radiol 2002; 12:1193–1202.
80. Santiago RC, Gimenez CR, McCarthy K. Imaging of osteomyelitis and musculoskeletal soft tissue infections: current concepts. Rheum Dis Clin North Am 2003; 29:89–109.
81. Peters AM. The use of nuclear medicine in infections. Br J Radiol 1998; 71:252–261.
82. Tumeh SS, Tohmeh AG. Nuclear medicine techniques in septic arthritis and osteomyelitis. Rheum Dis Clin North Am 1991; 17:559–583.
83. Oyen WJ, van H, Jr, Claessens RA, Slooff TJ, et al. Diagnosis of bone, joint, and joint prosthesis infections with In-111-labeled nonspecific human immunoglobulin G scintigraphy. Radiology 1992; 182:195–199.
84. Robiller FC, Stumpe KD, Kossmann T, et al. Chronic osteomyelitis of the femur: value of PET imaging. Eur Radiol 2000; 10:855–858.
85. Schmitz A, Kalicke T, Willkomm P, et al. Use of fluorine-18 fluoro-2-deoxy-D-glucose positron emission tomography in assessing the process of tuberculous spondylitis. J Spinal Disord 2000; 13:541–544.
86. Hovi I, Valtonen M, Korhola O, Hekali P. Low-field MR imaging for the assessment of therapy response in musculoskeletal infections. Acta Radiol 1995; 36:220–227.
87. Lewis VL, Jr, Bailey MH, Pulawski G, et al. The diagnosis of osteomyelitis in patients with pressure sores. Plast Reconstr Surg 1988; 81:229–232.
88. Capitano B, Leshem OA, Nightingale CH, Nicolau DP. Cost effect of managing methicillin-resistant Staphylococcus aureus in a long-term care facility. J Am Geriatr Soc 2003; 51:10–16.
89. Girou E, Loyeau S, Legrand P, et al. Efficacy of handrubbing with alcohol based solution versus standard handwashing with antiseptic soap: randomised clinical trial. BMJ 2002; 325: 362.
90. Girard R, Amazian K, Fabry J. Better compliance and better tolerance in relation to a well-conducted introduction to rub-in hand disinfection. J Hosp Infect 2001; 47:131–137.

91. Pittet D, Hugonnet S, Harbarth S, et al. Effectiveness of a hospital-wide programme to improve compliance with hand hygiene. Infection Control Programme. Lancet 2000; 356:1307–1312.

92. Rochon-Edouard S, Pons JL, Veber B, et al. Comparative in vitro and in vivo study of nine alcohol-based handrubs. Am J Infect Control 2004; 32:200–204.

93. Burks RI. Povidone-iodine solution in wound treatment. Phys Ther 1998; 78:212–218.

94. Mertz PM, Oliveira-Gandia MF, Davis SC. The evaluation of a cadexomer iodine wound dressing on methicillin resistant Staphylococcus aureus (MRSA) in acute wounds. Dermatol Surg 1999; 25:89–93.

95. Sundberg J, Meller R. A retrospective review of the use of cadexomer iodine in the treatment of chronic wounds. Wounds 1997; 9:68–86.

96. Gilchrist B. Should iodine be reconsidered in wound management? European Tissue Repair Society. J Wound Care 1997; 6:148–150.

97. Moberg S, Hoffman L, Grennert ML, Holst A. A randomized trial of cadexomer iodine in decubitus ulcers. J Am Geriatr Soc 1983; 31:462–465.

98. Grier N. Silver and its compounds. In: Block SS (ed) Disinfection, sterilization and preservation, 3rd edn. Philadelphia, PA: Lea & Febiger; 1983.

99. Hollinger MA. Toxicological aspects of topical silver pharmaceuticals. Crit Rev Toxicol 1996; 26:255–260.

100. Fox CL, Jr. Silver sulfadiazine—a new topical therapy for Pseudomonas in burns. Therapy of Pseudomonas infection in burns. Arch Surg 1968; 96:184–188.

101. Wright JB, Lam K, Burrell RE. Wound management in an era of increasing bacterial antibiotic resistance: a role for topical silver treatment. Am J Infect Control 1998; 26:572–577.

102. Wright JB, Lam K, Hansen D, Burrell RE. Efficacy of topical silver against fungal burn wound pathogens. Am J Infect Control 1999; 27:344–350.

103. Yin HQ, Langford R, Burrell RE. Comparative evaluation of the antimicrobial activity of ACTICOAT antimicrobial barrier dressing. J Burn Care Rehabil 1999; 20:195–200.

104. Ricketts CR, Lowbury EJ, Lawrence JC, et al. Mechanism of prophylaxis by silver compounds against infection of burns. BMJ 1970; i:444–446.

105. Demling RH, De Santi L. Effects of silver on wound management. Wounds 2001; 13(Suppl A):4.

106. Bader KF. Organ deposition of silver following silver nitrate therapy of burns. Plast Reconstr Surg 1966; 37:550–551.

107. Coombs CJ, Wan AT, Masterton JP, et al. Do burn patients have a silver lining? Burns 1992; 18:179–184.

108. Hall RE, Bender G, Marquis RE. In vitro effects of low intensity direct current generated silver on eukaryotic cells. J Oral Maxillofac Surg 1988; 46:128–133.

109. Paddock HN, Schultz GS, Perrin KJ, et al. Clinical assessment of silver coated antimicrobial dressing on MMPs and cytokine levels in non-healing wounds. Annual Meeting of the Pressure Wound Healing Society, 28 May 2002.

110. McCauley RL, Linares HA, Pelligrini V, et al. In vitro toxity of topical antimicrobial agents to human fibroblasts. J Surg Res 1989; 46:267–274.

111. Birringer R. Nanocrystalline materials. Mat Sci Eng 1989; A117:33–43.

112. Wright JB, Lam K, Buret AG, et al. Early healing events in a porcine model of contaminated wounds: effects of nanocrystalline silver on matrix metalloproteinases, cell apoptosis, and healing. Wound Repair Regen 2002; 10:141–151.

113. European Pressure Ulcer Advisory Panel. Guidelines on treatment of pressure ulcers. EPUAP Review 1999; 1:31–33.

17 Litigation

Courtney H. Lyder

Introduction

The development of pressure ulcers can often be viewed by the legal community as a violation in quality of care. Patients and/or family members may perceive their development as a failure in the healthcare system. When there is a lack of explanation as to its development and/or unavoidability patients and/or family members may seek legal remedies.

Many pressure ulcer cases are often settled through an inquiry by a health trust. However, when families are not satisfied, families may seek financial remedies. Coupled with this is the growing number of pressure ulcer cases (usually the worst cases) being publicized in local or national media as evidence of poor healthcare or a failing healthcare system.

Explanations in the media concerning their development may range from patients being exposed to untrained healthcare professionals to lack of appropriate nursing to patient–staff ratios. Often the media may give the lay community the perception that all pressure ulcers are avoidable. Thus, when pressure ulcers do develop, patients and/or families may have more incentive to pursue legal recourse.

This chapter will review several key factors that may place healthcare providers and healthcare systems at risk for litigation. It should be noted that the legal systems in various European countries may vary. However, the concept of proving negligence remains a universal principle. This chapter will also highlight essential documentation that could decrease healthcare provider exposure to litigation.

Litigation

A growing number of health professionals view the development of pressure ulcers as negligent care by a healthcare provider or healthcare system. One German study investigating 10,222 corpses found a pressure ulcer prevalence rate of 11.2%.[1] Although the majority of corpses were elderly, the investigators concluded that the majority of physicians did not correlate fatality (e.g. sepsis) with pressure ulcer development. These investigators further concluded that pressure ulcer prevalence rates are an excellent indicator to determine quality of nursing and medical care.

The increasing use of pressure ulcers as a quality indicator on nursing and medical care has led to increased litigation. Healthcare systems continue to place themselves unduly at risk of litigation due to lack of proactive pressure ulcer prevention. One retrospective study investigating hospital litigation in the United Kingdom found that there was a lack of comprehensive preventive measures implemented in UK hospitals. Because of the dearth of comprehensive pressure ulcer prevention strategies being used, amounts of £3500 to £12,500 were usually awarded, with a few cases receiving damages in excess of £100,000.[2]

Although Europe continues to have increasing litigation, it appears that the USA leads in awarding damages. Presently, throughout the USA plaintiff attorneys place advertisements on billboards, newspapers, and television seeking pressure ulcer cases. A retrospective study investigating typical pressure ulcer awards in the USA found that awards ranged from $5000 to $82,000,000, with a median award of approximately $250,000 reported.[3]

The following case study highlights elements of how healthcare providers and healthcare institutions can be easily exposed to litigation.

An 87-year-old woman was admitted to hospital with history of a closed stage 4 pressure ulcer on right hip, peripheral vascular disease, non-insulin dependent diabetes mellitus, left cerebral vascular accident, hypertension, and urinary incontinence. A pressure ulcer risk assessment scale was completed indicating that the patient was at mild risk for pressure ulcers. The patient was placed on a standard mattress, turned every two hours while in bed and chair. On day 2 of hospital admission, a nurse indicated an "erythematic" area on the right hip and heel. By day 5, a stage 2 pressure ulcer was noted on the right hip and heel. A hydrocolloid dressing was placed on the right hip and nothing was ordered for the heel. The charts noted that a tissue viability nurse would be consulted.

This case highlights some common errors made by the hospital staff. First, the patient was at high risk for pressure ulcers since she had multiple health conditions that placed her at risk (closed stage 4 pressure ulcer on right hip, peripheral vascular disease, non-insulin-dependent diabetes mellitus, left cerebral vascular accident, hypertension, and urinary incontinence). Moreover, the risk assessment tool placed her at mild risk. This is an important factor, indicating that the tool may have been completed incorrectly. It also highlights an important fact that no pressure ulcer risk assessment tool has 100% sensitivity and specificity.[4] Thus, independent of the risk assessment tool used, a patient may be at risk for pressure ulcers, so continuous assessments must be conducted. The patient was placed only on a standard mattress. Given the patient's high risk level, a dynamic surface (alternating air mattress or low-air-loss mattress) might have been preferable. Of concern, although erythematic areas were identified on the patient, no interventions were undertaken until the development of the stage 2 pressure ulcers. Clearly, at this point in time, the tissue was breaking down. The lack of intervention for both stage 1 pressure ulcers clearly placed the patient at greater risk for further development. Finally, of concern was the lack of treatment noted for the stage 2 pressure ulcer on her left heel. Although the heels can be difficult to manage, no off-loading was used to salvage the heel. In this case study, it was obvious that additional preventive measures were not instituted, nor was aggressive treatment used in a timely manner; thus these pressure ulcers might have been avoided. Given the paucity of information documented, both the hospital and healthcare providers are exposed to litigation.

Negligence

The above case study could occur anywhere in the world. Thus, any healthcare provider could be exposed to litigation when caring for a patient with a pressure ulcer. In the above case study, the plaintiff attorney may be able to demonstrate that the hospital was negligent in providing care to the patient. This is based on their lack of ability to complete an appropriate risk assessment and to follow it with appropriate preventive strategies and timely pressure ulcer interventions. Because of a dearth of documentation, the plaintiff attorney is left with many conjectures on the quality of care provided. A plaintiff attorney has to show that three major factors were met to prove negligence. These three factors are accountability, causation, and breach of standard of care.[5] When all three factors have been met, the verdict will usually be for the plaintiff.

Accountability

A breach of accountability must be proved in any negligence case. Thus, the plaintiff was owed a duty of care, and this duty of care was breached. Moreover, the breach of care resulted in permanent damage or injury, and the plaintiff is owed compensation due to the injury. This factor is easily acknowledged since any patient who enters a hospital, nursing home, or home care setting is owed a certain level of care by healthcare providers. If there is a violation of the healthcare system's policies and procedures or inconsistency in providing care not consistent with level of education of the healthcare provider, these may all be indications of breaching accountability. Further, since pressure ulcers can develop when preventive measures are not implemented or if an existing pressure ulcer exists but the medical team does not treat it adequately, it is very easy for the plaintiff to meet this standard.

Causation

Causation examines whether the harm suffered by the patient was a reasonable, foreseeable consequence of the breach of the duty of care. Most pressure ulcers do not result in death of the patient. In fact, it has been noted that only approximately 5% of pressure ulcers lead to osteomyelitis; however, they may expose the patient to cellulitis or pain.[6] Because there are numerous factors associated with pressure ulcer development, failure to recognize a risk factor (e.g. poor nutrition, immobility, etc.) and provide immediate remedies may make it possible for a plaintiff attorney to associate the failure with causation. Furthermore, when there is a dearth of documentation demonstrating interventions for prevention and/or treatment provided, this can make proving causation easy.

Standard of Care

The last key factor to prove in negligence is a breach of the standard of care by nursing and/or medical staff. It is important to note that the standard of care is not at the level of an expert, but rather that of an average healthcare professional. Most often, nursing and medical experts are used to determine the expected skill mix of the average healthcare provider related to wound care. Which healthcare experts are used to evaluate a medical record will be dictated by which discipline is implicated in the plaintiff case. Hence physician experts would comment on medical practice, whereas a nurse expert would appraise the nursing care provided. If national pressure ulcer prevention and treatment guidelines exist in a particular European country, often they will guide the healthcare expert/consultant opinions. A US retrospective study investigating the impact of implementing and complying with pressure ulcer practice guidelines in 49 plaintiff cases with compensations worth $14,418,770 estimated that if guidelines had been used, these could have saved the defendants $11,389,989 in litigation.[7]

Although the development and use of pressure ulcer guidelines has been prolific, their implementation can be costly. One British study found that costs for implementing support surface replacements could range from £100 for some foam overlays to over £30,000 for some bed replacements.[8] These costs do not take into account the continued maintenance of such support surfaces. This is especially challenging when the daily cost of managing a pressure ulcer ranges from £38 to £196.[9] Thus, the challenge for healthcare systems of allocating funds for prevention and/or treatment may strain a healthcare system. However, the alternative for healthcare systems would be greater exposure to pressure ulcer litigation.

Documentation to Reduce Litigation Exposure

Good and thoughtful documentation remains the single best measure to decrease a healthcare provider's exposure to litigation. Although it does not guarantee 100% that the healthcare provider will be litigation free, it does ensure that the healthcare provider will be better positioned to defend their practice. It is also important to note that most cases are not brought to trial for several years, so there is an increasing dependence on the medical record to reconstruct the care that was provided. Essential documentation should include the following, independent of healthcare setting.[10]

Prevention of Pressure Ulcers

1. Risk assessment tool (e.g. Waterlow, Norton, Braden scales)
2. Daily skin assessment
3. Repositioning (off-loading) and turning schedules
4. Use of support surfaces to address pressure redistribution (both bed and chair)
5. Moisture control from perspiration, and urinary and fecal incontinence
6. Nutritional assessment and supplementation when appropriate
7. Education of patient and/or family

Treatment of Pressure Ulcers

1. Regular assessment/reassessment of the wound (daily, weekly, etc.)
2. Characteristics of the ulcer
   (a) length
   (b) width
   (c) depth
   (d) exudate amount
   (e) tissue type
   (f) pain
3. Local wound care
   (a) wound bed preparation
4. Repositioning (off-loading) and turning schedules
5. Use of support surfaces to address pressure redistribution (both bed and chair)
6. Moisture control from perspiration, and urinary and fecal incontinence
7. Nutritional assessment and supplementation when appropriate
8. Use of adjunctive therapies (e.g. negative pressure wound therapy, electrical stimulation, etc.)
9. Education of patient and/or family

Conclusion

As healthcare consumers become more educated about pressure ulcers, healthcare providers will become increasingly exposed to litigation. Thus, it is vitally important for healthcare providers to document the quality of care that is delivered. More importantly, it is critical for healthcare providers to increase communication with patients and/or families to discuss the issue of avoidable and unavoidable pressure ulcers, which may temper the expectations of both patients and their families.

References

1. Tsokos M, Heinemann A, Puschel K. Pressure sores: epidemiology, medico-legal implications and forensic argumentation concerning causality. Int J Legal Med 2000; 113:283–287.
2. Franks PJ. Health economics: The cost to nations. In: Morrison MJ (ed) The prevention and treatment of pressure ulcers. Edinburgh: Mosby; 2001: 52–53.
3. Bennett RG, O'Sullivan J, DeVito EM, Remsberg R. The increasing medical malpractice risk related to pressure ulcers in the United States. J Am Geriatr Soc 2000; 48(1):73–81.
4. Lyder C. Exploring pressure ulcer prevention and management. JAMA 2003; 289:223–226.
5. Dimond B. Pressure ulcers and litigation. Nurs Times 2003; 99:61–63.
6. Lyder C. Pressure ulcers. In: Geriatric review syllabus: A core curriculum in geriatric medicine, 5th edn. New York: American Geriatrics Society; 2002: 202–209.
7. Goebel RH, Goebel MR. Clinical practice guidelines for pressure ulcer prevention can prevent malpractice lawsuits in older patients. J Wound Ostomy Continence Nurs 1999; 26:175–184.
8. NHS. 2002 (www.guideline.gov/summary).
9. Bennett G, Dealey C, Posnett J. The cost of pressure ulcers in the UK. Age Ageing 2004; 33:230–235.
10. Lyder C. Regulation and wound care. In: Baranoski S, Ayello E (eds) Wound care essentials: Practice principles. Springhouse, PA: Lippincott Williams & Wilkins; 2003: 35–46.

18 The Development, Dissemination, and Use of Pressure Ulcer Guidelines

R.T. van Zelm, Michael Clark, and Jeen R.E. Haalboom

Introduction

Clinical guidelines have been defined as "systematically developed statement(s) to assist practitioner and patient decisions about appropriate health care for specific clinical circumstances."[1] In this definition the use of "assist" clearly indicates that a successful guideline does not seek to compel practitioners to practice in a rigid, inflexible manner but rather that evidence-based or evidence-linked recommendations are offered to help reduce inequities in healthcare provision. While clinical guidelines are a relatively recent phenomenon, there are now a wide range of national and international clinical guidelines that address pressure ulcer prevention and/or management[2] beginning with the consensus guidelines developed in the Netherlands in 1985,[3] through the US Agency for Health Care Policy and Research guidance issued in the early 1990s (on prevention[4] and treatment[5]) to European guidelines developed by the European Pressure Ulcer Advisory Panel (EPUAP).[6,7] Recently the wheel has turned full circle with the development of new national guidelines in both the Netherlands and the UK under the respective auspices of the Dutch Institute for Healthcare Improvement (CBO),[8] and the National Institute for Clinical Excellence (NICE).[9] The CBO is an independent, not-for-profit organization advising on clinical guideline development across the whole spectrum of healthcare, while NICE was established as a Special Health Authority within England and Wales in April 1999. Working within the UK National Health Service, NICE seeks to deliver "authoritative, robust and reliable guidance" (www.nice.org.uk) regarding what constitutes best practice, with this information available to all consumers, be they patients, the public, or the health professionals.

The wealth of pressure ulcer guidelines has been developed using a variety of methods that seek to synthesize the available scientific and clinical knowledge available during each guideline's development. Early national guidelines, for example the Dutch guidelines of 1985 (prevention) and 1986 (treatment), were developed using informal consensus techniques. Later guidelines such as those of the US Agency for Health Care Policy and Research (AHCPR) were based on formal consensus techniques, with more recent guidelines seeking to be based solely upon the best practices of evidence-based medicine.

This chapter discusses the evolution of pressure ulcer guideline development using the new Dutch guidelines as examples of evidence-based national guidelines. Beyond guideline evolution aspects of their dissemination, implementation, and appraisal will also be considered.

The Evolution of Pressure Ulcer Guidelines

Consensus guideline development processes, using either informal or formal techniques, has until recently been the foundation of many pressure ulcer guidelines. Informal consensus methods such as those employed during the development of the EPUAP pressure ulcer prevention and treatment guidelines in the late 1990s rely upon the collective experience and knowledge of the guideline panel. There are no attempts to ensure that all the relevant literature is searched or appraised when deriving practice recommendations, leaving the guideline vulnerable to being driven by panel members with the greatest authority rather than the recommendations flowing from scientific evidence. To overcome this problem, formal consensus strategies have been used since the early 1990s with these introducing literature searches, the use of Delphi methods, and weighed consensus techniques. Usually, both informal and formal consensus guidelines are discussed in draft format within open public meetings with a panel established to sift the evidence and opinions presented and then derive the final recommendations.

Evidence-Based Pressure Ulcer Guidelines—the Development Process

In contrast to consensus driven guidelines, those that claim to be evidence-based explicitly seek to integrate the best available research evidence with both clinical expertise and patient preferences and values. These evidence-based guidelines, almost regardless of their country of origin, are typically developed following a clearly defined process that includes seven key stages:

1. Development of the guideline scope and purpose
2. Development of the draft guideline
3. External review of the draft
4. Endorsement of the revised guideline
5. Publication and dissemination
6. Implementation
7. Evaluation and updating

In the first step, the topic of the guideline is selected and defined; within NICE this process involves the creation of a scope document which sets out the limits of the guideline. For example, the recent NICE guideline on pressure-relieving support surfaces was preceded by a scope document that set out the technologies to be included in the review, the care settings to be considered, and the patient populations that the guideline was intended to cover. This scope document is circulated to registered stakeholders including professional bodies, patient groups, and the relevant healthcare manufacturers. Once a scope document is agreed, this limits the work of the guideline development group (GDG), who cannot stray outside the agreed limits of the guideline. Having established the scope of the guideline, then a GDG is formed and a chair identified. This group includes representatives from all parties likely to be affected by the guideline (excluding manufacturers) along with subject experts and technical support (literature reviewers, economists, for example), the key questions to be addressed by the GDG being already identified

> **Box 18.1** Preparation of the scope
>
> The development, or rather the revision, of the Dutch guideline started with a project aimed at developing clinical indicators for several topics, including pressure ulcers. A committee of pressure ulcer researchers was formed to develop clinical indicators for professionals; initially these were to be drawn from the CBO guideline on pressure ulcers—first revision (1992). During this process the committee came to view this guideline as being outdated given that the available scientific evidence on pressure ulcers was believed to have grown significantly since 1992. The original committee was then extended with clinical experts and started the development of the new guideline. The key questions were based on the previous guideline.
>   The questions were:
>
> - What is the most effective method for risk assessment?
> - Which are effective preventive measures?
> - What are the relevant aspects in diagnosing and staging of pressure ulcers?
> - What are effective treatments?

through the scope document. The definition of the guideline topic and the subsequent steps in its development are illustrated in the following text boxes using the new Dutch guideline as a specific example (Box 18.1).

The second stage is the creation of the draft guideline by the GDG with the recommendations based upon a systematic search of the literature and preexisting guidelines (Box 18.2). Technical reports will be produced to summarize the body of relevant research evidence and the draft recommendations based on this review. At this stage the recommendations will be weighted to reflect the strength of the evidence base that underpins each recommendation. The draft guideline will typically be circulated to all stakeholders for their comments.

The third step finalizes the external review by stakeholders (Box 18.3); all comments passed on the draft guideline will be considered and the text of the guideline revised if required. At this stage the revised guideline will be circulated once again to stakeholders to gain their acceptance of the revised document. While NICE tends to refine draft guidelines through written submissions from registered

> **Box 18.2** Development of draft guideline
>
> This phase started with a search for existing guidelines and for scientific literature in several databases including Cochrane, Medline, Embase, and Cinahl from 1992 through to July 2000. The literature was then appraised and graded, using a Cochrane-like grading system.
>   Based on the literature, recommendations were formulated to answer the key questions. The guideline committee met several times to discuss the conclusions and to finalize the draft guideline.

Box 18.3 External review/endorsement

The draft guideline has not been tested in practice but a consensus of experts was achieved during a national meeting in which over 500 professionals participated. Each participant received the draft guideline and a set of forms to give their written comments before the national meeting. Some of these comments were discussed during the meeting; the rest of the comments were addressed by the committee in two meetings after the national meeting. Finally, based on the discussions during the national meeting and on the written comments, the final version of the guideline was drawn up.

stakeholders, this review process can also be undertaken through open (national) meetings. In some cases a pilot implementation phase may be adopted to explore the use of the draft guideline in clinical practice. Once external review is complete, then the final version of the guideline will be formally endorsed by the organization(s) responsible for creating the guideline; this endorsement may be explicit or implied through the publication of the guideline by organizations such as NICE.

The final version of the guideline is then widely disseminated to all groups that may implement the guideline (Box 18.4). This dissemination may take many forms, with the guideline often available in versions for clinicians and patients and as a full technical report including information about the details of the methods used to identify and appraise evidence. Increasingly dissemination of clinical guidelines occurs through the availability of PDF versions of the documents available over the internet.

Once a guideline is disseminated the next stage lies with achieving its implementation into practice (Box 18.5). Although this step has traditionally been seen as the responsibility of health professionals and their workplace, there has been a growing trend towards guideline developers suggesting appropriate intervention strategies and tactics.

The final step completes the development cycle by evaluating the impact of the guideline in clinical practice and using the fruit of this evaluation to refine the scope and content of the guideline as new evidence emerges (Box 18.6). These processes involve monitoring compliance with the recommendations of the guide-

Box 18.4 Publication and dissemination

The guideline has been published as a book and on the internet (www.cbo.nl) in Portable Document Format (PDF). Furthermore, three copies of the guideline have been sent to all Dutch acute care hospitals. A number of articles summarizing the guideline have been published. Sending copies of clinical guidelines to acute care hospitals is a standard mode of guideline diffusion used by the CBO. However, many other relevant care settings (e.g. nursing homes) did not receive the guideline, leaving staff in these sectors having to search for the guideline on the internet or to order it directly from the CBO.

> **Box 18.5** Implementation
>
> To facilitate implementation, two related products were developed. In the first a summary card showing the key recommendations for risk assessment, prevention, classification, and treatment was developed. The second project developed a set of clinical indicators. For each activity (assessment, prevention, classification, and treatment) process and outcome indicators were identified. For example, when considering risk assessment, the process indicator is the percentage of patients assessed using a formal risk assessment. The outcome measure is the incidence of patients developing pressure ulcers despite the formal risk assessment having been performed. There has been pilot implementation of these indicators in nine institutes.[12]

line, evaluating the change in the processes and outcomes of care that flow from guideline implementation, and planning scheduled reviews of the evidence base— in this last case many guidelines have scheduled review dates. However, how many of these are actually reviewed at the "due date" following changes in heath priorities and policies is unclear.

The above description of the processes involved in developing, disseminating, and implementing evidence-based guidelines in pressure ulcer prevention and management highlights that this is not a simple process and requires the coordinated effort of many individuals and professional groups. Traveling from defining the scope of the guideline to its evaluation in practice may take several years and this exacting process highlights the extent of the evolution of pressure ulcer guidelines from the early informal consensus documents to today's evidence-based guideline industry.

Removing Barriers to the Dissemination, Implementation, and Monitoring of Pressure Ulcer Guidelines

Given that the dissemination of clinical guidelines forms part of their development process, what about implementation? For if this step is not undertaken then regardless of the rigor of the development process the guideline will effectively sit on a shelf, and not contribute to improving the care of patients.

There are many steps towards guideline implementation and one of these lies in the recognition of barriers to guideline use. Clark[10] reported the five key barriers to

> **Box 18.6** Evaluation and updating
>
> There has not yet been an evaluation of the guideline although indicators are available for this evaluation to be performed. The guideline proposed that revision of its recommendations may be required by a "due date" in 2007. If revision is considered necessary in 2007 a new guideline development group will be formed to undertake the revision.

wound care guideline use in the United Kingdom—lack of resources, lack of aware-ness of the guideline content, a lack of acceptance of the recommendations, uncer-tainty as to how to monitor successful implementation, and the perceived failure of the guideline to identify best practice. There are many tactics available to help over-come some of these barriers—in particular, the use of implementation aids, clini-cal indicators, and protocols or integrated care pathways deserves mention. Implementation aids are intended to help professionals to easily access and act upon the guideline and can take the form of summary cards or quick reference sheets, decision algorithms or electronic devices such as clinical support systems or handheld computer (PDA/palmtop) versions of the guideline. Clinical indicators are used to measure the degree of compliance to the guideline based on the guide-line recommendations and can be used to give feedback to the professionals on their performance in a specific care process. For example, one guideline recom-mendation may be to use a visual analog scale (VAS) to assess a patient's level of pain associated with their pressure ulcer(s). The clinical indicator in this case would be the percentage of patients whose pain level was assessed using a VAS.

Guidelines while often developed at the international or national level need to be implemented locally. Clark[10] reported that 42% ($n = 200$) of respondents to a questionnaire on wound care guideline development used locally derived versions of national or international guidelines. These translations from the macro to the micro level help to associate evidence-based guidelines with local resources; for example, a guideline recommendation on prevention of hip fractures might involve the use of hip protectors. The (local) protocol based on this guideline will have to specify the brand, type, or name of the hip protector that is used in the specific care facility.

International Developments

Recently there has been increasing interest in forging international collaborations and consensus upon guideline development and implementation. Two interna-tional initiatives in this regard deserve mention; firstly the AGREE instrument (Appraisal of Guidelines for Research and Evaluation).[11] This tool was developed by an international group of researchers to assess the quality of clinical guidelines and was field-tested using 100 guidelines developed across 11 countries. The final version of the AGREE instrument consists of 23 items divided into six domains:

1. Scope and purpose—the overall aim of the guideline, the specific clinical ques-tions considered, the care settings, and the patient populations reflected in the guideline.
2. Stakeholder involvement—the extent to which the guideline represents the views of its intended users.
3. Rigor of development—the process used to gather and synthesize the evidence, the methods to formulate the recommendations and to update them.
4. Clarity and presentation—the language and format of the guideline.
5. Applicability—the (potential) organizational, behavioral, and cost implications of applying the guideline.
6. Editorial independence—the extent to which the guideline committee were independent of pressures that might bias the guideline recommendations.

The criteria mainly concern the methods used for developing the guideline and the quality of the reporting rather than the clinical content of the guideline recommendations. Currently, many guideline developers across the world use the AGREE instrument as a checklist in the development of new guidelines.

The second recent development is the foundation of the Guidelines International Network (GIN) in 2002. GIN is an international not-for-profit association of organizations and individuals involved in clinical practice guidelines. GIN has now grown to more than 50 member organizations from 26 countries. The network seeks to improve the quality of healthcare by promoting systematic development of clinical practice guidelines and their application into practice, through supporting international collaboration (www.g-i-n.net). Their website contains a guideline library, which provides the ability to search and review the guideline programs of all member organizations. The library also includes development tools and resources about techniques and instruments for developing evidence-based guidelines, training materials on producing and using clinical practice guidelines, and patient/consumer resources from GIN members. The AGREE Instrument and the establishment of GIN could be considered as the result of a growing consensus about the methodology of evidence-based guideline development. While this focus upon guideline development is to be welcomed, there remains much to do to improve the utilization of pressure ulcer and other clinical guidelines in practice.

References

1. Effective Health Care. Implementing clinical practice guidelines. Can guidelines be used to improve clinical practice? University of Leeds, 1994.
2. Clark M. Developing Guidelines for Pressure Ulcer Prevention and Management. J Wound Care 1999; 8(7):357–359.
3. Dutch Health Care Improvement Institute. The Dutch Consensus Prevention of Bedulcers. CBO, Utrecht, 1985.
4. Panel for the Prediction and Prevention of Pressure Ulcers in Adults. Pressure ulcers in adults: prediction and prevention. Clinical practice guideline number 3. Rockville, MD: Agency for Health Care Policy and Research, Public Health Service, US Department of Health and Human Services, AHCPR Publication No. 92–0047, 1992.
5. Bergstrom N, Bennett MA, Carlson CE, et al. Treatment of pressure ulcers. Clinical practice guideline, number 15. Rockville, MD: US Department of Health and Human Services. Public Health Service, Agency for Health Care Policy and Research. AHCPR Publication No 95–0652,1994.
6. European Pressure Ulcer Advisory Panel. Pressure ulcer prevention guidelines. Br J Nurs 1998; 7(15):888–889.
7. European Pressure Ulcer Advisory Panel. Guidelines on treatment of pressure ulcers. EPUAP Review 1999; 1(2):31–33.
8. Kwaliteitsinstituut voor de Gezondheidszorg CBO. Richtlijn decubitus—tweede herziening (Guideline on pressure ulcers—second revision). Utrecht: CBO; 2002.
9. National Institute for Clinical Excellence. Pressure ulcer risk management and prevention (Inherited Guideline B). National Institute for Clinical Excellence, 2001.
10. Clark M. Barriers to the implementation of clinical guidelines. J Tissue Viability 2003; 13(2):62–64, 66, 68 passim.
11. The AGREE Collaboration. Development and validation of an international appraisal instrument for assessing the quality of clinical practice guidelines: the AGREE project. Qual Safety Health Care 2003; 12:18–23.
12. Van Zelm RT. Improving quality of pressure ulcer care using an evidence based guideline and clinical indicators. Second International Conference on Best Practice Guidelines, Toronto, Canada, 5–6 June 2003.

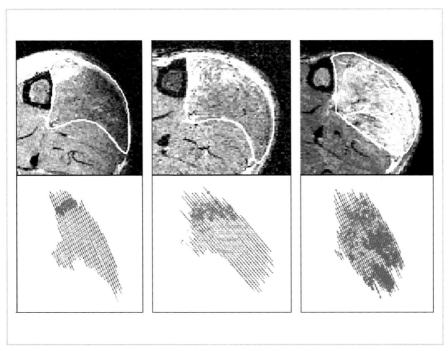

Figure 3.8 Damage in transverse histological slices (below) and MR images (above) beneath an indenter caused by loading tissue for 2 hours. Each pair of images represents a separate experiment.

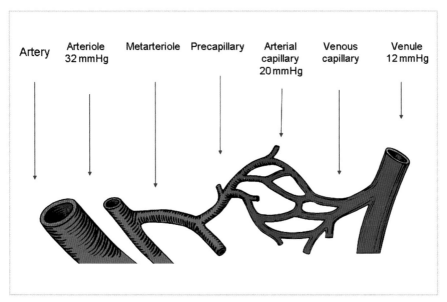

Figure 4.1 The microcirculation is especially prone to damage by extrinsic local pressure and shearing forces. (From: Collier M. Fundamental concepts. Resource file: Beds and mattresses. *Journal of Wound Care* 1999: 1–8. Reproduced by kind permission of Huntleigh Healthcare Ltd.)

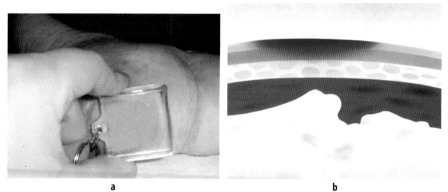

a   **b**

Figure 5.1 A grade 1 pressure ulcer. (Part **b** reproduced by kind permission of Huntleigh Healthcare Ltd.)

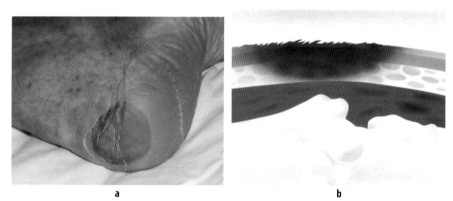

a   **b**

Figure 5.2 A grade 2 pressure ulcer. (Part **b** reproduced by kind permission of Huntleigh Healthcare Ltd.)

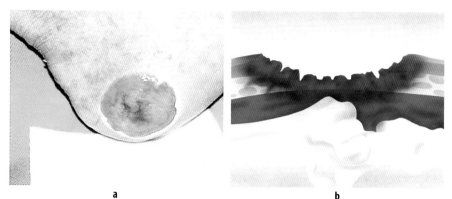

Figure 5.3 A grade 3 pressure ulcer. (Part **b** reproduced by kind permission of Huntleigh Healthcare Ltd.)

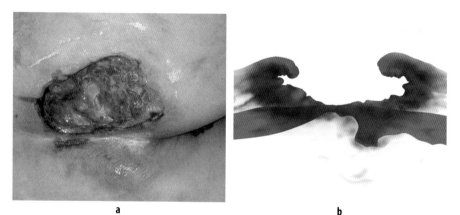

Figure 5.4 A grade 4 pressure ulcer. (Part **b** reproduced by kind permission of Huntleigh Healthcare Ltd.)

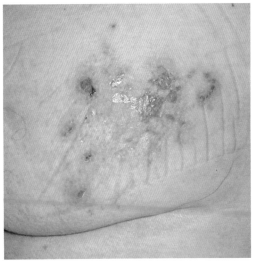

Figure 5.5 An incontinence lesion.

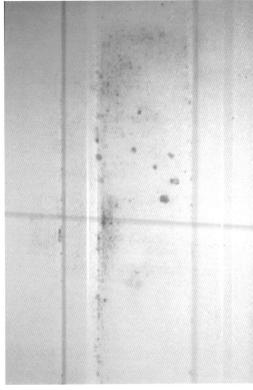

Figure 7.1 Mold on a bed frame.

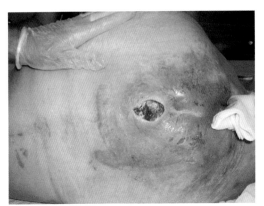

Figure 9.1 Surrounding skin irritation due to fecal incontinence in a sacral pressure ulcer.

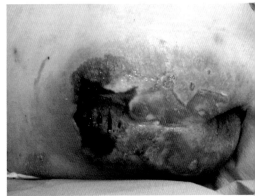

Figure 9.2 Extensive deterioration of surrounding skin due to excessive moisture in a lower back pressure ulcer.

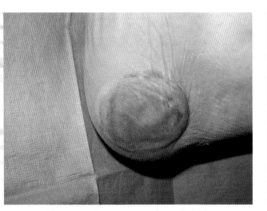

Figure 11.1 A stage 2 pressure ulcer on the heel.

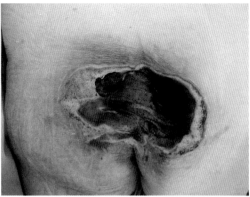

Figure 11.2 Different color tones in a sacral pressure ulcer, reflecting different wound tissues.

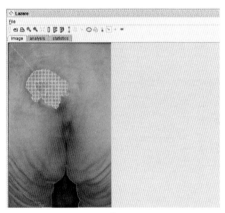

a

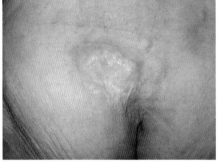

b

Figure 11.3 (**a** and **b**) Computerized planimetric evaluation of pressure ulcer.

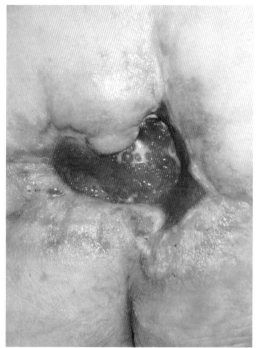

Figure 13.1 Sacral pressure ulcer. Clean granulating wound.

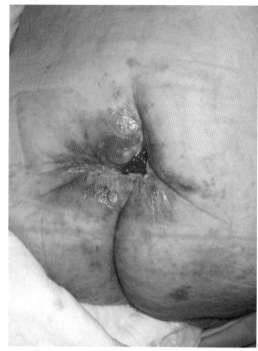

Figure 13.2 Sacral pressure ulcer (the same as in Figure 13.1), treated with advanced dressing. Result after 10 weeks.

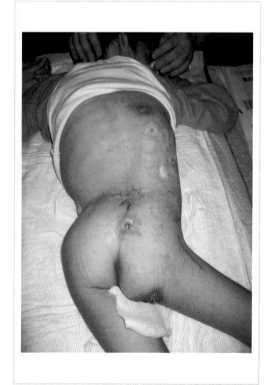

Figure 13.3 Eight-year-old boy, multiple pressure ulcers at different sites.

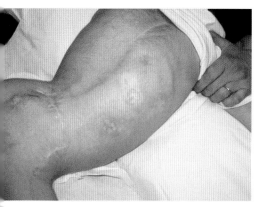

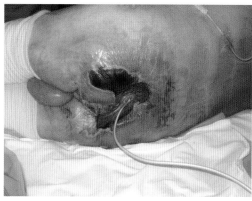

Figure 13.4 Same case as Figure 13.3, result after 6 months. Treatment with pressure relief and control with advanced dressings.

Figure 13.5 Topical negative pressure treatment in a sacral pressure ulcer.

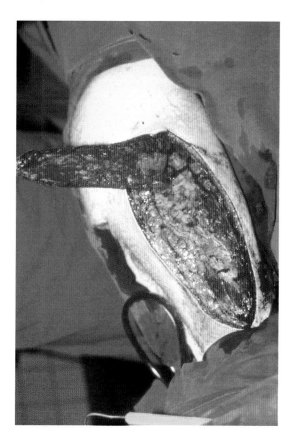

Figure 14.1 Hamstring flap. The flap has been raised in full muscle length to allow for reuse at recurrence.

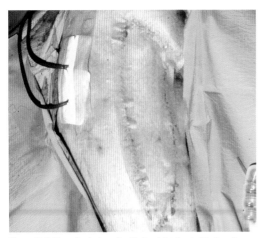

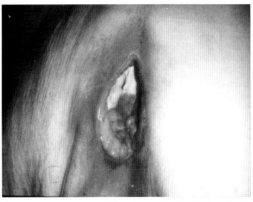

Figure 15.1 Pressure ulcer with fatty tissue and tendon sheath; no devitalized tissue present. Debridement is contraindicated.

Figure 14.2 Tensor fasciae latae flap. The freed distal part of the long flap can easily be folded or transposed to cover a trochanteric pressure ulcer.

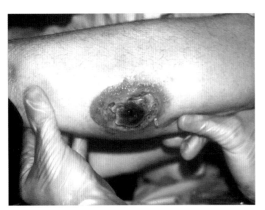

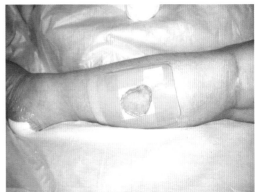

Figure 15.2 Pressure ulcer on calf prior to debridement.

Figure 15.3 Larvae in place under dressing.

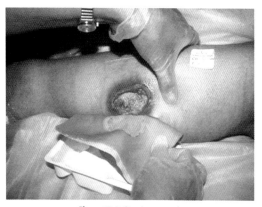

Figure 15.4 Dressing removal.

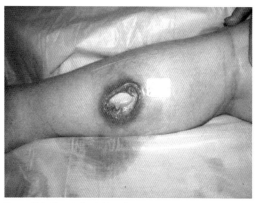

Figure 15.5 Wound after 3 days of treatment with maggot debridement therapy.

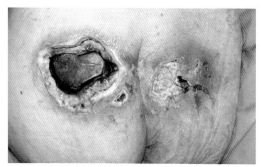

a

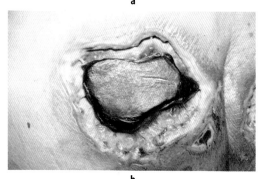

b

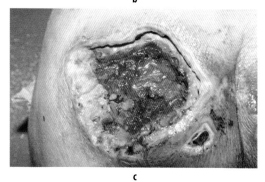

c

Figure 16.2 Eschar debridement. **a** and **b** Necrotic tissue should be debrided to decrease bacterial burden and to allow for an accurate assessment of the depth and extension of the wound.

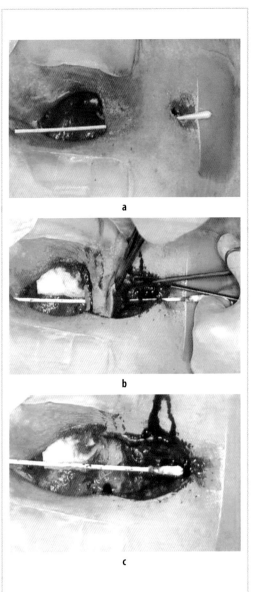

a

b

c

Figure 16.3 De-roofing of stage 4 ulcer. **a** Preliminary probing demonstrating communication between ulcers. **b** Removal of bridge overlying the ulcerated area. **c** Full visualization of the wound bed upon completion of de-roofing.

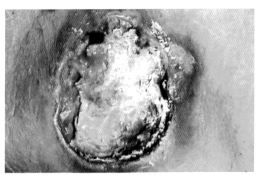

Figure 16.4 Slough. Moist necrotic tissue is an excellent breeding ground for bacteria.

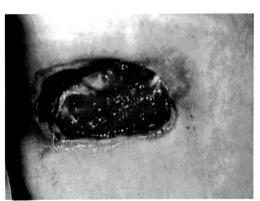

Figure 16.5 Bright red granulation tissue indicates poor capillary neoformation secondary to increased bacterial burden. Note that tissue is friable, and that the wound bleeds easily.

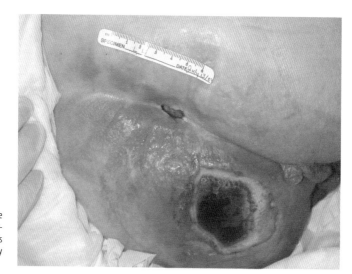

Figure 16.6 Cellulitis. Note erythema and edema surrounding the eschar on this stage "x̌" ischeal tuberosity pressure ulcer.

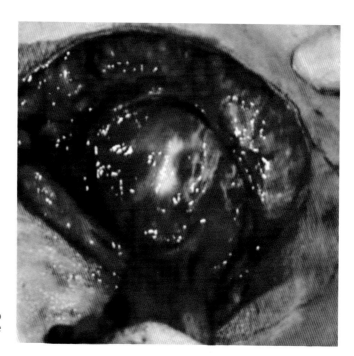

Figure 16.7 Probing to bone. Stage 4 ulcer with bone exposure.

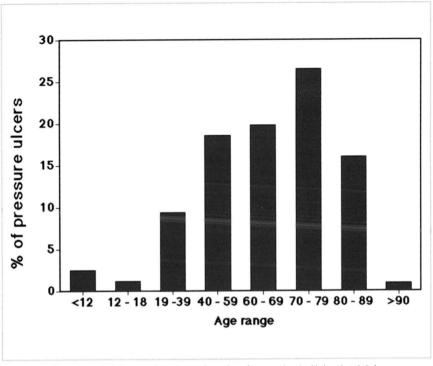

Figure 20.1 Graph demonstrating an increase in numbers of pressure ulcers in elderly patients in Italy.

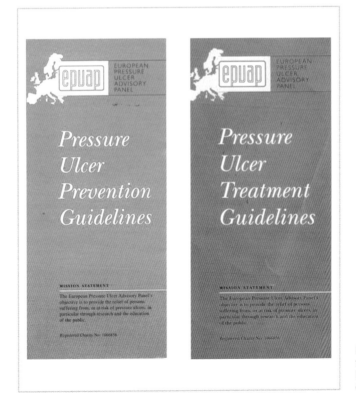

Figure 20.3 EPUAP prevention and treatment guidelines published in a number of European languages.

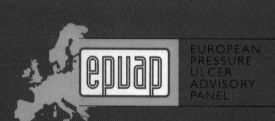

Nutritional Guidelines for Pressure Ulcer Prevention and Treatment

MISSION STATEMENT

The European Pressure Ulcer Advisory Panel's objective is to provide the relief of persons suffering from, or at risk of pressure ulcers, in particular through research and the education of the public.

Registered Charity No: 1066856

Figure 20.4 EPUAP nutrition guidelines.

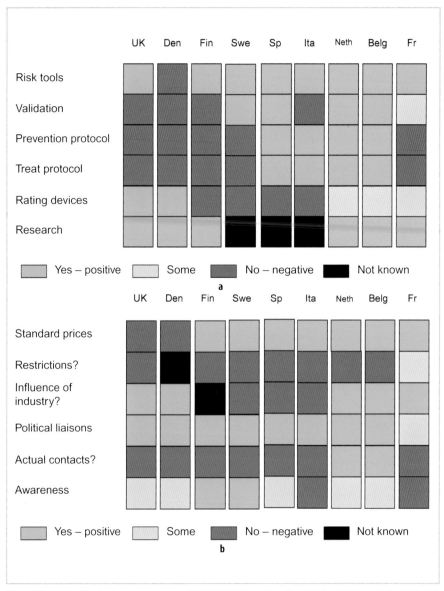

Figure 20.5 (**a** and **b**) Results of questionnaire sent in 1998 designed to assess the policy and tools used in pressure ulcers in nine different European countries. (*Source:* J. Haalboom, Utrecht, the Netherlands.)

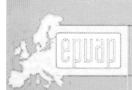

EUROPEAN PRESSURE ULCER ADVISORY PANEL

Volume 1, Issue 1, 1998, pages 1–24

epuap *Review*

CONTENTS

	page
• Trustees and executive committee of the EPUAP	1
• Letter from the President	2
• Welcome to the *EPUAP Review*	3
• EPUAP research award	4
• Introduction to the executive committee members	5
• First EPUAP guideline – the prevention of pressure ulcers	7
• Future EPUAP meetings	9
• Pressure ulcers in Italy	10
• The Swedish Wound Healing Society	11
• National pressure ulcer groups – the UK Wound Care Society and the UK Tissue Viability Society	12
• Selected abstracts from the first EPUAP open meeting, 1997	13
• Membership list	19
• Membership application form	23

Published by the European Pressure Ulcer Advisory Panel
Editor: Michael Clark, PhD, (Cardiff, UK)
Editorial Assistant: Christine Cherry, DSR/R), (Oxford, UK)
Editorial Office: EPUAP Business Office, Department of Dermatology
The Churchill Hospital, Old Road, Headington, Oxford, OX3 7LJ
Telephone: +44 (0)1865 228264/69
Telefax: +44 (0)1865 228233
E-mail EuropeanPressureUlcerAdvisPanel@compuserve.com
Registered Charity No. 1066856

1·1

ISSN 1464-7796

Figure 20.6 EPUAP Review – in-house journal.

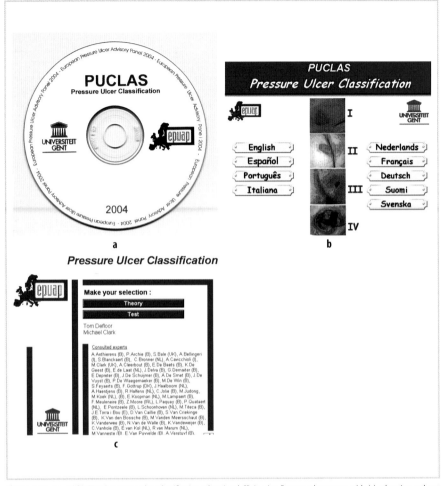

Figure 20.7 (**a** and **b**) EPUAP pressure ulcer classification educational CD in nine European languages, with (**c**) education and test assessment.

19 Developing a Research Agenda

Denis Colin

In recent years much has been written and done throughout the world concerning the prevention and treatment of pressure ulcers, particularly in terms of education. However, it is widely recognized that the level of evidence underpinning guidelines or good practice recommendations is fairly poor. The majority of pressure ulcer prevention and care is derived from expert opinion rather than empirical evidence. The scientific basis in this area must certainly be improved and the European Pressure Ulcer Advisory Panel (EPUAP) is convinced that this is a worthwhile challenge. All research programs are expected to use a rigorous and efficient design including methodology that maximizes their validity, reliability, reproducibility, and usefulness in clinical situations. Research needs to be grounded in the realities of clinical practice and address caregiver needs; it also needs to have a clear theoretical framework and to analyze pertinent literature data. A multidisciplinary research approach also needs to be developed since it is widely recognized that it is a realistic approach to pressure ulcer management. We should include appropriate outcome measures such as quality of life, satisfaction with care, and resource use (e.g. institutional care, length of stay, equipment or drug costs). We certainly need fundamental research but this research has to be directly linked to clinical research in order to improve our daily practice; this research must help us to find new ways of prevention in terms of techniques, materials, and drugs. Lastly we have also to consider all the means allowing us to translate theoretical concepts into practice.

A research agenda must be focused on key areas of uncertainty, which are numerous. Considering that it would probably be unrealistic to treat all aspects of pressure ulcers in a short period of time, we have to select some of the priorities. For this reason a pragmatic approach is adopted. A research agenda must be followed by concrete decisions and lead to real improvements in clinical results. Several priorities have been selected and will be scheduled and later debated over the next five years.

Epidemiology: Prevalence, Incidence, Mortality

There is an absolute necessity to standardize an accurate way of measuring pressure ulcer prevalence and incidence. This is the only way of taking into account the importance of pressure ulcers in terms of health priority. It is generally acknowledged that incidence provides information about the factors contributing to the development of pressure ulcers and leads to the interventions of prevention.

Prevalence does not provide this information but prevalence studies contribute to our knowledge of the problem of pressure ulcers. Prevalence is of value when the determination of the magnitude of a problem (in this case pressure ulcers) is concerned.[1-3] Prevalence studies have shown that pressure ulcers occur more often than was assumed. The value of prevalence may be considered as limited. For insight into the factors influencing the development of pressure ulcers the best method is continuous registration, that is the use of incidence.[4,5] However, there are not enough validated incidence methods known. The development of sufficient incidence methods for use in all types of institutions is needed. Incidence should be an integral part of the regular quality reports to the health authorities.

Moreover there is another key issue: the number of deaths arising from pressure ulcers is unknown.[6,7] We certainly need to emphasize this aspect and develop the principle of evaluating precisely mortality in the European countries.

How Much Do Pressure Ulcers Cost?

The reported costs of pressure ulcers vary widely from study to study.[8-11] There is no real consensus in pressure ulcer cost evaluation although this topic seems fundamental. Existing information is rather poor and sometimes controversial. A methodology allowing a pragmatic and precise evaluation of the economical impact of pressure ulcers has obvious advantages:

- giving relevant information to the health authorities;
- better allocation of resources inside hospitals or community;
- proving (if necessary) that prevention is less expensive than treatment.

It seems essential to find a reproducible methodology that could be used by health authorities.

Do We Know All the Mechanisms of Pressure Ulcer Occurrence?

Despite considerable input from many scientific organizations and educational initiatives in numerous countries, pressure ulcer incidence remains at an unacceptably high level. This observation may partly be due to limited knowledge about the precise mechanisms of pressure ulcer occurrence. Although it is generally assumed that pressure and shear are major components of tissue breakdown,[12] our understanding of the basic pathways whereby mechanical loading leads to soft tissue breakdown is less clear. The relationships between external pressure and/or shear applied to tissues and their impact on microcirculation,[13] soft tissue deformation, cell damage and dysfunction are not clearly understood.[14,15] We certainly need a better understanding of the physiological impact of these mechanical factors. In practice, identification and prevention of pressure ulcers focus mainly on skin tissue, even though the underlying muscle tissue may be more susceptible to mechanical loading.

A research program could investigate the relationships between

- the global mechanical stress at skin level;
- the resulting mechanical conditions within the soft tissue extending from skin to muscle and bone;

- the pathophysiological response to loading of all these tissues including tissue deformation and tissue biological consequences.

This research could lead to objective ways of assessing all the tissue units involved in soft tissue breakdown: the cells, the interstitial space, blood and lymph vessels. This research should provide fundamental knowledge about the etiology of pressure ulcers which could result in effective prevention and early identification of pressure ulcers.

Pressure-Relieving Devices[16–19]

Evaluation of support surfaces needs to be based on a scientific approach. We do not know for certain how to assess technically and clinically low pressure devices. There is no strong evidence that an alternative mode is more efficient than a static mode in air devices. There is also no strong documented evidence of low-air loss principle interest, even if pathophysiological theories are often used as clinical demonstrations. Investigation is obviously needed in terms of quality of life of individuals and caregivers. Prospective evaluation of the impact and effectiveness of support surfaces in specific areas such as acute care settings, community or elderly groups should be done. Comparisons of support surface efficiency including ethical aspects may be proposed.

Diagnosing Early Pressure Ulcers; Imaging Early Tissue Damage

Evaluation, in clinical wards, of the early damage to soft tissues is difficult. There is certainly still a need for early diagnosis of pressure ulcers occurring in soft tissues. Is there a place for techniques such as nuclear magnetic resonance (NMR) or ultrasonography? Could they provide the potential for non-invasive examination of these underlying tissues? We know that parameters relevant to pressure ulcers, such as ischemia, edema, and inflammatory responses, have previously been examined for other purposes using NMR. Some authors have examined inflammatory responses to encapsulated foreign bodies using NMR, and found that some NMR parameters were correlated strongly with blood activation studies and histology.[20] Others[21] have evaluated the viability of skin flaps using magnetic resonance spectroscopy. This process could generate a normative database and document the natural history of the pressure ulcer from an entirely unseen perspective. It seems essential to continue this research activity in order to identify new strategies for prediction, early identification, and prevention of pressure ulcers.

Living with a Pressure Ulcer

What is the lived experience of patients with pressure ulcers? Little is known of the impact of pressure ulcers on an individual's quality of life. In one qualitative study,[22] the authors reported that pressure ulcers had a profound impact on the lives of sufferers. They suggested that a larger study was required to obtain a greater understanding of the patient's experience of living with a pressure ulcer.

Other authors[23] studied the experience of five patients who had had grade 4 pressure ulcers that were healed or nearly healed. The patients in this study were relatively young with an age range of 30 to 64 years. This is by no means representative of patients with pressure ulcers as a whole as the majority have been found to be over 65 years of age in a number of surveys. For example, Whittington et al.[24] surveyed 17,560 acute patients and found an incidence rate of 7%; of these 73% were aged over 65 years. Also the majority of patients in Langemo et al.'s study[22] had spinal cord injury and it was difficult to separate the impact of this injury from the impact of the pressure ulcer.

It is proposed that the EPUAP builds on current research by undertaking a further qualitative study in a range of countries across Europe, collecting data from a variety of people of different age groups and with different underlying pathologies. It is considered that the evidence obtained from such a study will provide valuable supporting information regarding the impact of pressure ulcers on people living in Europe. This evidence could be used when seeking grants from the European Commission to support the work of EPUAP.

Assessment of Pressure Ulcer Healing

Several methods of wound healing assessment are described and used.[25] However, there is no real consensus and there is often a lack of accuracy. An important research objective would be to find methods for accurate and repeatable evaluation of wound healing.

Despite the considerable improvement of medical knowledge and its impact on the domain of health in the past 30 years, pressure ulcers remain a major healthcare preoccupation. Efficient research programs closely linked to clinical practice are probably the most effective way of reducing the incidence of pressure ulcers. Numerous gaps remain in our understanding of effective pressure ulcer prevention and treatment. Moreover, the majority of pressure ulcer management is derived from expert opinion rather than scientific evidence. Thus further research is vital in order to reduce the incidence of this severe disease and improve quality of life for our patients. We also need broad financial support for research; it is our responsibility to promote pressure ulcer as a major health problem. The financial investment in this area is actually very low. Beyond our technical involvement, which is our responsibility, there is also a political challenge, which depends on our credibility with politicians and health authorities.

References

1. Barrois B, Allaert FA, Colin D. A survey of pressure sore prevalence in hospitals in the greater Paris region. J Wound Care 1995; 4(5):234–236.
2. Bours G, Halfens RJ, Abu-Saad, Grol R. Prevalence, prevention and treatment of pressure ulcers; descriptive study in 89 institutions in the Netherlands. Res Nurs Health 2002; 25(2):99–110.
3. Clark M, Defloor T, Bours G. A pilot study of the prevalence of pressure ulcers in European hospitals. In: Clark M (ed) Pressure ulcers; Recent advances in tissue viability. Salisbury: Quay Books; 2004; 8–22.
4. Robinson C, Gloekner M, Bush S, et al. Determining the efficacy of a pressure ulcer prevention program by collecting prevalence and incidence data: a unit-based effort. Ostomy Wound Manage 2003; 49(5):44–46, 48–51.

5. Benbow M. Pressure ulcer incidence reporting. Nurs Stand 2004; 18(32):57–60, 62, 64.
6. Kiely DK, Flacker JM. Resident characteristics associated with mortality in long-term care nursing homes: is there a gender difference? J Am Med Dir Assoc 2000; 1(1):8–13.
7. Baudoin C, Fardellone P, Bean K, et al. Clinical outcomes and mortality after hip fracture: a 2-year follow-up study. Bone 1996; 18:149S–157S.
8. Gebhardt KS. Cost-effective management of pressure relieving equipment in a large teaching trust. J Tissue Viability 2003; 13(2):74–77.
9. Cho SH, Ketefian S, Barkauskas VH, Smith DG. The effects of nurse staffing on adverse events, morbidity, mortality, and medical costs. Nurs Res 2003; 52(2):71–79.
10. Harding K, Cutting K, Price P. The cost-effectiveness of wound management protocols of care. Br J Nurs 2000; 9(19 suppl):S6, S8, S10.
11. Lyder C. Cost-effectiveness of wound management in long term care. Director 2002; 10(3):100–102.
12. Nixon J. The pathophysiology and aetiology of pressure ulcers. In: Morrison MJ (ed) The prevention and treatment of pressure ulcers. Edinburgh: Mosby; 2001: 55–74.
13. Knight S, Taylor R, Polliack A, Bader DL. Establishing predictive indicators for the status of loaded tissues. J Appl Physiol 2001; 90:2231–2237.
14. Bouten CV, Oomens CW, Baaijens FP, Bader DL. The etiology of pressure ulcers: skin deep or muscle bound? Arch Phys Med Rehabil 2003; 84(4):616–619.
15. Houwing R, Overgoor M, Kon M, et al. Pressure-induced skin lesions in pigs: reperfusion injury and the effects of vitamin E. J Wound Care 2000; 9:36–40.
16. Rithalia SV. Evaluation of alternating pressure air mattresses: one laboratory-based strategy. J Tissue Viability 2004; 14(2):51–58.
17. Collins F. Russka pressure-relieving low air-loss mattress system. Br J Nurs 2004; 13(6 Suppl): S50–S54.
18. Shelton F, Lott JW. Conducting and interpreting interface pressure evaluations of clinical support surfaces. Geriatr Nurs 2003; 24(4):222–227.
19. Wolsley CJ, Hill PD. Review of interface pressure measurement to establish a protocol for their use in the assessment of patient support surfaces. J Tissue Viability 2000; 10(2):53–57.
20. Alikacem N, Stroman PW, Marois Y, et al. Non-invasive follow-up of tissue encapsulation of foreign materials. A magnetic resonance imaging and spectroscopy breakthrough. ASAIO J 1995; 41(3): M617–M624.
21. Klein HW, Gourley IM. Use of magnetic resonance spectroscopy in the evaluation of skin flaps. Ann Plast Surg 1988; 20(6):547–551.
22. Langemo DK, Melland H, Hanson D, et al. The lived experience of having a pressure ulcer: a qualitative analysis. Adv Skin Wound Care 2000; 13(5):225–235.
23. Fox C. Living with a pressure ulcer: a descriptive study of patients' experiences. J Wound Care 2002; 11(6):10–22.
24. Whittington K, Patrick M, Roberts JL. A national study of pressure ulcer prevalence and incidence in acute care hospitals. J Wound Ostomy Continence Nurs 2000: 27(4):209–215.
25. Bolton L, McNees P, van Rijswijk L, et al; Wound Outcomes Study Group. Wound-healing outcomes using standardized assessment and care in clinical practice. J Wound Ostomy Continence Nurs 2004; 31(2):65–71.

20 The European Pressure Ulcer Advisory Panel: A Means of Identifying and Dealing with a Major Health Problem with a European Initiative

George W. Cherry

Introduction: The Problem

Pressure ulcers are a major health problem worldwide. Historically and even today they have not had a high profile when compared to other medical conditions such as cardiovascular disease and cancer. However, awareness of the extent and cost of the problem is growing. Factors contributing to this are an increase in the aging population in developed countries as well as in developing countries, immuno-compromising diseases such as HIV and AIDS, and trauma such as burns leading to an increased susceptibility of pressure-related wounds.[1] Figure 20.1 (see color section) illustrates how pressure ulcers particularly affect the elderly population.

The financial burden on healthcare systems is also increasing due to treatment costs, up to £1.4–2.1 billion (4% annual NHS expenditure) per year in the National Health Service in the United Kingdom, and in the USA it has been estimated to be even higher, particularly with the indirect effect of litigation.[2]

Pressure ulcers have been a major medical problem since the beginning of civilization. In the nineteenth century.[3] William Heberdeen in a presentation to the College of Physicians in London in 1815 gave a description of a bed frame that would aid in the treatment of these wounds (Figure 20.2). He summarized his presentation by stating:

> As the ultimate object of the medical art is the removal or alleviation of those evils to which the human body is exposed, I make no scruple of laying before the College of Physicians some account of a contrivance from which I have lately experienced great benefit; though strictly speaking the calamity be no disease and the remedy no medicine. There is no-one in the habit of attending the sick but must have had reason to deplore the wretched condition of those who, being bedridden through accident or infirmity, have contracted sores of a very painful and dangerous kind by long pressure. Especially if the patient lie in the wet and filth of his own body which he is unable to restrain.

Development of the European Pressure Ulcer Advisory Panel (EPUAP)

The organization of the EPUAP began in Amsterdam at the 6th European Conference of the Wound Management Association in October 1996 when a few of the participants were approached by Dr Willi Jung of Germany to meet with

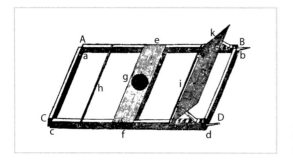

Figure 20.2 Bed frame designed by William Heberdeen Jr in 1815 for the treatment and prevention of pressure sores.

representatives of the National Pressure Ulcer Advisory Panel (NPUAP) from the USA to determine if a similar organization could be established in Europe. Following this meeting an inaugural meeting of the EPUAP was held in London in December 1996 with representatives from more than 13 European countries who had an interest in pressure ulcers. Though it was thought that many of the organizational aspects of the NPUAP were relevant, it was generally agreed that the EPUAP should be unique in its structure, reflecting the differences in the healthcare systems between the USA and Europe.

The EPUAP was formally established after that meeting and a public announcement was published in the *Lancet* at the beginning of 1997.[4] The advisory panel was registered as a charity in the UK but with activities throughout Europe with the following mission statement:

> The European Pressure Ulcer Advisory Panel's objective is to provide the relief of persons suffering from or at risk of pressure ulcers, in particular through research and the education of the public.

Development of EPUAP Through Annual Open Meetings

The publicity of the launch of the EPUAP in the *Lancet* was followed by the first open meeting, which was held in Oxford in September 1997. This first meeting was well attended by delegates from throughout Europe and other parts of the world and led to a number of important initiatives, in particular the formation of the EPUAP's pressure ulcer prevention guidelines through the interactive input led by our first president, Professor Keith Harding (Figure 20.3—see color section). This interaction was particularly useful in having participants openly debate statements which would become part of the guidelines. A working committee came up with the final guidelines based on levels of evidence similar to those used by the NPUAP (Table 20.1).

The success of the panel was also ensured by the support of our annual meetings by the EPUAP corporate sponsors. In addition, the content of the first meeting and those that followed was ensured by the late Professor Gerry Bennett who was the first Recorder and a major contributor to the inaugural meeting held in London in 1996.

Table 20.1. Levels of evidence

A	Results of two or more randomized, controlled trials in pressure ulcers in humans
B	Results of two or more controlled clinical trials in humans or, where appropriate, results in two or more controlled trials in an animal model provide indirect support
C	This rating requires one or more of the following: (1) results of one controlled trial (2) results of at least two case series/descriptive studies on pressure ulcers in humans, or (3) expert opinion

The second annual open meeting was held in Oxford with its theme "Learning from each other—the European experience." Again this was well attended and a major outcome was the publication of the EPUAP pressure ulcer treatment guidelines (Figure 20.3—see color section). Ownership of both of the guideline documents was established with the input from the delegates attending these meetings.

Recently nutritional guidelines for pressure ulcer prevention and treatment were published and presented at the 2nd World Union of Wound Healing Societies Meeting in Paris in July 2004. Again the formation of these guidelines followed the same protocols as the prevention and treatment guidelines in their development (Figure 20.4—see color section).

The EPUAP guidelines have been translated into a number of European languages and more than 100,000 individual brochures have been distributed to clinicians throughout Europe. They are also available on the EPUAP website (www.epuap.org).

An early achievement of the EPUAP led by Professor Jeen Haalboom, our second president, was highlighted in another article published in the *Lancet* in 1998 on the need for establishing a uniform method in Europe to deal with the prevention and treatment of pressure ulcers.[5] From the answers to questionnaires sent to EPUAP representatives in different countries, he was able to highlight how information concerning such items as basic registration of pressure ulcers and related aspects of management was lacking (Figure 20.5a and b—see color section).

Further annual open meetings were held in Amsterdam (the Netherlands), Pisa (Italy), Le Mans (France), Budapest (Hungary), Tampere (Finland), and Aberdeen (Scotland), each with a specific theme ranging from "Technology in the new millennium" to "Pressure ulcers; back to basics—the fundamental principles." The annual meetings are a major educational opportunity and the Recorder and the scientific committee play an important role in the success of these events. Dr Michael Clark has been Recorder since the Budapest meeting in 2002, where the theme was "Pressure ulcers—a quality of care indicator." At this meeting a major focus of the program was dedicated to work that the EPUAP itself had carried out, with the results of the Prevalence of Pressure Ulcers in Europe study being an important aspect of the Budapest program.

Additional Education Activities

The EPUAP has been producing its own journal, the EPUAP Review, three times per year, under the editorship of Dr Michael Clark published through the EPUAP Business Office (Figure 20.6—see color section). The Review has served as a forum for debates on issues about pressure ulcers. One item that stimulated considerable discussion was an article written by Professor Joe Barbenel and S. Hagisawa: "The limits of pressure sore prevention."[6] The Review is also published on our website www.epuap.org, which was established shortly after the Panel was established.

A major recent educational project has been carried out under the leadership of Professor Tom Defloor of the University of Ghent, Belgium, who produced the computer CD PUCLAS (pressure ulcer classification system), which is available in nine languages (Figure 20.7a, b, and c—see color section).

Educational grants have been set up through contributions from industry, which have led to a number of studies including the major European pressure ulcer prevalence study as well as the development of the nutritional guidelines.

In addition to ascertaining the extent of the problem of pressure ulcers throughout Europe, we thought that it would be important to determine the effectiveness and impact of our guidelines and a baseline of the problem was necessary. The importance of having such information has recently been emphasized in the work of the NPUAP in the USA, where shortly after the panel was established in 1989 they set as a national goal to reduce the incidence of pressure ulcers by 50% by the year 2000.[7] This organization has recently published its progress in reaching that goal in "Pressure ulcers in America: Prevalence, incidence and implications for the future," where they state that the major problem in assessing this goal has been inconsistency in the initial figures presented on incidence and inconsistencies in methodology. The EPUAP prevalence study was designed to reduce or eliminate these obstacles in order to assess the problem as well as benefits from interventions that arise from the work of the EPUAP.

Education of the Public and Government

Education is a major part of our mission statement and educating the public as to the extent of pressure ulcers and their cost to health budgets is extremely important. The role of litigation following pressure ulcers, although not as extensive as in the USA, is beginning to be publicized in European countries. This awareness has been further highlighted in popular television medical dramas where the development of pressure ulcers and their consequences have been emphasized.

The EPUAP has made a major effort in pointing out the problem of pressure ulcers to government, though not to the same successful extent as has been done in the Netherlands where economic studies revealed that the costs of prevention and treatment of pressure ulcers approach those of cardiovascular disease and cancer.[5] To make governments aware of the problem the EPUAP has written to Members of Parliament in the UK as well as to the European Parliament emphasizing the extent and cost of pressure ulcers.

Summary

The European Pressure Ulcer Advisory Panel (EPUAP) is an example of how a dedicated organization from a number of countries can approach a major chronic wound healing problem such as pressure ulcers through education, research, and dissemination through a cooperative program.

References

1. Romanelli M. Pressure ulcer prevention and management in Italy. In: Cherry GW (ed) Concepts in pressure relief – importance in the prevention and treatment of pressure ulcers. Oxford: Positif Press; 2004: 18–19.
2. Bennett G, Dealey C, Posnett J. The cost of pressure ulcers in the UK. Age Ageing 2004; 33(3): 230–235.
3. Bedsores over the centuries. In: Parish LC, Witkowski JA, Crissey JT (eds) The decubitus ulcer in clinical practice. Berlin, Heidelberg: Springer-Verlag; 1997: 3–8.
4. EPUAP. European Pressure Ulcer Panel launched. Lancet 1997; 349:262.
5. Haalboom JRS. Pressure ulcers. Lancet 1998; 352(15 August): 581.
6. Barbenel J, Hagisawa S. The limits of pressure sore prevention. J R Soc Med 1999; 92:576–578; reviewed in the EPUAP Review 2000; 2(2):43–44.
7. National Pressure Ulcer Panel. Cuddingan J, Ayello EA, Sussman C (eds) Pressure ulcers in America: Prevalence, incidence and implications for the future. Reston, VA: NPUAP; 2001.
8. Clark M, Bours G, Defloor T. The prevalence of pressure ulcers. in Europe. Hospital Decisions 2003/2004; Winter: 123–129.

21 Pressure Ulcer Prevention and Management in the Developing World: The Developed World Must Provide Leadership

Terence J. Ryan

This is not a review of pressure ulcers in the developing world because there are insufficient data to write one. The pressure ulcers that I have seen there, in the terminally ill and in the paraplegic, mostly come for treatment after great delay and the patients are very sick. There is a case of need and the solutions must come in part from the developed world and none better than the US National Pressure Ulcer Advisory Panel and the European Pressure Ulcer Advisory Panel.

The pathogenesis of the pressure ulcer is no different in the developing world from that in the developed world. It is due to pressure and occurs in the sick. There are two major subgroups: those who are systemically sick who depend on carers to manage their predisposition to develop pressure sores and to heal them, and a second group such as the paraplegic who with self-help can both prevent and heal their pressure sores.

It was Ludwig Guttman who with passion persuaded the world that the paraplegic need not develop pressure sores. He came to Oxford during the Second World War as a refugee and, in a third world setting of the country wartime hospital the Radcliffe Infirmary at a time of great deprivation, he worked on severely injured soldiers and civilians. Nearby in the equally third world conditions of a wonderfully antique Radcliffe Observatory, the Spanish surgeon Joseph Trueta worked on crush injury. Two decades later I collaborated with Trueta on an exhibition on blood supply of skin and bone and I was a registrar at Stoke Mandeville where Ludwig Guttman proved that pressures sores were preventable and repairable. This experience did not employ high technology. It was very basic.

The prevention of pressure sores begins with detailed attention to preventing the impairment of blood supply due to pressure and includes maneuvers at the scene of an accident such as removing solid objects like car keys from a hip pocket upon which the patient is lying and, on the ward, nurses turning the patient. At Stoke Mandeville we healed large pressure sores with low-cost wet dressings and frequent turns. We had none of the water or air-filled beds now used in the developed world and our usual wetting agent was the now much maligned Eusol and paraffin.

One of the most celebrated sufferers from paraplegia of recent times was Christopher Reeve, or one time "Superman." He did much for the advocacy of "best practice." Interestingly he was especially an advocate for research into stem cells with which to repair the spinal cord injury.[1] This is high technology and it is both costly and questionable whether it will ever be affordable in the developing world. It illustrates a dilemma. How much attention should be given to costly research which may benefit only an elite and wealthy few? Where safety is unproven how much should the advice of the scientist or the marketing needs of the pharmaceutical and devices industry be allowed to throw doubt on cheap solutions? There are many examples in the field of pressure sore management and they include Eusol, gentian violet, honey, and maggot therapy, none of which would be available if their critics had been listened to.

The European Pressure Ulcer Advisory Panel (EPUAP)

The story since 1995 of the progress of the EPUAP is described[2] as first asking the question "what are we talking about?" It led to the discussions on definitions and classifications. Then there were the discussions on the size of the problem and on "what does it cost?" A great service was done by sorting out incidence from prevalence. The next stage was the registration of all known preventive and therapeutic interventions as well as the level of evidence for their effectiveness. The Panel then applied "Marks of Quality" to devices.[3] The final steps were the production of educational material and the identification of the army of workers that should read them.

Under the heading of Health Services Research and terms such as "access" one can debate whether investment in increasing the knowledge of the carer in the developing world should be at the level of postgraduate training of doctors or of allied health professionals or at the level of family members of the patient. My experience has been that the greatest disappointments come from training doctors in the developing world, especially if they are male. They emigrate and they take up full-time private practice, where there is no public health ethos. If while overseas they are any good at research they do not return to their country of origin.

There is thus the need for a further stage of development for organizations such as the EPUAP and that is applying "Quality Marks" to the carer. It should be based on availability, commitment, cost, and their belief in the possibility of prevention and healing of pressure ulcers. Barbenel and Hagisawa[4] alarmed the EPUAP by substituting realism for a range of views from pessimism to optimism. They suggested that not all ulcers are preventable. What has not been measured is whether more ulcers are healed when the carer expects them to heal.

Aging

It is often said that our increasing life expectancy will create an aged population without the young carers to look after them. By the year 2030 half the population of Europe will be over 30 years of age and will expect to live a further 40 years. In the UK there will be approaching a quarter of a million people over 100 years of age. At the same time declining fertility will reduce the young population.

Recently it has been argued[5] that this aged population is not only fitter but is more capable of doing a carer's job perhaps even into their nineties. Issues of access require that this population is helped to be more effective and to be more knowledgeable. Early retirement at around age 50 should be followed by encouragement to take on community projects for at least 20 years.

In the meantime the AIDS epidemic in the developing world is reducing life expectancy and increasing the number of chronic sick with heightened vulnerability to pressure ulcers.

The Family

There is some debate whether in the twenty-first century the family is more dysfunctional than before. Especially in urban developments the older members of the family cannot expect their young to give up their employment to look after them unpaid. Others[5] argue that there is preservation of and maybe an increase in a sense of responsibility for care of elderly relatives. Increasingly the bond with the elderly is strengthened by the greater role they play in managing the daily demands of a family out at work when the children are out of school. It is poverty that is the main concern because the elderly need financial support for themselves and it is common for all their dwindling resources to be spent on the needs of an extended family, perhaps orphaned as a result of AIDS.

A threat to rational management is the discovery by families and their lawyers that there is money to be made by suing hospitals for allowing pressure ulcers to happen in one of their relatives. A complaint that enriches a lawyer is far less desirable than one that improves the health service. Scott[6] stated that some lessons are too big to learn. It takes a Ludwig Guttman or perhaps an EPUAP to give the master class that breaks bad habits, and also demonstrates that errors are a consequence of problems not their cause.

Information Technology

Information technology is one way forward but writing in the sand may require less backup.

During the past decade I have visited on several occasions villages near Pondicherry in southern India, where there is great poverty and illiteracy. An experiment led by the Swaminathan Foundation supported by the Canadian government has provided internet to these villages. Information comes to them in their own language and important messages are vocalized. A majority of the village inhabitants become computer literate and many of the women retrieve health information. Such experiments are being undertaken in many other parts of the developing world.

At conferences devoted to pressure ulcers no one doubts that knowledge exists but a familiar cry is that it is not getting to where it is needed. Sharing knowledge has never been easier. The expert patient is now a potential replacement for the apathetic one. One area of knowledge that has not been widely disseminated is that of nutrition, which is well described in the literature on pressure ulcers in the developed world. This needs rewriting for the developing world, where even in hospital the patient's food is provided unsupervised by the family away from the cheaper resources of their home support. This requires someone to understand the family background before giving advice. Thus for the developing world "poverty alleviation" has to be to the fore. Often the visitor to healthcare projects in the developing world will be first shown the private hospitals of a not insubstantial middle class. But even their best practice and gold standards are replaced by silver plate. It must be the role of leaders such as the EPUAP to become partners with the poor. "Macroeconomics and Health"[7] demand that such an organization representing best practice in the developed world should set aside time to boost their own reputation and finance by providing good advice to donors and governance globally and not just to their own parish. It will be advice in a language of gold standards, "evidence based medicine," "low technology transfer," and "cost effectiveness" for much needed National Commissions. It must make sure that the support given to the middle class raises the standard of care given to the poor and at the same time the poor are real beneficiaries of their intervention.

Rewards and Awards

Where the patient is too sick to play a leading role in self-help there is a great problem of the need for and provision of a devoted carer. Such people need respite and rewards. A fraction of the costs of wound healing research directed at examining ways to encourage care would go a long way to improving the wellbeing of the chronically sick.

At the top of the pyramid, a National Commission will focus on the leading medical and nursing schools in tertiary hospitals. The focus should not be on pathogenesis alone, but should have education of lower tiers in the pyramid as a main objective. At the lowest level encouragement of the carer and of self-help requires more than knowledge of wound healing. It requires especially experience in leadership and rewards and awards. These will be influenced by community needs, poverty, and cultural differences.

The developing world is most unlikely to generate the knowledge it needs by itself. The remarkable achievements of the EPUAP in its first five years could not have happened in the developing world but they could now be copied there; but the copy will need to be culturally sensitive.

Skin Assessment

Pressure ulcers are a skin problem and skin observation and assessment is central to diagnosis and intervention. Ulcers are a huge economic burden that should justify the focus of the custodians of the skin namely the dermatologist. During the last few decades dermatology departments have created wound healing units, such as that from which this chapter is written, journals, and societies. The majority of dermatologists have, however, steered clear of being expert in the management of pressure ulcers. Hopefully the concept of the wound healing team will allow the dermatologist to select a field of interest and share, most likely with a skin-care nursing profession, areas that are a weighty burden. So far the leading policy-makers such as the World Health Organization or major funding bodies such as the Melinda and Bill Gates Foundation have not perceived skin care as a priority. Sadly the majority of dermatologists see no role for themselves in this respect. At a recent international workshop on the Intensified Control of Neglected Diseases,[8] "skin failure" was not on the agenda. In due course maybe the importance of absent skin and ulceration will be recognized. Furthermore "the wound healers" will have promoted models of the prevention of non-communicable disease that demonstrate the importance of examining the skin. They will also have promoted models that organize the patient within the context of a team that includes the community. This is something demanding leadership and the kind of organization demonstrated by the European Pressure Ulcer Advisory Panel. This is knowledge that has to be taken into the "general health services" and not just to a few leading tertiary hospitals in the developing world. It is appropriate for it to be transported there with other knowledge of the skin such as common infections, wounds and burns, leprosy, lymphatic filariasis, and several other conditions all requiring the same basic interventions of skin care when first seen in a rural health center.

Looking at the skin and seeing the subtleties of what is there needs a new curriculum that is less dermatology orientated. What is required is less naming of patterns with Latin names but a greater skill at recognizing poor health and early skin failure and potential vulnerability. We must teach the examination of the skin for loss of barrier function, failure of reflex hyperemia, or early sensory loss, so early signs of skin failure are picked up as well as most physicians recognize heart failure.

The largest healthcare profession is nursing and pressure ulcers are given prominence in their practice. The professions involved in early diagnosis of skin failure in disorders such as leprosy, the diabetic foot, or lymphedema are not small. Until recently dermatologists have not been invited to be writers of their guidelines, because they have not been interested. Fortunately this is now changing. No one caring for the skin can ignore the developing knowledge base of dermatology. Fortunately the concept of team management and collaboration is encouraging this knowledge base to be a contributor to all aspects of the management of skin failure. The development of a skin-care nursing profession points the way to a better future.

The International Foundation for Dermatology

Directing attention from the range of interests usually shown by the urban-based private practitioner to a broader curriculum that includes skin care where it is needed in the general health services has been the focus of the International Foundation for Dermatology. It has made a point of including wounds and burns in its program because these are skin problems commonly presenting at a health center. This kind of dermatology also embraces sexually transmitted disease. The empires built for dermatology on syphilis in the nineteenth century are now potentially being re-established mostly by other branches of medicine, but with a focus on HIV/AIDS. The recognition of physical signs in the skin embracing the early signs of AIDS and much else besides, such as tropical diseases like leprosy, leishmaniasis, onchocerciasis, the lymphedema of lymphatic filariasis, and of course wounds and burns. In taking the management of these into the general health services one is aiming to teach skin signs to the allied health professionals that manage health centers. It is appropriate that in looking at the skin they should recognize the signs presaging pressure ulcers. Furthermore if they are to manage ulcers due to venous disease or diabetes or leprosy it is appropriate that they should also manage pressure ulcers.

Increasingly the AIDS epidemic is a prevailing influence. It provides the sick but also inhibits healing. In one study[9] of skin grafting in burns, healing in HIV patients was 22% compared to 69% in non-HIV patients. In the developing world effective management is so costly that those affected return to traditional health systems and mostly these do not fail to give welcome support and a degree of effectiveness unrealized in the developed world. Of course there is quackery and there are roadside sellers with no expertise. There are also traditional healers or practitioners of Chinese medicine or Indian systems of medicine who are expert. Breathing, posture or movement, so effective for lymphedema, are better understood by Asian systems of medicine than by practitioners of biomedicine. One should not forget when examining the prescription of herbal medicines that plants developed before the animal kingdom, and many have antiseptic, antioxidant, and antihistamine properties, and much else besides.

It is in terminal illness that the management of pressure ulcers poses difficult questions, since in a dying patient with falling blood perfusion pressure, death of tissue may be unavoidable. Expectations of healing may be irrelevant and wound bed preparation unacceptably invasive. Pain relief becomes a priority. As with anyone so sick, issues of hydration and nutrition require fine judgment.

Getting Management of Pressure Ulcers into the Curriculum

At all levels of the health service the curriculum is overloaded. The medical student who must become a safe doctor and the nurse who may have to survive overnight solely responsible for an intensive care unit have to know an enormous amount. They are also increasingly under observation in case mistakes made are worthy of litigation. Every branch of medicine will have advocates for including their interests in the curriculum. How to decide on priorities for each discipline is increasingly difficult, as more and more knowledge becomes available to us. The prevalence and cost of pressure sores is such that a strong case can be made for ensuring that it is understood by every doctor and nurse and indeed that it becomes public knowledge under the heading of public health.

Fifteen years ago there were 25 countries in Africa without anyone to advise government or universities about skin priorities. Since then at the Regional Dermatology Training Centre in Tanzania 120 allied health professionals have undergone 2 years of additional training about the skin. With a university qualification they have enlarged the knowledge base of 14 countries. Recently in Mali, and previously in Guatemala, the International Foundation for Dermatology focused on one-day courses for nurses. The curriculum was determined by the case of need. Taking the commonest diseases and observing how misdiagnosis would lead to wrong, ineffective, and costly prescribing, it was not difficult to establish priorities. It was important to eliminate the roadside seller but it was equally important to examine high utilization of traditional medicine. Such utilization is of public health significance and should not be ignored in training a doctor or nurse. It must be made safe, but its efficacy, sustainability, local availability, and low cost must not be undervalued. Wherever there is a break in the surface continuity of skin, traditional therapy will have a role to play and agents such as honey or larvae therapy must not be downplayed.

Recently in India I have helped to initiate three programs. India is a nation without a substantial body of nurses interested in the skin. In January 2004 a new "Skin-Care Nursing Group" was inaugurated at the annual Indian Dermatology Congress in Bombay. There have been a number of wound healing programs also inaugurated in India and in neighboring Sri Lanka. So far these have been mostly for the benefit of a substantial but minority middle class and their private hospitals. It has to be said that if best practice exists anywhere, it may raise standards and filter through to the majority.

India is a nation with large government-supported "Indian Systems of Medicine." They are of especial importance for the rural poor. Taking lymphatic filariasis as a condition highly prevalent in rural areas, I have initiated in Kerala a program of management supported by the Cochrane body in the UK and by international ethics foundations.

Recently it has become evident that China has developed its cities at the expense of the rural peasant. A plan to retrain 5 million "village doctors" is being examined. Their curriculum must be worked on. Maybe here too the EPUAP could give advice. It is my hope that a younger generation of dermatologists will perceive their role as part of a team sharing responsibility for skin failure and that their orientation will include poverty alleviation. Such a focus will identify pressure ulcers as a high priority.

References

1. Cherry GW. Letter from the editor. Eur Tissue Repair Soc Bull 2004; 11:48.
2. Haalboom JRE. Pressure ulcer management in Europe. The Oxford wound healing course handbook. Oxford Wound Healing Institute; 2002.
3. Haalboom JRE. Quality marks, a European dream. EPUAP Review 2002; 4:6–7.
4. Barbenel JC, Hagisawa S. The limits of pressure sore prevention. J R Soc Med 1999; 92:576–578.
5. Harper S. Ageing society. Oxford Today 2004; 16–18.
6. Scott H. Education-sharing our experiences. Can complaint change culture? EPUAP Review 2001; 3:90–92.
7. Morrow RH. Macroeconomics and health. BMJ 2002; 325:53–55.
8. International control of neglected diseases. Report of an International Workshop, Berlin, December 2003 (further information from: neglected.diseases@who.int).
9. Mzezewa S. Burns in Zimbabwe. Epidemiology, immunosuppression, infection and surgical management. Doctoral dissertation. Department of Plastic Surgery, Malmo University Hospital, Sweden, 2003.
10. Ryan TJ. Pressure sores: prevention management and future research--a medical perspective. Palliat Med 1989; 3:249–525.

22 Innovation in Pressure Ulcer Prevention and Management

Keith G. Harding and Michael Clark

Introduction

For many practitioners achieving successful pressure ulcer prevention and management has long been regarded as a straightforward task albeit one that is often not achieved. This view was succinctly described in the first paper presented at the first UK pressure ulcer conference back in 1975 when Roaf[1] commented that "we know how to avoid bed sores and tissue necrosis—maintain the circulation, avoid long continued pressure, abrasions, extremes of heat and cold, maintain a favourable micro-climate, avoid irritating fluids and infection. The problem is the logistics of this programme." So now, thirty years after this seminal meeting on pressure ulcers, does such a statement still hold true and have we really achieved significant innovations in our research and practice which have helped resolve the logistical challenges in service delivery? There are four key dimensions where pressure ulcer innovations might be encountered—in clinical practice, research, the organization and logistics of service delivery, and finally in society's views on the significance of pressure ulceration. Each dimension clearly overlaps with its neighbors but will be treated separately in this chapter both to tease out advances and to identify the challenges that remain.

Innovations in Clinical Practice?

In the early 1980s pressure ulcer management differed significantly from today. There were no specialist nursing positions, with the first wave of UK tissue viability nurses appointed in 1986–1987; by 1992, 23 tissue viability nurse specialists were in post;[2] today the precise number is unclear but is likely to be over 400. This explosion in the number of specialist nursing posts has created a demand for targeted education in tissue viability to enable the new cadres to be competent practitioners with the specific competencies having been defined in recent years.[3] Such courses extend from informal company-delivered seminars through to formal academic training such as the MSc in Wound Healing and Tissue Repair organized by the Wound Healing Research Unit. For medical colleagues, there remains a scarcity of education (and interest) in pressure ulcer prevention and treatment. Bennett[4] surveyed the wound care training delivered by the 27 medical schools in the UK; of the 19 respondents only 13 delivered any formal teaching on pressure ulcer management; and of these schools pressure ulcer preventive care was covered by 10, the use of wound dressings by 10, and pressure-redistributing devices by 8, with on average 6 hours of content delivered (range 0 to 35.5 hours). If such a survey were to be repeated today across Europe would training of medical practitioners in pressure ulcer prevention and management be commonplace or would this remain a topic that relatively few medical schools would consider to be relevant?

Not only have the numbers and training of health professionals changed over the past twenty years, the use of resources has evolved significantly. For example, in 1983 David and colleagues[5] surveyed the care received by 961 patients with pressure ulcers across 132 hospitals in England and Wales. The vast majority ($n = 599$; 62.3%) were nursed upon standard hospital mattresses. Since 1983 the diffusion of pressure-redistributing mattresses within healthcare has significantly expanded— in 2001 the European Pressure Ulcer Advisory Panel (EPUAP) completed a pilot survey of pressure ulcer prevalence across 26 hospitals located in five European countries.[6] Of the 5947 patients included in the pilot survey; 52.1% ($n = 3099$) had been allocated a pressure-redistributing mattress. The expanded use of pressure-redistributing beds and mattresses was particularly marked within some countries; for example, in the UK only 53 patients considered to be vulnerable to pressure ulcer development were nursed on standard mattresses, with the use of such devices extended into the patient population considered to be at minimal risk of pressure ulcers (1234 (84.3%) of 1464 patients not at risk were allocated a pressure-redistributing mattress).

These trends towards enhanced diffusion of interventions have recently been augmented by the introduction of partnerships between equipment suppliers and the health service leading to the initiation of total bed management (TBM) where a supplier is selected to supply all pressure-redistributing surfaces for a healthcare provider usually within a limited defined budget. These schemes offer an example of true partnership between the commercial sector and the health service and it is probable that one future trend will be the spread of such schemes across the expanded European Union. However, there remains a lack of evidence that any of these structural and process changes in the prevention and management of pressure ulcers have helped to reduce the size of the problem. This point will be considered in depth when reviewing innovation at the organizational and societal levels.

What about Innovation in Research?

It is without question that pressure ulcer research lies at the unglamorous end of the research spectrum—attracting little attention from funding bodies and career scientists alike. Much of the available research on pressure ulcers has benefited from commercial support and without this source of income pressure ulcer studies would be relatively scarce. While commercial support has been important and will probably continue to be the largest single sponsor of pressure ulcer studies, the need to obtain data in a timescale attractive to industrial sponsors has limited many studies—studies are frequently underpowered with little long-term follow-up of subjects. These weaknesses have been compounded by the common belief that it is somehow impossible to conduct blinded pressure ulcer intervention studies. This belief often relates to the investigation of devices such as beds and mattresses—how can those involved in studies be blinded to such visible devices? Eliminating this false belief poses a clear challenge for the pressure ulcer research community, with the use of photographic and video records presented to panels independent of the study presenting one solution.

The end-product of the myriad weaknesses in the design, conduct, and reporting of many pressure ulcer studies has been to limit their value in determining the most appropriate clinical interventions. Pressure-redistributing mattress use is widespread but there remains little clear evidence that any system is more effective than its competitors—low pressure foam mattresses have been clearly shown to reduce the incidence of pressure ulcers compared with standard mattresses[7] but this remains one of the very few outcomes from pressure ulcer research that may directly benefit patients.

Pressure ulcer research is often focused upon intermediate or surrogate outcome measures such as reductions in wound size and changes in the mechanical loads imposed on vulnerable anatomical sites. The measurement of contact (or interface) pressure has been the most common approach taken to evaluate patient support surfaces and the technique was well represented in papers presented during the first UK pressure ulcer conference.[8] In the intervening quarter of a century, while the measurement tools have evolved to today's pressure mapping systems that can display the pressure applied to all parts of the body in contact with the support surface, fundamental problems remain unsolved. There is currently no general agreement upon how contact pressures should be measured and reported. The EPUAP began to tackle this issue through seeking consensus among European researchers with a summary report published in 2002.[9] This discussion needs to be continued upon a broader basis involving colleagues both within and beyond Europe for without agreement upon how to measure contact pressure it is unlikely that we will achieve an answer to the key question—do changes in measured contact pressures translate into different clinical outcomes? At present much is made of relatively small differences between the contact pressures exerted by different support surfaces but do differences of 5 mmHg, 10 mmHg, or 50 mmHg have any clinical significance?

The clinical significance of other surrogate outcomes also deserves mention. In the past few years there has been growing speculation regarding the role of ischemia–reperfusion injuries within the etiology of pressure ulcers. For example, Peirce and colleagues[10] reported how increased numbers of cycles of ischemia followed by reperfusion produced more skin damage in a rat model compared with constant loading. In a series of elegant experiments mobile rats were subjected to externally applied loads of 50 mmHg induced by placing an external magnet over an implanted steel sheet. Skin blood flow during compression was evaluated using laser Doppler flowmetry and the area of necrotic tissue following loading was visually assessed. The key finding was that five cycles of ischemia and reperfusion (total ischemic period of 10 hours) produced more skin damage than 10 hours of continuous loading. If this result could be replicated in appropriate human studies then it would appear to call into question two fundamental pressure ulcer preventive strategies—manual repositioning and the use of dynamic mattresses—if intermittent loading caused more tissue damage than constant loading. Although investigation of ischemia–reperfusion may shed new insights into what is happening to the soft tissues during repetitive loading, the clinical significance of such observations may be questionable, for the majority of the (admittedly weak) randomized controlled trials show no difference between constant and dynamic support surfaces when used either to prevent or to help heal pressure ulcers,[11] with no study favoring the constant pressure device.

There remains much scope for innovation in pressure ulcer research—with many studies being poorly designed or with undue emphasis upon surrogate outcome measures. The challenge for pressure ulcer researchers lies with building appropriate networks at national and international levels to enable appropriately powered clinical studies to be undertaken. However, the funding that will be required to support and fully harness the potential for sound pressure ulcer studies may only be forthcoming when the final two dimensions—organizational and societal perspectives on pressure ulcers have been successfully tackled.

Organization and Logistics of Service Delivery

Beyond pressure ulcer epidemiology studies, research has not (to date) provided either a solid foundation or justification for the rapid changes in clinical practice observed over the past twenty years. These practice changes appear to have resulted from organizational issues and (albeit minor) political pressure. Taking the United Kingdom as an example, the first local policy tackling pressure ulcer management was published in 1986[12] and the publicity surrounding this policy played a significant role in creating the demand for pressure-redistributing devices due to the inclusion of a list of devices that would be required by a 2000 bed hospital. Some time later parliamentary questions prompted attention to the costs of pressure ulcers[13,14] and the use of pressure ulcers as an indicator of the quality of care delivered.[15] All of these initiatives fueled the attention to pressure ulcers at a local level with the consequent dissemination of pressure-redistributing devices and the growth of specialist nursing roles.

But have these changes achieved reductions in the number of people with pressure ulcers? Unfortunately this is a question that cannot be answered for there are no comparable epidemiological data that span the past twenty years. This flows from the wide variety of methods used to collect pressure ulcer occurrence data—prevalence, incidence, or more recently incidents. There is an urgent need for formal guidance upon the most appropriate form of pressure ulcer audit.[16] Increasingly healthcare providers are being asked to provide data on the numbers of people with pressure ulcers but are such requests reasonable when no guidance is offered on how the information should be collected? The potential for inappropriate comparisons—for example between facilities that include grade 1 pressure ulcers and a facility that excludes such wounds—is high and effectively devalues the drive towards recording pressure ulcers that can now be seen across different countries and healthcare settings. Systematic audit can be developed, as was shown by the pilot prevalence survey conducted by the EPUAP in 2001, and there is now a need to explore how incidence or incidents data can be collected in a valid but cost-effective manner.

Developing effective audit tools is important but so is providing guidance on when to audit and when to stop! Many providers undertake serial prevalence surveys but given that the data from successive surveys are not adjusted in light of changes in the patient population then interpretation of any variations in pressure ulcer occurrence over time is challenging. Collecting incidence data can be time-consuming and there may need to be a pragmatic trade-off between extending the period of data collection and the manpower and resources available to conduct the survey. It may be that routine valid and reliable incidence data will remain an unattainable goal until such time as data can be captured directly into a provider's electronic records.

How should the audit guidance required to effectively monitor trends in the occurrence of pressure ulcers be best developed? Perhaps this is a key role for the professional bodies that have emerged to provide leadership and support to those working on pressure ulcer prevention and management? There are now a multitude of organizations with overlapping remits—from the European level (EPUAP) through to national groups such as the Tissue Viability Society in the UK. Unfortunately many countries appear to have several national groups that hold pressure ulcers within their remit. In England and Wales at present there are three national organizations that may consider pressure ulcers—the Tissue Viability Society, the Wound Care Society, and the Tissue Viability Nurses Association. Do we really need such a profusion of national bodies? And could we be more effective working together? These are profound organizational issues that require discussion to ensure that effort is not duplicated and scarce resources wasted. While such discussion is required it is not unreasonable to predict that the future will see the closer working together of national groups and, where feasible, amalgamation into larger, and perhaps more effective organizations.

While not research per se, the development of pressure ulcer organizations at the international level has delivered benefits in a relatively short timescale; the US National Pressure Ulcer Advisory Panel (NPUAP) initially set the scene with consensus definitions of pressure ulcer grading, the role of reverse staging and alternatives such as the PUSH tool,[17] and more recently the identification of early pressure ulcers in darkly pigmented skin along with the growing role of litigation as a driver for pressure ulcer prevention and treatment. The European Pressure Ulcer Advisory Panel (EPUAP) have contributed strongly with guidelines on pressure ulcer prevention and management, comments upon support surface evaluation, and the audit of pressure ulcer occurrence. Recently the EPUAP has taken the lead in developing a specific guideline for the management of nutrition in both pressure ulcer prevention and treatment[18] and has explored the identification of early pressure ulcers and their discrimination from lesions arising from patient incontinence. These organizational achievements illustrate what can be gained from closer collaboration at the international level; what more could be gained through closer relationships at the national level?

Society and Pressure Ulcers

What of pressure ulcers at the societal level? This is perhaps the area where least has occurred over the past decades. How do we educate the public to the likelihood that they or their relatives might experience pressure ulcers? With almost 20% of hospital patients having one or more pressure ulcers, it is likely that most people will encounter this wound directly or at second hand during their lives. Regardless of how common pressure ulcers are, they are a decidedly unglamorous aspect of healthcare. This lack of glamour associated with pressure ulcers along with the public focus upon key health problems such as heart disease and cancers appears to limit how pressure ulcers can be brought to the attention of the general public.

One would have expected that a condition that affects up to 20% of hospital patients would have gained the attention of politicians—the EPUAP recently contacted all 635 UK Members of Parliament to inform them that 1 in 5 hospital patients might have pressure ulcers. Of the body of politicians only five replied—and these all sent standard responses noting that they had received our information. How then do we make an impact upon policy-makers? For the health professional, gains have been made—the development of international bodies such as the EPUAP and the growth of national organizations such as the UK Tissue Viability Society have expanded the access to information on pressure ulceration as a significant component of the jigsaw that is healthcare. The challenge now is to make the voice of each organization stronger—through organic growth or even through the amalgamation of existing groups into more powerful national organizations. While for the professional the information to help improve pressure ulcer care is available, the next major innovation in pressure ulcer prevention and management is likely to flow from attempts from national and international bodies to place pressure ulcers firmly among the priorities of healthcare policy-makers and the general public.

References

1. Roaf R. The causation and prevention of bed sores. In: Kenedi RM, Cowden JM, Scales JT (eds) Bedsore biomechanics. London: Macmillan Press; 1976: 5–9.
2. Watts S, Clark M. Pressure sore prevention: a review of policy documents. Final report to the UK Department of Health. Nursing Practice Research Unit, University of Surrey, Guildford, 1993.
3. Finnie A. An exploration of competency frameworks developed and implemented for Clinical Nurse Specialists in Community, Acute and Academic settings and their potential applicability to future specialist practice within Scotland. Proceedings of NBS Research Dissemination Conference, Dundee, 2001.
4. Bennett G. Medical undergraduate teaching in chronic wound care (a survey). J Tissue Viability 2003; 13(4):150–152.
5. David JA, Chapman RG, Chapman EJ, Lockett B. An investigation of the current methods used in nursing for the care of patients with established pressure sores. Final report to the UK Department of Health. Nursing Practice Research Unit, Northwick Park, London, 1983.
6. Clark M, Defloor T, Bours G. A pilot study of the prevalence of pressure ulcers in European hospitals. In: Clark M (ed) Pressure ulcers: Recent advances in tissue viability. Salisbury: Quay Books; 2004: 8–22.
7. Cullum N, McInnes E, Bell-Syer SEM, Legood R. Support surfaces for pressure ulcer prevention (Cochrane Review). In: The Cochrane Library, Issue 3, 2004. Chichester, UK: John Wiley & Sons.
8. Kenedi RM, Cowden JM, Scales JT (eds) Bedsore biomechanics. London: Macmillan Press; 1976.
9. McLeod A. Draft guidelines for the laboratory evaluation of pressure-redistributing support surfaces. EPUAP Review 2002; 4(1).
10. Peirce SM, Skalak TC, Rodeheaver GT. Ischemia-reperfusion injury in chronic pressure ulcer formation: a skin model in the rat. Wound Repair Regen 2000; 8(1):68–76.
11. University of York, NHS Centre for Reviews, Dissemination, University of Leeds, Nuffield Institute for Health. The prevention and treatment of pressure sores: how effective are pressure-relieving interventions and risk assessment for the prevention and treatment of pressure sores? Eff Health Care 1995; 2(1). 16p.
12. Hibbs P. Pressure area care policy. City and Hackney Health Authority, London, 1986.
13. Clark M, Watts S, Chapman RG, et al. The financial costs of pressure sores to the National Health Service: A case study. Final report to the UK Department of Health. Nursing Practice Research Unit, University of Surrey, Guildford, 1993.
14. Touche Ross. The cost of pressure sores. London: Touche Ross & Company; 1993.
15. Department of Health. Pressure sores: a key quality indicator. London: The Stationery Office; 1993.
16. Clark M, Orchard H. Do we take pressure ulcers seriously enough? (Editorial). J Tissue Viability 2004; 14(1):2.

17. Stotts NA, Rodeheaver GT, Thomas DR, et al. An instrument to measure healing in pressure ulcers: development and validation of the pressure ulcer scale for healing (PUSH). J Gerontol A Biol Sci Med Sci 2001; 56(12):N797–N799.
18. Clark M, Schols JMGA, Benati G, et al. Pressure ulcers and nutrition: a new European guideline. J Wound Care 2004; 13(7):267–274.

Index

Acetic acid, 143
Acid mantle, 96
Acinetobacter calcoaceticus, 151
Acticoat, 156
Actisorb, 156
Africa, 194
Agency for Health Care Policy and Research,
        USA (AHCPR), 169
Aging, 190–191
    of skin, 78
AGREE. *See* Appraisal of Guidelines for Research
        and Evaluation
AHCPR. *See* Agency for Health Care Policy and
        Research, USA
AIDS, 191, 193
Albumin, 32–33, 101
Alcohol hand rinses, 154
Alginate, 135
Allogeneic constructs. *See* Bioengineered skin
Alternating pressure mattress, 7, 8
Antibiotics, 111
Antibody labeling scanning, 153
Antimicrobials, 155
Antioxidant vitamins, 85, 87
Antiseptics, 142–143
    alcohols and, 142
    biguanides and, 142
    dressings and, 135
    for enzymatic debridement, 134
    halogen compounds and, 142
    iodine and, 143
    organic acids and, 143
    peroxides and, 143
    tinctures and, 143
Apligraf®, 115
Appraisal of Guidelines for Research and
        Evaluation (AGREE), 174
Aquacel-AG, 156
Arginine, 85, 87
Arglaes, 156
Autolytic debridement, 134–135
    alginate dressings and, 135
    cellulose dressings and, 135
    hydrocolloids and, 134
    hydrogels and, 134
    occlusive dressings and, 135

polyacrylates and, 135
Ringer's solution and, 135

Bacitracin zinc, 155
Bacteremia, 145
Bacteria. *See* Infection
Benzoyl peroxide, 155
Betadine, 143
Bioengineered skin, 104
    keratinocyte sheets and, 104
    neonatal foreskin cells and, 104
Biopsy
    of bone, 153
    of tissue, 149
Birty Pressure Risk Assessment scale, 53
Blanching hyperemia, 29
Bone scintigraphy, 153
Braden Q scale, 53
Braden scale
    parameters of, 50–51
    validation studies on, 51–52
Braden score, 3, 45

Cadexomer iodine, 135, 154–155
Capillary closure pressure, 11, 29
Case mix method, 4
CBO. *See* Dutch Institute for Healthcare
        Improvement
Cellular deformation
    in muscle tissue, 21, 23
    pathogenesis and, 20
Cellular senescence, 103
Cellulose, 135
Cetrimide, 143
Charcot foot, 148
China, 195
Chlorhexidine, 142
Classification, 37–40
    controversies in, 38
    dark skin assessment for, 39
    EPUAP systems for, 3, 37–38
    grade 1 ulcers and, 38–39
        criteria for, 39
        definitions of, 38
        erythema and, 38
        reactive hyperemia and, 38

Classification (*continued*)
    incontinence lesion identification for, 40
    inter-rater reliability of, 37
    NPUAP system for, 37
    PUCLAS and, 40
    reverse grading and, 39–40
    Stirling Grading System for, 37
Clinical practice guidelines (CPG), 44–45, 86,
    169–175
    barriers to, 173–174
        clinical indicators and, 174
        implementation aids and, 174
    consensus-based, 170
        Delphi methods for, 170
        literature searches for, 170
        weighed consensus techniques for, 170
    evidence-based, 170–173
        draft of, 171
        evaluation of, 172–173
        external review of, 171–172
        implementation of, 172–173
        publication and dissemination of, 172
        scope of, 170–171
    international development of
        AGREE and, 174
        GIN and, 175
    national development of
        AHCPR and, 169
        CBO and, 169
        EPUAP and, 169
        NICE and, 169
    on nutrition, 86
Collagen, 22, 30, 32, 77
Collagenase, 133
Compression. *See* Pressure
Computed tomography, 153
Computerized planimetry, 93
Confocal laser scanning microscopy, 21
Contreet Foam, 156
Contreet -HC, 156
Cornell Ulcer Risk Score, 53
Costs, 183, 186
C-reactive protein, 153
Cryopreserved skin, 115
Cubbin-Jackson scale, 53
Culture-grown fibroblasts, 115
Culture-grown keratinocyte, 115
Culture-grown skin, 115
Cutaneous flaps, 121
Cytokines, 101

Dakins, 142
Damage law, 23
Data collection, 1
Debridement, 129–136, 144–145
    antiseptic dressings for, 135
        cadexomer iodine for, 135
        honey for, 135
        hypochlorite solutions for, 135
        silver for, 135
    autolytic method of, 134–135

        alginate dressings and, 135
        cellulose dressings and, 135
        hydrocolloids and, 134
        hydrogels and, 134
        occlusive dressings and, 135
        polyacrylates and, 135
        Ringer's solution and, 135
    bacteremia and, 145
    contraindications for, 130–131
        black heels and, 130
        obliterative arterial disease, 130
        pyoderma gangrenosum and, 131
        terminally ill patients and, 130
    enzymatic method of, 133–134
        antiseptics and, 134
        collagenase use for, 133
        deoxyribonuclease use for, 134
        fibrinolysin use for, 134
        papaina use for, 134
    eschar and, 129
    maggot method of, 132–133
        antibacterial effects of, 133
        propylene glycol and, 133
        proteolytic enzymes and, 133
    necrotic tissue and, 129
    perfusion and, 131
    sharp method of, 131–132
        complications with, 132
        contraindications for, 132
    slough and, 129
    TIME concept and, 103–104, 140, 144
    wound bed preparation and, 103
Decubitus Ulcer Potential Analyzer, 53
Dental impression materials, 94
Deoxyribonuclease, 134
Dermagraft®, 115
Dermatitis, 80
Dermatology, 192–194
Dermis. *See* Skin
Developing world, 189–195
    access of, 190
    Africa and, 194
    aging and, 190–191
    China and, 195
    dermatology in, 192–194
        signs of early skin failure and, 193
    encouraging care in, 192
    EPUAP and, 189–190
    family and, 191
    HIV/AIDS in, 191, 193
    India and, 194–195
    inexpensive treatment solutions for, 190
    information technology in, 191–192
    International Foundation for Dermatology
        and, 193
    litigation and, 191
    medical curricula in, 194
    NPUAP and, 189
    poverty and, 191
    skin assessment in, 192
Devitalized tissue. *See* Debridement

Dressings, 111–114. *See also* Debridement
  adsorbents for, 111
  antibiotics for, 111
  antiseptics for, 111, 135
  gauzes for, 111
  granulation encouraging products for, 112
  growth factor group of, 115
  guidelines for, 113
  hydrocolloids for, 112
  hydrogels for, 112
  interactive methods for, 113, 114
    cultured cell group of, 115
    metalloprotease inhibitor group of, 115
    skin substitute group of, 115
    surgical group of, 115
  non-allopathic types of, 113
  philosophy of, 112
  polyurethane films for, 112
  polyurethane foams for, 112
  proteolytic enzymes for, 111–112
  technical devices for, 113
    hydrotherapy related, 116–117
    topical negative pressure therapy related,
      114, 116
    warming therapy related, 117, 118
Dutch Institute for Healthcare Improvement
    (CBO), 169

EGF. *See* Epidermal growth factor
Ek scale, 48–49
Elastography, 20
Engineered derma, 115
Enzymatic debridement, 133–134
  antiseptics and, 134
  collagenase use for, 133
  deoxyribonuclease use for, 134
  fibrinolysin use for, 134
  papaina use for, 134
Epidermal growth factor (EGF), 104
Epidermis. *See* Skin
Epithelial cancer, 92
EPUAP Review, 86–87, 185–186
Equipment, 59–65
  efficacy of, 59
  pressure reduction with, 60
    powered systems for, 60
    static systems for, 60
  pressure relief with
    air fluidized systems for, 60–61
    alternating pressure mattresses for, 60
  selection of, 61
    aesthetics and, 64
    alarm systems and, 64
    cleaning and, 64
    contraindicated conditions and, 62
    electrical power sources and, 63
    exudate levels and, 62
    financial considerations for, 64
    handling requirements and, 62
    home care and, 62–64
    mattress height and, 62

  resuscitation and, 62
  storage and transportation for, 64
  temperature control and, 62
  weight limits and, 63
Erythema, 38, 146–147
Erythrocyte sedimentation rate, 153
Eschar, 129
Ethyl alcohol, 142
Etiology
  capillary closure pressure and, 11
  interface pressures and, 11–12
  pressure and, 27–30
    blanching hyperemia and, 29
    at capillary closure, 29
    capillary occlusion and, 29
    formula for calculation of, 27
    friction and, 28
    in healthy capillary bed, 29
    humidity and, 28
    nonblanching hyperemia and, 29
    perfusion and, 30
    shear and, 27–28
    tissue collagen levels and, 30
    transmission of, 28–29
  prolonged pressure and, 11
  shear forces and, 11
European Pressure Ulcer Advisory Panel
    (EPUAP), 183–186, 201
  classification systems by, 3, 37–38
  CPGs and, 169
  definition of pressure ulcers by, 2
  developing world and, 189–190
  development of, 183–184
  educational initiatives of
    EPUAP Review and, 185–186
    PUCLAS and, 40, 186
  guidelines by
    nutritional, 185
    prevention, 8, 184
    treatment, 8, 185
  Marks of Quality and, 190
  NPUAP and, 184
  open meetings of, 184–185
  survey by, 2–3
  website of, 185
Eusol, 142, 189–190
Exudate
  enzyme levels in, 82
  maceration from, 82
  peri-wound skin protection from
    barrier preparations for, 82
    corticosteroids for, 82
    dressings for, 82
  wound bed preparation and, 102

Fasciocutaneous flaps, 122
FEA. *See* Finite element analysis
FGF. *See* Fibroblast growth factor
Fibrin, 105
Fibrinogen, 101
Fibrinolysin, 134

Fibroblast growth factor (FGF), 104
Fibroblasts, 102, 115
Finite element analysis (FEA), 18
Flamazine, 156
Fluorodeoxyglucose-positron emission
     tomography, 153
Free flaps, 124
Frequency, 1
Full-thickness skin grafts, 121
Fusidin ointment, 155

Gene therapy, 104–105
   gene gun injection for, 104–105
   naked plasmid DNA and, 104–105
   viruses for, 104–105
Gentamicin, 155
Gentian violet, 143, 190
GIN. See Guidelines International Network
Glycerol skin, 115
Gosnell scale, 48–49
Grafts, 115
Growth factors
   dressings and, 115
   hypoxia and, 102
   trapping of, 101
   for wound bed preparation, 104
Guidelines. See also Clinical practice guidelines
   for control of infection, 140
   for dressings, 113
   by EPUAP, 8, 184–185
   litigation and, 166
   for management of incontinence, 81
Guidelines International Network (GIN), 175

Heterologous culture-grown skin, 115
History, 183
HIV, 191, 193
Honey, 135, 190
Hyalograft 3D®, 115
Hyalograft 3D KC®, 115
Hyalomatrix®, 115
Hydrocolloids, 112, 134, 156
Hydrogels, 112, 134–135
Hydrogen peroxide, 143
Hydrotherapy, 116–117
   high-pressure microjet technology for, 117
   hydromassage for, 117
   immersion pools for, 116
   irrigation pressure in, 117
   syringe method of, 117
Hygeol, 142
Hyperemia, 29, 38
Hypoalbuminemia, 33
Hypochlorite solutions, 135
Hypothermia, 117
Hypoxia, 102, 151

Incidence rates, 1–6, 177
Incontinence, 79–81
   dermatitis from, 80

fecal, 79–80
   guidelines for management of, 81
   healthcare institutions and, 79
   maceration from, 80
   parous women and, 79
   skin-care product use for, 81
   skin pH levels and, 80
   soap use for, 80
   urinary
      overflow induced, 79
      stress induced, 79
      urge induced, 79
India, 194–195
Indian Dermatology Congress, 194
Infection, 139–158
   antiseptics for, 142–143
   assessment of, 145–148
      covert infections and, 148
      discoloration and, 146
      erythema and, 146–147
      infrared thermometry for, 148
      pain and, 146
      purulent discharge and, 146
      symptoms list for, 147
      warmth and, 146–147
   bacterial species in, 150–152
      aerobic, 150
      anaerobic, 150
      Gram-negative, 150
      Gram-positive, 150
      predictable progression of, 150–151
      relevance of, 151
      synergistic effects of, 151
   bacterial tests for, 148–150
      MRSA and, 148
      neutrophils and, 148
      swab technique for, 150
      tissue biopsy and, 149
      VRE and, 148
   debridement and, 144–145
      bacteremia and, 145
      foreign material, 145
   guidelines for control of, 140
   host resistance and, 139
   local wound care for, 144
      TIME concept and, 144
   MRSA vectors and, 153
   nonhealable ulcers and, 142
   organism numbers and, 139
   organism virulence and, 139
   osteomyelitis and, 152–153
      bone biopsies for, 152
      imaging studies of, 153
      laboratory tests for, 153
      sterile probe use on, 152
   patient-centered concerns regarding, 141
   treatment of, 153–158
      infection control measures for, 153–154
      iodine use for, 154–155
      nanocrystalline silver use for, 157–158

Infection (*continued*)
  silver preparations for, 155–157
  topical antimicrobials for, 155
Infrared spectroscopy, 20
Infrared thermometry, 148
Innovations, 197–202
  in clinical practice, 197–198
    with pressure-redistributing mattresses, 198
    with tissue viability nurse specialists, 197
    with total bed management, 198
  in logistics, 200–201
    from EPUAP, 201
    from NPUAP, 201
    with pressure ulcer audit, 200
    using prevalence surveys, 200
  in research, 198–199
    on interface pressure, 199
    on ischemia-reperfusion cycles v. constant
      loading, 199
    on pressure-redistributing mattresses, 199
  in societal views, 201–202
Integra®, 115
Interface pressures, 11–13
  incorrect threshold for, 11–12
  pressure monitoring systems and, 12
    FSA and, 12
    Novel and, 12
    Oxford Mk I/II, 12
    Talley Pressure Monitoring system and, 12
    Talley-Schimedics single cell system and, 12
    Tekscan and, 12
  pressure profiles and, 12–13
  relationship of interstitial pressures and,
    18–19
Internal mechanical environment, 18–20
  bony prominences and, 18–19
  computational modeling of, 18–19
    elastography and, 20
    FEA and, 18
    infrared spectroscopy, 20
    MRI and, 20
    MRI/MRS and, 20
    ultrasound and, 20
  global external loads' effect on, 18
  material properties of soft tissue and,
    19–20
  subcutaneous tissues and
    mechanical integrity of, 18
    thickness of, 18
    tone of, 18
  wick catheter and, 18
International Foundation for Dermatology,
  193–194
Interstitial pressures, 18–19
Iodine, 143
Ischemia, 20, 199. *See also* Etiology; Pressure
Isopropyl alcohol, 142

Keratinocyte growth factor-2, 104
Keratinocytes, 104, 115

Larval debridement. *See* Maggot debridement
Laser Skin®, 115
Laser triangulation scanner, 94
Lateral lying position, 70
Leishmaniasis, 193
Leprosy, 193
Leukocytes, 153
Litigation, 163–167
  in developing world, 191
  documentation and, 166–167
    prevention measures with, 166
    treatment measures with, 167
  negligence and, 165
    accountability and, 165
    causation and, 165
    standard of care and, 166
  pressure ulcer guidelines and, 166
  prevalence rates and, 163
  typical awards from, 164
Loading
  hierarchical modeling of, 21
  postoperative care and, 125
  research on, 199
  tissue status under
    Doppler fluxmetry and, 13
    metabolite levels and, 15
    reflective spectrophotometry and, 13
    transcutaneous oxygen tensions and, 13–14
Lymphatic filariasis, 193

α-2 macroglobulin, 101
Maggot debridement, 132–133, 190
  antibacterial effects of, 133
  propylene glycol and, 133
  proteolytic enzymes and, 133
Magnetic resonance imaging (MRI)
  internal mechanical environment and, 20
  of muscle tissue, 23
  for osteomyelitis, 153
Magnetic resonance spectroscopy (MRS), 179
  internal mechanical environment and, 20
  muscle tissue and, 23
Malnutrition. *See* Nutrition
Matrix metalloproteinases, 102
Mattresses. *See also* Equipment
  alternating pressure, 7, 8
  pressure-redistributing, 198–199
  quality of life and, 7
  research on, 199
  viscoelastic, 68
McClemont cone of pressure, 28
Melinda and Bill Gates Foundation, 192
Mercurochrome, 143
Metalloprotease inhibitors, 115
Methicillin-resistant staphylococcus aureus
  (MRSA), 148, 151, 153, 155
Metronidazole, 155
Minimum physiological mobility requirement
  (MPMR), 31
Mortality rates, 178

MPMR. *See* Minimum physiological mobility
    requirement
MRSA. *See* Methicillin-resistant staphylococcus
    aureus
Mupirocin, 155
Muscle-sparing perforator flaps, 124
Muscle tissue
    cellular deformation in, 21, 23
        dead cell distribution from, 23
    compression-induced cellular breakdown in,
        21–23
        agarose gel construct and, 21
        cell membrane disintegration and, 21
        collagen scaffold and, 22
        confocal laser scanning microscopy and, 21
        contractile protein disintegration and, 21
        damage threshold model of, 22
        histological examination for, 23
        inflammation and, 21
        MRI and, 23
        MRS and, 23
        nuclear pyknosis and, 21
    damage law for, 23
        cell tolerance parameter and, 23
        damage evolution parameter and, 23
        dimensionless strain energy density
            parameter and, 23
        material parameters and, 23
    pathogenesis and, 20
    reperfusion and, 23
Myocutaneous flaps, 122–123

Nanocrystalline silver, 156–158
National Institute for Clinical Excellence, UK
    (NICE), 169
National Pressure Ulcer Advisory Panel, USA
    (NPUAP), 201
    classification system by, 37
    developing world and, 189
    EPUAP and, 184
Necrotic tissue, 129. *See also* Debridement
Negative pressure therapy. *See* Topical negative
    pressure therapy
Negligence, 165–166
    accountability and, 165
    causation and, 165
    standard of care and, 166
Neutrophils, 148, 153
NICE. *See* National Institute for Clinical
    Excellence, UK
Nonblanching hyperemia, 29
Nonresponse rate, 4
Norton scale, 45
    derivatives of, 48–49
    limits of, 48
    parameters of, 47
    validation studies on, 48
Nova-4 scale, 48–49
NPUAP. *See* National Pressure Ulcer Advisory
    Panel, USA
Nuclear magnetic resonance, 179

Nuclear pyknosis, 21
Nutrition, 32–33, 85–89
    assessment of, 87–88
    CPGs on, 86
    decision tree on, 88
    intervention with, 87–88
    oral feeding and, 85, 87
    protein and, 87
    risk factors related to
        collagen production and, 32
        hypoalbuminemia and, 33
        muscle wasting and, 32
        odds ratio assessments for, 33
        relative risk assessments for, 33
        serum albumin levels and, 32–33
    screening for, 87–88
    supplements for, 87
    tube feeding and, 85, 87

Odds ratio assessments
    for age, 32
    for mobility, 31
    for nutrition, 33
Osteomyelitis
    bone biopsies for, 152
    imaging studies of, 153
    laboratory tests for, 153
    sterile probe use on, 152

Papaina, 134
Pathogenesis
    cellular deformation and, 20
    interstitial transport and, 20
    ischemic damage and, 20
    lymphatic system and, 20
    muscle tissue and, 20
    pressure-induced ischemia and, 20
    reperfusion damage and, 20
PDGF. *See* Platelet-derived growth factor
Perfusion
    subcutaneous pressure and, 30
Perfusion MRI, 23
Peri-wound skin, 82
pH
    skin and, 80
    wound assessment and, 96–97
Photogrammetry, 93
Platelet-derived growth factor (PDGF), 102, 104
Platelet gels, 115
Polyacrylates, 134–135
Polymyxin B sulfate, 155
Polyurethane, 112
Povidone iodine, 154
Pressure, 27–30
    blanching hyperemia and, 29
    at capillary closure, 11, 29
    capillary occlusion and, 29
    formula for calculation of, 27
    friction and, 28
    in healthy capillary bed, 29
    humidity and, 28

Pressure (*continued*)
  nonblanching hyperemia and, 29
  perfusion and, 30
  relief of
    equipment for, 60–61, 179, 198–199
    surgical treatment and, 125
  shear and, 27–28
    avulsion of capillaries from, 28
    regional stretching from shear, 28
    vascular occlusion from, 27
  tissue collagen levels and, 30
  transmission of, 28–29
    McClemont cone of pressure and, 28
Pressure-redistributing mattress, 198–199
Pressure ulcer classification system (PUCLAS),
      40, 186
Pressure ulcer risk assessment scales. *See* Risk
      assessment scales
Prevalence rates, 1–6
  by body site location, 2
  in children, 2
  by country, 3
  by grade, 3
  as healthcare quality indicator, 163
  litigation and, 163
  research on, 178
Prevention
  costs of, 178
  EPUAP guidelines for, 8, 184
  litigation and, 166
  quality of life and, 7–8
  risk assessment scales for, 43
Promogran®, 115
Prone lying position, 70
Propylene glycol, 133
Protein, 87
Proteolytic enzymes
  dressings and, 111–112
  maggot debridement and, 133
Pseudomonas aeruginosa, 150–151, 155
PUCLAS. *See* Pressure ulcer classification system

Quality of life, 7–9, 179–180
  auxiliary devices and, 7
  economical treatments and, 8
  mattresses and, 7
  nurses and, 7
  pain treatment and, 7
  physiotherapists and, 8
  prevention of ulcers and, 7–8
    spinal cord injuries and, 7
    young patients and, 7
  skin condition and, 7
  sleep and, 7
  wound care and, 7
Quantitative microbiology, 149

Radiolabeled leukocytes, 153
Rates, 1–6
  calculation of, 3–4, 5
    Braden score and, 3

case mix method and, 4
  cutoff points and, 3–4
  nonresponse rates and, 4
  risk group definition and, 3–4
of incidence, 1–6
litigation and, 163
of mortality, 178
of prevalence, 1–6
  by body site location, 2
  in children, 2
  by country of origin, 3
  in geriatric patients, 5
  by grade, 3
prevalence v. incidence, 3, 5
  multiple pressure sores and, 3, 5
  progression to higher grades and, 3, 5
research on, 177–178
time period and, 2
Reeve, Christopher, 189
Regranex®, 115
Relative risk assessments
  for mobility, 31
  for nutrition, 33
Reperfusion
  muscle tissue and, 23
  pathogenesis and, 23
Repositioning, 67–72
  frequency of, 68–69
    research on, 68
  pressure-reduction with, 69–70
    adapted repositioning scheme for, 70
    lateral lying position for, 70
    prone lying position for, 70
    semi-Fowler 30° position for, 69–70
    supine lying position for, 69
  upright-sitting position and, 70
    bending and stretching in, 71
    chair type for, 71
    optimal posture for, 71
    pressure-reducing cushions for, 71
Research, 11–23, 177–180, 198–199
  capillary closure pressure and, 11
  on costs of prevention and treatment, 178
  on diagnostic imaging techniques, 179
  on incidence rates, 177
  incorrect measures and, 11
  on interface pressure, 199
  interface pressures and, 11–12
  on ischemia-reperfusion cycles v. constant
      loading, 199
  on mortality rates, 178
  on patient quality of life, 179–180
  on physiological response to mechanical
      factors, 178–179
  on pressure-redistributing mattresses, 199
  on pressure relieving devices, 179, 198–199
  on prevalence rates, 177–178
  on wound healing, 180
Ringer's solution, 135
Risk assessment scales, 43–59
  Braden scale

Risk assessment scales (*continued*)
    parameters of, 50–51
    validation studies on, 51–52
  characteristics of, 46–47
    applicability and, 47
    definite criteria and, 47
    ease of use and, 47
    predictive value and, 47
    sensitivity and, 46
    specificity and, 46
  CPG recommendations about, 44–45
  for intensive care patients, 53
  Norton scale, 45
    derivatives of, 48–49
    limits of, 48
    parameters of, 47
    validation studies on, 48
  for pediatric patients, 53
  preventative measures based on, 43
  systematic review of, 46
  Waterlow scale
    appraisals of, 50
    parameters of, 49
    validation studies on, 50
Risk factors, 30–34
  age and, 31–32
    odds ratio assessments for, 32
    pathological skin changes and, 32
  mobility and, 30–31
    MPMR and, 31
    odds ratio assessments for, 31
    relative risk assessments for, 31
    spontaneous nocturnal movement and,
      31
  nutrition and, 32–33
    collagen production and, 32
    hypoalbuminemia and, 33
    muscle wasting and, 32
    odds ratio assessments for, 33
    relative risk assessments for, 33
    serum albumin levels and, 32–33
  reference table of, 34
  tissue tolerance and, 30

Scale. *See* Risk assessment scales
Semi-Fowler 30° position, 69–70
Sensate myocutaneous flaps, 123–124
Sharp debridement, 131–132
  complications with, 132
  contraindications for, 132
Shear, 11
  avulsion of capillaries from, 28
  regional stretching from shear, 28
  vascular occlusion from, 27
Silvadene, 156
Silver, 133, 135, 155–158
  adsorbed, 156
  allergic sensitization to, 156
  minimum inhibitory concentrations of, 157
  nanocrystalline, 157

preparations of, 156
salts, 156
Silver-calcium-sodium phosphates, 156
Silver charcoal, 156
Silver coated foam, 156
Silver combined with hydrocolloid, 156
Silver nitrate, 156
Silver-sodium carboxymethylcellulose, 156
Silver sulfadiazine, 156
Sinus tracts, 92
Skin, 75–82
  acid mantle, 80
  aging of
    drying during, 78
    elasticity loss during, 78
    fatty layer reduction during, 78
    thinning during, 78
  bioengineered, 104
  dark colored, 39
  dermal layer of
    collagen fibers in, 77
    elastin fibers in, 77
    ground substance of, 77
    lymph vessels in, 77
    nerve endings in, 78
    sebaceous glands in, 78
    sweat glands in, 78
    tissue mast cells in, 77
    tissue microphages in, 77
  epidermal layer of
    basal layer of, 77
    clear cell layer of, 77
    dermal junction with, 77
    granular layer of, 77
    horny layer of, 76
    prickle cell layer of, 77
  failure of, 193
  functions of, 75–76
    protection, 76
    sensation, 76
    thermal regulation, 76
    vitamin D production, 76
  grafts of, 120–123
  incontinence and, 75, 80–81
  peri-wound, 82
  pH levels of, 80
  quality of life and, 7
  wound assessment and, 92
Skin bank, 115
Skin flaps, 121
Slough, 129
Sodium hypochlorite, 142
Spectrophotometry, 13
Split-thickness skin grafts, 120–121
SSD Cream, 156
Staphylococcus aureus, 150–151, 152, 155
Stem cell therapy, 105
  fibrin use for, 105
  pluripotentiality of, 105
Stereophotogrammetry, 93–94

Stereophotography, 93–94
Stirling Grading System, 37
Stratum basale, 77
Stratum corneum, 76, 81, 82, 96
Stratum granulosum, 77
Stratum lucidum, 77
Stratum spinosum, 77
Streptococci, 150, 153, 155
Sunderland scale, 53
Supine lying position, 69
Surgical treatment, 119–125
  debridement during, 120
  patient selection for, 119–120
  postoperative care after, 124–125
    diet during, 125
    load conditioning during, 125
    physical training during, 125
    pressure relief during, 125
  reconstruction with
    direct closure for, 121
    fasciocutaneous flaps for, 122
    flaps without skin coverage for, 123
    free flaps for, 124
    full-thickness skin grafts for, 121
    muscle-sparing perforator flaps for, 124
    myocutaneous flaps for, 122–123
    sensate myocutaneous flaps for, 123–124
    skin flaps for, 121
    split-thickness skin grafts for, 120–121
    tissue expansion for, 124
  staff for, 119
Swaminathan Foundation, 191
Sweat, 78. See also Tissue biochemistry

T2-weighted MRI, 23
Tagging MRI, 23
TGF-β1. See Transforming growth factor-β1
TIME. See Tissue debridement,
    infection/inflammation, moisture
    balance, edge effect
Tissue biochemistry, 14–18
  carbon dioxide levels and, 16–17
  metabolite levels under loading and, 14–15
  oxygen levels under, 16–17
  sweat lactate levels and, 15, 16–17
  sweat metabolite constituents and, 14
  sweat purines and, 16
  sweat urea levels and, 16
Tissue debridement, infection/inflammation,
    moisture balance, edge effect (TIME),
    103–104, 140, 144
Topical negative pressure therapy, 114, 116
  contraindications for, 116
  duration of, 116
  indications for, 116
  target pressure of, 116
  Vacuum Assisted Closure device for, 114, 116
Transcutaneous oxygen tension, 13–14, 102
Transforming growth factor-β1 (TGF-β1), 101,
    102

Ultrasound, 20, 153, 179
Upright-sitting position, 70–71

Vacuum Assisted Closure, 114, 116
Vancomycin-resistant enterococcus (VRE),
    148
Vascular endothelial growth factor (VEGF),
    102
VEGF. See Vascular endothelial growth factor
Viscoelastic mattresses, 67, 68
Vitamins, 76, 85, 87
VRE. See Vancomycin-resistant enterococcus

Warming therapy, 117–118
  blood flow and, 117
  hypothermia and, 117
Waterlow pressure ulcer risk scores, 33
Waterlow scale
  appraisals of, 50
  parameters of, 49
  validation studies on, 50
World Health Organization, 192
Wound assessment, 91–97
  area and volume measurements in, 91, 93–94
    computerized planimetry for, 93
    dental impression materials for, 94
    image processing for, 93
    laser triangulation scanner use for, 94
    metric grid use for, 93
    photogrammetry use for, 93
    sheet tracing for, 93
    stereophotogrammetry use for, 93–94
    stereophotography use for, 93–94
    three-dimensional scanner use for, 94
  exudate and, 92
  infection and, 92–93
  odor and, 92
  pH measurements in, 96–97
    colorimetric technique for, 96
    flat glass electrode use for, 96
    pH transistor technology for, 97
  surrounding skin and, 92
  tissue density measurements in, 94–95
    echogenicity values and, 95
    ultrasonography use for, 94–95
  tissue perfusion measurements in, 95–96
    laser Doppler flowmetry use for, 95
    laser Doppler imaging use for, 96
  undermining tissue and, 92
  viable tissue quantity and, 92
  wound edges and, 92
Wound bed preparation, 99–105
  bacterial burdens and, 100
  bioengineered skin and, 105
  biofilms and, 101
  debridement and, 103
  gene therapy for, 104–105
  growth factors for, 104
    PDGF and, 104
    sequential treatment with, 104

Wound bed preparation (*continued*)
  growth factor trapping and, 101
  hypoxia and, 102
    fibroblast proliferation and, 102
    growth factors and, 102
  impaired healing and, 100
  phenotypic wound cell alteration and,
      102–103
    cellular senescence and, 103

  healing capacity and, 103
  stem cell therapy for, 105
  TIME concept for, 103–104
  wound fluid and, 101–102
    exudate levels and, 102
    matrix metalloproteinases and,
      102

X-rays, 153